EVIDENCE-BASED PRACTICE FOR HEALTH PROFESSIONALS

An Interprofessional Approach

Bernadette Howlett, PhD
Director of Research
Bingham Memorial Hospital
Affiliate Faculty Member
Institute of Rural Health
Idaho State University

Ellen J. Rogo, RDH, PhD
Associate Professor
Department of Dental Hygiene
Idaho State University

Teresa Gabiola Shelton, MPAS, PA-C
Physician Assistant
Cache Valley, Utah

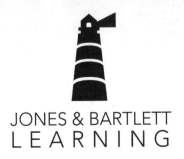

JONES & BARTLETT
LEARNING

World Headquarters
Jones & Bartlett Learning
5 Wall Street
Burlington, MA 01803
978-443-5000
info@jblearning.com
www.jblearning.com

Jones & Bartlett Learning books and products are available through most bookstores and online booksellers. To contact Jones & Bartlett Learning directly, call 800-832-0034, fax 978-443-8000, or visit our website, www.jblearning.com.

Substantial discounts on bulk quantities of Jones & Bartlett Learning publications are available to corporations, professional associations, and other qualified organizations. For details and specific discount information, contact the special sales department at Jones & Bartlett Learning via the above contact information or send an email to specialsales@jblearning.com.

Production Credits
Publisher: William Brottmiller
Senior Acquisitions Editor: Katey Birtcher
Associate Editor: Teresa Reilly
Production Manager: Julie Champagne Bolduc
Production Assistant: Stephanie Rineman
Marketing Manager: Grace Richards
Manufacturing and Inventory Control Supervisor: Amy Bacus
Composition: Laserwords Private Limited, Chennai, India
Cover Design: Scott Moden
Cover Image: © Costock Images/Thinkstock
Printing and Binding: Edwards Brothers Malloy
Cover Printing: Edwards Brothers Malloy

To order this product, use ISBN: 978-1-4496-5277-7

Library of Congress Cataloging-in-Publication Data
Howlett, Bernadette
 Evidence-based practice for health professionals : an interprofessional approach / by Bernadette Howlett, Ellen J. Rogo, and Teresa Gabiola Shelton.
     p. ; cm.
 Includes bibliographical references and index.
 ISBN 978-1-4496-1163-7—ISBN 1-4496-1163-X
 I. Rogo, Ellen J. II. Shelton, Teresa Gabiola. III. Title.
 [DNLM: 1. Evidence-Based Practice. 2. Health Personnel. 3. Interprofessional Relations. 4. Patient Care Team. WB 102.5]

 362.1—dc23
                          2012035123
6048
Printed in the United States of America
17 16   10 9 8 7 6 5

Contents

Preface

The concept for this book was born of the need for a text to accompany a course in evidence-based medicine and biostatistics. These topics are taught early in many health professional training programs across the country and around the world. Although useful and informative resources are available on these topics, many of them are geared toward experienced clinicians or designed to prepare students to perform biomedical research. The content and organization of this book emerged and solidified over years of teaching physician assistant, public health, nursing, and dental hygiene students.

This entry-level textbook for health professional students explores the basic concepts of evidence-based practice with a clinical emphasis. The text utilizes cases and examples derived from primary care. A pragmatic strategy is employed in this book, teaching the skills needed to access, interpret, evaluate, and apply evidence to interprofessional, patient-centered healthcare decisions. Practice exercises are included to provide applied learning experiences. These activities engage students in communication about evidence-based practice with other health professionals, patients, families, and professionals in related fields, including pharmaceutical representatives.

One of the most frequent encounters healthcare providers experience with healthcare-related evidence is through the pharmaceutical sales pitch. This textbook gives readers the knowledge and tools to make self-informed, evidence-based decisions and to communicate effectively with professionals in the pharmaceutical and other healthcare-related industries. The book also reviews common biomedical research and statistics terminology. A glossary of terms is also included.

OBJECTIVES AND THE NEED FOR THIS TEXT

Evidence-based practice (EBP) is a powerful tool for healthcare providers. This book is designed to help readers achieve two objectives related to EBP: (1) to locate, interpret, evaluate, and apply research to the care of individual patients and (2) to communicate effectively about research to patients, colleagues, and other professionals. Many books and resources are available to help practitioners understand the array of sophisticated concepts involved with EBP. Too often, however, these resources focus on statistics and research, emphasizing how to design and conduct clinical studies. Although these skills are important for researchers, they are less relevant for healthcare students and educational programs whose interests focus on quality clinical practice.

Other EBP resources with a more clinical emphasis have been written outside of the United States. The concepts, language, and examples in these texts do not fit with the healthcare system in the United States. Lastly, other books on EBP remain highly abstract, offering no applied learning experiences. This textbook provides meaningful learning activities through communications such as writing a letter to an insurance company, explaining the evidence regarding treatment to a patient, selecting a diagnostic tool, and designing community-based educational materials. These brief applied-learning experiences, along with clinical case studies, help students bridge the gap from the abstract concepts of research, statistics, and technical jargon to the concrete skills of healthcare decision making and communications.

INTENDED AUDIENCE

This book was developed for teaching EBP to college students who have a basic science and statistics background. We have written with medical, dental, physician assistant, nursing, dental hygiene, pharmacy, rehabilitative professions, and public health programs in mind. This textbook is intended to be incorporated into the larger curriculum of entry-level training programs. It is designed to accompany a semester-long course in EBP. We presume the readers of this book also have a set of primary textbooks and other references appropriate for their training programs.

ACCREDITATION AND PROFESSIONAL STANDARDS

Satisfaction of accreditation standards is just one reason for programs to teach EBP. It was also one of the reasons this book was written. For example, accrediting bodies for schools of allopathic medicine,

osteopathic medicine, physician assistant studies, dental hygiene, and nursing require the teaching of EBP. Here are a few examples of accreditation standards related to EBP and evidence-based nursing.

The Liaison Committee on Medical Education (LCME) is the national accrediting authority for medical education programs leading to the MD degree in the United States and Canada. Its education standard number 6 states:

> The curriculum of a medical education program must incorporate the fundamental principles of medicine and its underlying scientific concepts; allow medical students to acquire skills of critical judgment based on evidence and experience; and develop medical students' ability to use principles and skills wisely in solving problems of health and disease. (www.lcme .org/functions2010jun.pdf)

Predoctoral osteopathic schools of medicine are accredited by The American Osteopathic Association's Commission on Osteopathic College Accreditation (COCA). The core competencies of the COCA state:

> At minimum, a graduate must be able to: (1) Demonstrate basic knowledge of osteopathic philosophy and practice and osteopathic manipulative treatment; and, (2) Demonstrate medical knowledge through one or more of the following: passing of course tests, standardized tests of the NBOME, post-core rotation tests, research activities, presentations, and participation in directed reading programs and/or journal clubs; and/or other evidence-based medical activities. (www.do-online .org/pdf/SB03-Standards_of_Accreditation _July%201,%202010.pdf)

The Commission on Collegiate Nursing Education (CCNE) accredits nursing programs. The CCNE's standards call for nursing programs to incorporate guidelines from the AACN (American Association of Critical-Care Nurses). The AACN includes a host of expectations related to evidence-based nursing, which are too lengthy for purposes of this discussion. However, we include one of the AACN statements here regarding baccalaureate nursing education:

> *Professional nursing practice is grounded in the translation of current evidence into practice. Scholarship for the baccalaureate graduate involves identification of practice issues; appraisal and integration of evidence; and evaluation of outcomes. As practitioners at the point of care, baccalaureate nurses are uniquely positioned to monitor patient outcomes and identify practice issues. Evidence-based practice models provide a systematic process for the evaluation and application of scientific evidence surrounding practice issues . . . . Dissemination is a critical element of scholarly practice; baccalaureate graduates are prepared to share evidence of best practices with the interprofessional team. (www.aacn.nche.edu)*

Physician assistant (PA) programs are accredited by the Accreditation Review Commission on Education for the Physician Assistant (ARC-PA). Regarding the PA curriculum, the most recent ARC-PA standards state:

> *The curriculum establishes a strong foundation in health information technology and evidence-based medicine and emphasizes the importance of remaining current with the changing nature of clinical practice.*

The ARC-PA holds PA programs to the following standard:

> *The program curriculum must include instruction to prepare students to search, interpret and evaluate the medical literature, including its application to individualized patient care. (www.arc-pa.org)*

Acknowledgements

The three lead authors would like to thank all of the people who contributed to this text, both directly and indirectly. We want to thank our contributing authors Gloria A. Jones Taylor, DSN, RN; Barbara J. Blake, PhD, RN, ACRN; and D. Dennis Flores, BSN, ACRN.

It took 3 years to fully realize this book, and 14 years of education for this project. As such, my husband, Richard, and my sons, Jacob and Calvin, have committed as much of their lives to this book as did I. The writing of this book was, in some ways, similar to competing in a professional car race. If a racecar driver alone tried to compete, he or she could not get past the starting line. The car and the race require a team. My team included my co-authors, my immediate and extended family, my friends, many of my colleagues, my students, and the teachers whose classes I took during my education. Ellen Rogo has been a colleague, mentor, and friend for many years. I wish to thank her for everything she has taught me. Teresa Shelton was once a student who took an EBP course from me and has since become both a friend and valued colleague. My family members were unwavering in their confidence in me throughout this project, as were my colleagues and students. I will be forever grateful to the students who have taken my EBP courses—they are the reason I wanted to write this book. I wish to acknowledge Teri Peterson, the statistician for the Division of Health Sciences at Idaho State University. Through my work with Teri on countless research projects over the years I gained a deep understanding of research and appreciation for the importance of a team approach to research. I want to thank Kate Erickson, Rebecca Hall, Jessica Fullmer, and Kathy Evans. They are exceptional students, researchers, and scholars from Idaho State University who worked closely with me throughout the process of developing this book. I wish to thank the teachers and staff at Holy Spirit Catholic School, in Pocatello, ID, whose demonstration of outstanding education and steadfast support of my family has been a constant inspiration to me. I am sorry I cannot identify by name everyone who has been by my side throughout this process. I hope you all know how very grateful I am.

Bernadette Howlett, PhD

Life for me has been a journey surrounded by individuals who have loved and supported me in my professional pursuits. During my younger years, my parents, Audrey and James Spangler, my brother,

Jim, and my grandparents provided unconditional love and ongoing support as a valuable gift to me throughout my journey. My grandmother Mary, as a spiritual icon, helped me realize the many blessings in my life, and to live life by values that are important. My own family has been a significant inspiration for my professional endeavors. To my husband, Paul Rogo, I appreciate your ability to keep me grounded in reality and for the adventures that provided relaxation during my scholarly pursuits. My son Paul Marco, I thank you for your support and being proud of my accomplishments, as I am proud of yours. To Jason, my youngest son, I am eternally grateful for your ongoing computer and technical support to complete this project; your talents continue to impress me. My mother-in-law, Ruth Rogo, has always been proud of my accomplishments as a working mother and I thank her for her support. To my grandsons, Braxton and Gunner, I wish you a lifetime of love, happiness, and success. It has been an honor and a privilege to work with Bernadette Howlett. Her wealth of knowledge of evidence-based practice and her dedication and commitment to the writing of this textbook are noteworthy. I cherish the hours we spent together and the laughs we had. To Teresa Shelton, thank you for your valuable insights into the pharmaceutical industry.

Ellen J. Rogo, RDH, PhD

First, I wish to acknowledge my co-authors. To Bernadette Howlett, thank you for educating me on the relevance of types of scientific evidence and further expanding my knowledge and use of medical statistics. Thank you for creating this book, and inviting me to be a part of the project. The health professional students that receive this EBP text in place of four separate books deserve this all-in-one tool for learning. Most of all, I am grateful for your guidance and friendship during my PA training and beyond. I look forward to more spirited conversations with you in the future. To Ellen Rogo, your expertise, time, and extensive commitment to creating this textbook are incredibly appreciated. Other thanks go to past and present colleagues in the pharmaceutical and physician assistant professions, including Gregg Luke, RPh, for performing chapter reviews and for generously advising me on drug therapy in my clinical practice; to the pharmaceutical industry, for training me on the basics of therapeutics, as well as for creating medications that improve patients' quality of life; and to my preceptors and mentors of clinical medical practice who have shown me how they practice EBP and further teach me to think critically when making important treatment decisions with patients. Finally, I express infinite gratitude to my friends and family who have supported me in my medical career; especially my husband Brett, for being my source of courage and encouragement. You are a true partner. To Zane and Kepa, thank you for the joy of being our greatest creations and inspiration.

Teresa Gabiola Shelton, MPAS, PA-C

About the Authors

Bernadette Howlett, PhD, is the director of research for a rural Critical Access Hospital (Bingham Memorial Hospital, Blackfoot, Idaho) and was formerly an associate professor and research coordinator for a physician assistant (PA) studies program. She is currently an affiliate faculty member with the Institute of Rural Health at Idaho State University contracted to design and teach courses in evidence-based practice as well as interprofessional practice. She has taught evidence-based medicine for 9 years and was the coordinator for a cumulative evaluation and a capstone assessment course in a physician assistant graduate program. She is an accomplished researcher and has a doctorate in adult and organizational learning. She is also an expert in online education.

In addition to teaching in a graduate PA program, Dr. Howlett has also taught graduate-level classes for nurse practitioner, dental hygiene, and public health programs. She also taught a freshman seminar course for more than 10 years. Dr. Howlett has coordinated and designed clinical trials, and has written numerous publications, national paper presentations, and international conference presentations. She is a recipient of the John L.V. Bobell Award for Outstanding Dedication and Devotion to the Field of Adult Learning from the American Society of Training and Development.

Ellen J. Rogo, RDH, PhD, is currently an associate professor in the Department of Dental Hygiene at Idaho State University in Pocatello, Idaho, and was previously an associate professor at Fairleigh Dickinson University College of Dental Medicine, Division of Dental Hygiene. She has been a dental hygiene educator for more than 30 years, with administrative leadership positions as the coordinator of a degree completion program and department chairperson. Her experience includes teaching courses in research methodology and evidence-based practice to undergraduate students as well as supervising dental hygiene research, literature analysis and synthesis, and thesis research for graduate students. Dr. Rogo also mentors graduate students and faculty in their research, grant writing, and manuscript-preparation endeavors. Her accomplishments include numerous national and international presentations and publications in a variety of professional journals. In addition, she has authored several book chapters and has received a number of research grants. Dr. Rogo has designed and conducted quantitative and qualitative research investigations on clinical and educational topics.

Teresa Gabiola Shelton, MPAS, PA-C, is a physician assistant residing in Cache Valley, Utah. She holds a master's degree in physician assistant studies, a national license to practice family medicine with the National Commission on Certification of Physician Assistants (NCCPA), and is currently licensed to practice in Utah. Her undergraduate degrees are in foreign languages and business.

For the past 10 years, her career focus has been in the pharmaceutical and medical fields. She has combined her knowledge of medical Spanish and Hispanic culture as well as pharmacology and medical practice training for the provision of services in a family practice setting. In her current position at a rural community health center, Teresa provides health care to a population of medically underserved people in northern Utah and southeastern Idaho.

Contributors

Barbara J. Blake, PhD, RN, ACRN
Associate Professor of Nursing
WellStar School of Nursing
Kennesaw State University
Kennesaw, Georgia

D. Dennis Flores, BSN, ACRN
Grady Health System
Atlanta, Georgia

Gloria A. Jones Taylor, DSN, RN
Professor of Nursing
WellStar School of Nursing
Kennesaw State University
Kennesaw, Georgia

Reviewers

R. David Doan III, MS, PA-C
Evidence Based Medicine Instructor
Physician Assistant Program
Western Michigan University
Kalamazoo, Michigan

Claudia Leiras-Laubach, PhD
Director of Research, College of Health
    Professions
Assistant Professor, Physician Assistant Studies/
    Allied Health Studies
Grand Valley State University
Grand Rapids, Michigan

Eric C. Nemec, PharmD, BCPS
Clinical Assistant Professor
College of Pharmacy
Western New England University
Springfield, Massachusetts

Howard Straket, EdD, MPH, PA-C
Assistant Professor
Director, Community Medicine
Department of Physician Assistant Studies
The George Washington University
Washington, District of Columbia

Adam J. Thompson, PhD, LAT, ATC
Professor
Director of Athletic Training Education
Indiana Wesleyan University
Marion, Indiana

Eric Vangsnes, PhD, PA-C
Chair and Program Director Physician Assistant
    Department
Western Michigan University
Kalamazoo, Michigan

Linda J. Vorvick, MD
Medical Director
MEDEX Northwest Division of Physician Assistant
    Studies
Department of Family Medicine
University of Washington School of Medicine
Seattle, Washington

Evelyn Wilson, MHS, NREMT-P
Assistant Professor
Western Carolina University
Gaffney, South Carolina

Becky Wolff, MSN, RN, MA
Assistant Professor
University of South Dakota
Vermillion, South Dakota

Supakit Wongwiwatthananukit, PharmD, PhD
Associate Professor of Pharmacy Practice
College of Pharmacy
University of Hawaii at Hilo
Hilo, Hawaii

Marla Wonser, MSOT, OTR/L
Program Director
Casper College
Casper, Wyoming

Christine E. Wright, PhD, LOTR
Assistant Professor, Program in Occupational
    Therapy
Louisiana State University Health Sciences
    Center – Shreveport
Shreveport, Louisiana

Stephen W. Wyatt, DMD, MPH
Dean and Professor
University of Kentucky
Lexington, Kentucky

Y. Tony Yang, ScD, MPH
Assistant Professor
George Mason University
Fairfax, Virginia

Catherine L.E. Young, PhD
Visiting Assistant Professor of Biology and Public
    Health
Ohio Northern University
Ada, Ohio

FOUNDATIONS OF EVIDENCE-BASED PRACTICE

INTRODUCTION

This text is divided into two major sections: Part I, "Foundations of Evidence-Based Practice," and Part II, "Applications of Evidence-Based Practice." In the first six chapters of this text, we address the foundational concepts for evidence-based practice (EBP) as well as the interprofessional approach to patient-centered care. In Part II, we explore concrete applications of EBP.

In Chapter 1, we define EBP and explain how it works. In Chapter 2, we explore the various types and methods of healthcare publications. These first two chapters introduce much of the basic vocabulary of the subject matter and situate EBP into clinical practice. The next two chapters examine the various types and modes of health communication (Chapter 3), with an emphasis on patient education, as well as instructions on how to locate relevant evidence to answer focused clinical questions (Chapter 4). Part I closes with two chapters on statistics: descriptive statistics (Chapter 5) and inferential statistics (Chapter 6). These two chapters are primarily review of material you are expected to have studied previously.

Throughout this text we refer to the overarching concept of **Interprofessional Collaborative Practice (ICP)**. ICP provides the philosophical underpinnings for the approach to EBP presented in this book. As such, we provide here an introduction to ICP, which is:

> The development of a cohesive practice between professionals from different disciplines. It is the process by which professionals reflect on and develop ways of practicing that provides an integrated and cohesive answer to the needs of the client/family/population.[1]

ICP is designed to ensure high-quality, comprehensive care. The Interprofessional Education Collaboration explains interprofessional values and ethics as "grounded in a sense of shared purpose to support the common good in health care, and reflect a shared commitment to creating safer, more efficient, and more effective systems of care."[2]

The concept of ICP represents a recent shift from independent silos of health care to an integrated approach to providing patient-centered care. Traditionally, healthcare organizations, as well as individual practitioners, have operated separately, making decisions without complete information about a patient, such as the patient's condition, care provided in other settings, and medications prescribed by others.[3]

Consensus reports completed by the Institute of Medicine (IOM) in the early 2000s identified widespread patient errors in hospitals associated with significant preventable morbidity and mortality. These publications described major issues related to quality of care as well as costly care delivery systems. The reports recommended retraining of the healthcare workforce in "new ways of relating to patients and each other"[3] through interprofessional learning and approaches. The 2001 IOM report stated:

> The U.S. healthcare delivery system does not provide consistent, high-quality medical care to all people. Americans should be able to count on receiving care that meets their needs and is based on the best scientific knowledge—yet there is strong evidence that this frequently is not the case. Health care harms patients too frequently and routinely fails to deliver its potential benefits. Indeed, between the health care that we now have and the health care that we could have lies not just a gap, but a chasm.[3]

The IOM proposed in its 2001 report 10 rules for redesign of the healthcare system, many of which require interprofessional collaborative practice, as well as EBP. The 10 rules are as follows:

1. *Care is based on continuous healing relationships.*
2. *Care is customized according to patient needs and values.*
3. *The patient is the source of control.*
4. *Knowledge is shared and information flows freely.*
5. *Decision making is evidence-based.*
6. *Safety is a system property.*
7. *Transparency is necessary.*
8. *Needs are anticipated.*
9. *Waste is continuously decreased.*
10. *Cooperation among clinicians is a priority.*[3]

The IOM report led to the convening of an expert panel, sponsored by the American Association of Colleges of Nursing, the American Association of Colleges of Osteopathic Medicine, the American Association of Colleges of Pharmacy, the American Dental Education Association, the Association of American Medical Colleges, and the Association of Schools of Public Health. The work of the panel resulted in the formation of an organization called the Interprofessional Education Collaboration (IEC),[2] which was charged with developing a common set of core competencies and learning experiences to meet these competencies.

The IEC linked the competencies it developed with the competencies for health professionals developed by the IOM,[4] dividing the core IEC competencies into four domains:

1. *Values/ethics for interprofessional practice*
2. *Roles/responsibilities*
3. *Interprofessional communication*
4. *Teams and teamwork*

Thus, with the IOM rules and IEC core competencies in mind, the goals in this textbook regarding interprofessional practice are as follows:

1. *Apply EBP procedures to address questions in a variety of health professions.*
2. *Recognize the value of the team approach to EBP.*
3. *Develop awareness of other professions' information resources and how to use them.*
4. *Communicate interprofessionally in a patient/population-centered manner.*

REFERENCES

1. D'Amour D, Oandasan I. Interprofessionality as the field of interprofessional practice and interprofessional education: An emerging concept. *J Interprof Care*. 2005;19(Suppl 1):8–20.
2. Interprofessional Education Collaborative. Core competencies for interprofessional collaborative practice: Report of an expert panel. 2011. Available at: www.aamc.org /download/186750/data/core_competencies.pdf. Accessed September 3, 2012.
3. Institute of Medicine. *Crossing the quality chasm: Report brief*. March 2001. Washington DC: National Academies Press. Available at: www.iom.edu/ ~ /media/Files/Report % 20 Files/2001/Crossing-the-Quality-Chasm/Quality % 20Chasm % 202001 % 20 % 20report % 20brief.pdf. Accessed September 3, 2012.
4. Peterson C. Institute of Medicine. Health professions education: A bridge to quality. [Executive Summary]. *Tar Heel Nurse*. 2003;65(4):12.

What Evidence-Based Practice Is and Why It Matters

Bernadette Howlett, PhD

INTRODUCTION

When you are choosing a diagnostic test, performing a treatment, or looking for drug interactions, you will base your decisions on many sources of information. You will rely on your accumulated knowledge of biology, biochemistry, physiology, pathology, and health care. However, vast sources of information are available to improve on that knowledge. How will you decide which sources to use and which ones are trustworthy? This text will provide you with the skills to answer that question.

Today, many sources of healthcare information are available and innumerable authorities offer recommendations. The sources are as varied as they can be contradictory: textbooks, medical journal articles, specialty organizations, the gray-haired doctor, the actor in a drug commercial, the pharmaceutical representative, health professional faculty members, supervising clinicians, brochures, websites, friends, family,

and neighbors. You, your patients, and your organization might turn at times to many of these sources.

For students in health professional education programs, textbooks, healthcare-related journals in the library or in online databases, and instructors are the main sources of knowledge. These sources are sometimes presumed to be infallible. It is not uncommon for practitioners to use the phrase, "That's how it was taught in *my* program" in defense of a treatment choice. The statement implies that a choice is correct based purely on the instruction of a faculty member, regardless of how long ago the practitioner graduated. There is a tendency to assign authority to certain sources of information. A quote from a reputable journal, for example, can carry great weight with practitioners and patients alike. However, premature or misleading information can be reported, even by the most trustworthy of sources. The story of thalidomide exemplifies this point.

In the late 1950s, it became common practice in Europe to prescribe a drug called **thalidomide** (a sedative-hypnotic drug) as a treatment for morning sickness and to help pregnant women sleep.[1,2,3] It was accepted practice in more than 50 countries. Articles about the drug were published in 1959 and 1960 in sources that included the *British Medical Journal,* the *American Journal of Psychiatry,* the *British Journal of Pharmacology and Chemotherapy,* and the *American Journal of Obstetrics and Gynecology.*[4]

Many newborns of mothers who had taken thalidomide were afflicted with **phocomelia** (also known as "seal limb"). Thalidomide not only caused limb deformities, but also deafness, blindness, cleft palate, and other internal problems. Most frequently phocomelia affected the formation of the arms, which ended up looking like flippers. The condition was caused by failure of the long bones of the arm to develop. In some instances, fingers grew from an infant's shoulders (**Figure 1–1**).

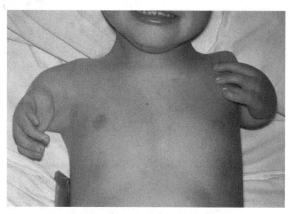

Figure 1–1 Thalidomide Baby
© Wellcome Images/Custom Medical Stock Photo

The drug was marketed as "completely safe" by its manufacturer, the German company Chemie Grünenthal. However, the drug did not receive approval from the FDA when a company by the name of Richardson-Merrell applied to market it in the United States years after it had been introduced in Europe. Nonetheless, the company distributed millions of doses of the drug to U.S. physicians while it performed animal studies on the safety and efficacy of the drug. This practice was legal at the time. It is estimated that some 20,000 patients in the United States received the drug.

The first articles questioning thalidomide's safety came out in June of 1960. However, the use of thalidomide in pregnant women was not banned until 1962, after more than 10,000 cases (40 in the United States) of birth defects had been reported.[1,2] Approximately 40% of these infants died within their first year of life. Today in some parts of the world women continue to take thalidomide and give birth to children with phocomelia. While the drug is dangerous to fetuses, it is known to be effective in the treatment of leprosy and certain forms of cancer. It is now approved for these uses under strict guidelines.

The story of thalidomide demonstrates the hazard of selecting a treatment without sufficient research. It also reveals the persistence of a treatment choice despite great hazards once it becomes a common practice. Although such severe examples are rare, they provide a lens through which to view healthcare decision making.

The purpose of this discussion is not to cause you to distrust sources of healthcare information. More than likely, reputable journals, your textbooks, and your instructors will be correct the vast majority of the time. You should trust them—just not unquestioningly. You should have the skills to discern if information is indeed accurate and applicable in each case. It is essential, in fact, that you develop this skill for the sake of your patients and the longevity of your career.

As a member of a healthcare team, comprised of practitioners in your profession as well as other professions, you will eventually be responsible for the care of patients, either directly or indirectly. You will be making decisions without your preceptors or clinical faculty. You will make judgments in many different situations. For example, you will face clinical questions that do not have entries in the indexes of your textbooks. You might discover that a diagnostic tool is not as accurate as you thought it was. You are likely to encounter a patient who does not respond to the usual treatment protocol.

You might be asked by a clinic manager to develop a standard of care for your practice. You could be called upon to write letters to insurance companies explaining why they should cover the treatment you want for your patients. Terminal patients will ask you how long they have to live. You might be approached repeatedly by pharmaceutical representatives offering you samples and asking you to prescribe their products. You might even be asked to give a lecture in the very program from which you graduated. In all of these situations, and more, you will need to interpret and critically evaluate healthcare information. This chapter introduces you to a set of critical thinking skills that will enable you to engage in this activity, called *evidence-based practice*.

LEARNING STRATEGIES FOR SUCCESS IN HEALTH PROFESSIONAL EDUCATION PROGRAMS

Evidence-based practice (EBP) is a translational form of critical thinking. By **translational critical thinking** we mean that the theoretical skills and concepts of critical thinking are translated into real-world applications. As such, several learning strategies native to critical thinking can be applied to EBP. These strategies include the ability to solve ill-structured problems, self-awareness, self-direction, and

active engagement. EBP is also a lifelong learning activity. You will engage in this process throughout your career.

Solving Ill-Structured Problems

Solving ill-structured problems is described by the Association of American Colleges (AAC) as, "knowing that the world is far more complex than it first appears." The AAC goes on to explain that students, "must make interpretive arguments and decision-judgments that entail real consequences for which they must take responsibility and from which they may not flee by disclaiming expertise."[5] Patient care often requires practitioners, as well as health professional students, to make healthcare decisions in the face of limited or contradictory information. To make a decision, they must take into account current research, patient preferences, cost, availability of resources, legal ramifications, local standards of care, and even religion and culture. It is rare for a patient care decision to be a simple binary (right/wrong) choice. In school, students will often be faced with questions that have more than one correct answer, in which the best choice depends on a variety of situational factors. Your comfort with making decisions under these circumstances will determine your success in solving these ill-structured problems, and hence your success in your degree program.

Self-Awareness

In order to engage in critical thinking, individuals need to be aware of their own knowledge, skills, and beliefs. Practitioners need to recognize the limits of their knowledge and abilities; reflect on their successes, as well as their mistakes; have the curiosity to seek new knowledge, and possess the humility to admit they need that knowledge. We need the ability to accept mistakes so that we can learn from them. We need to be able to articulate our values and know how they interact with our knowledge and decisions. It takes self-awareness to meet these needs. It takes self-awareness, and perhaps even a little courage, to engage in critical thinking.

We say this because there is a common fear that critical thinking can cause people to become indecisive or lose their core values. There is a saying that goes, "Don't be so open minded that your brain falls out." What this saying implies is that consideration of multiple perspectives can cause you to believe there is no right answer and, hence, forever vacillate between choices. Self-awareness will prevent this from happening. Furthermore, such vacillation by definition is not critical thinking. Critical thinking is about using information to make choices. Indecision is caused by fear, not by information. Self-awareness will allow you to recognize this fear and be able to use information to choose a course of action.

Self-Direction

Critical thinking requires self-direction, which is also referred to as *independent thinking*. Reliance on experts as the sole source of knowledge makes practitioners and students *dependent* thinkers. Self-direction leads to independence. This does not mean rejecting authoritative sources, but rather questioning them in order to provide the best quality care. Self-direction means seeking to expand your knowledge and skills. It means being intrinsically motivated by a desire to learn and continuously improve. Independent thinkers seek knowledge without the provocation of an external reward. This trait is evident in clinicians who participate in continuing education beyond the minimum required hours to retain their licenses or who learn about topics outside of their specialties. Self-direction is evident in students who do more than the required readings and seek knowledge beyond the facts communicated in lectures.

Active Learning

The final key component for critical thinking, as it relates to health professional education, is active learning. Active learning focuses the responsibility for learning on the student, rather than on the instructor. It requires that students do something beyond merely listening to a presentation. Students are actively learning when they ask questions, take notes, or complete assigned readings prior to lecture (and take notes related to the readings). Active learning includes completing case studies, participating in small groups, writing papers, or giving presentations. Active learning takes many forms, but the key ingredient is student accountability.

When students approach learning as *their* responsibility they become actively engaged in the learning. Regardless of what teaching strategy is employed, students can choose to be active or passive (independent or dependent). You can merely listen to a lecture, which is passive, or you can take notes and ask questions, which is active. You can passively let other small group members complete an assignment, or you can actively do your part as well as engage your group members with their parts.

One area where this trait is most evident is in exam behaviors. You can passively expect exams to include only the facts presented in lecture, or actively anticipate that exams will address relevant knowledge and skills to the course subject area. In health profession programs, active learners recognize not only that they are responsible for seeking information, but that they are also responsible for demonstrating their command of that information on an exam, even for concepts not presented in a lecture.

THE CASE OF MR. MARTINEZ

Let's look at an example. Later in the chapter we will provide brief explanations about some of the medical concepts within this example.

> Mr. Martinez, a 45-year-old male of Hispanic descent, visits his primary care provider for a routine employment-screening physical. He has been hired as a home construction site manager for a local company that requires a medical release in order for him to start his job. Mr. Martinez appears to be well, although overweight (height: 70 inches, weight: 202 pounds, waist: 38 inches).* He has no health complaints. When asked about his family history, he reports that his father died recently at the age of 65 from a heart attack. Further questioning

reveals that Mr. Martinez is quite concerned about his own heart health. He has a wife and two teenage sons. He does not want his family to lose him at a young age. Lab tests reveal that he has abnormal lipid levels: total cholesterol = 222 mg/dL; HDL = 30 mg/dL; LDL = 160 mg/dL; triglycerides = 160 mg/dL. He also admits to smoking one pack of cigarettes per day for the last 25 years. On physical exam he is found to have a heartbeat with regular rate and rhythm, without murmurs, rubs, or gallops. His pulse is 78 beats per minute. His blood pressure is 136/88 mm Hg. His lungs are clear to auscultation bilaterally.

* The CDC define overweight[6] in adults as those with a body mass index (BMI)[7] between 25 and 29.9.

As part of Mr. Martinez's primary care team, you have several immediate questions to address. What will you report to his employer? Is he healthy enough for the job? Should he be treated for overweight? Should he be treated for high cholesterol? Which types of treatments are most effective?

There are other questions you also need to consider. Is the cholesterol test accurate? What types of screening tools provide the best information and at what cost? What risk does Mr. Martinez have for diabetes, heart attack, lung cancer, or other illnesses? How might his gender, ethnicity/race, age, and lifestyle affect treatment choices? What are his needs and preferences?

The list of questions could fill an entire book. In healthcare practice, questions are as prevalent as their answers. This chapter introduces a process for contending with the questions healthcare providers ask and evaluating the answers to them. This process is known as *evidence-based practice*.

In this chapter, we introduce the fundamental concepts of evidence-based practice and provide a framework for the process. We explain its definition and purpose in light of two types of clinical outcomes: surrogate outcomes and outcomes that matter. We provide a brief history of EBP in order to help you understand what it is and why it matters. The main focus of the chapter is the process of EBP, including explanations of three different approaches

(prospective, concurrent, and retrospective) and clinical categories in which it is applied (epidemiology, diagnosis, prevention, treatment, prognosis, harm, and patient education).

Healthcare research is traditionally broken into so-called *levels of evidence*, for which there are numerous naming systems. In this chapter, we discuss several of these evidence-level systems, such as the one used by the **U.S. Preventive Services Task Force** (**USPSTF**). The chapter concludes with sample evidence-based practice questions and an exercise in writing focused questions based on the case of Mr. Martinez.

OVERVIEW OF EVIDENCE-BASED PRACTICE

Definition

Evidence-based practice (EBP) is the process of combining the best available research evidence with your knowledge and skill to make collaborative, patient- or population-centered decisions within the context of a given healthcare situation.

In the definition of evidence-based practice, there are four key concepts to consider:

- *Best available research.* The highest-quality, most recent research available should be consulted whenever possible. Study design and funding sources are key considerations. Critiquing healthcare research publications is a critical skill, as is locating applicable research.
- *Knowledge and skill.* Your clinical knowledge and skills, which you continuously assess and develop as a lifelong learner, form the basis for every decision you make. Critical thinking is the key competency to this aspect of healthcare decision making. It is well worth your time as a student to learn more about critical thinking and to endeavor to grow in this area. Many health professional training programs are

designed to develop critical thinking skills in students. Although this topic is beyond the scope of this text, we encourage you to learn as much as you can about critical thinking. It will not only improve your clinical effectiveness, but it will help you communicate with patients and with other professionals.

- *Collaborative, patient-centered decisions.* Even the best-quality research might not apply to a given patient. Research deals with representative samples, but individual patients each have unique needs and responses to treatment as well as individual desires and circumstances. Every decision must be a collaborative process between the practitioner and the patient. This patient-centered concept will emerge many times throughout your health professional education and your career. **Figure 1–2** shows the elements of patient-centered decisions, how they interact as well as how they relate to one another.

- *Context of a given clinical situation.* Many situational factors influence health decisions, such as the specialties of clinical team members, the setting in which the patient is seen (a rural family practice versus an urban trauma center, for example), available resources (such as access to equipment or labs), urgency of the patient's complaint, the patient's ability to pay, and the preferences of the patient and the patient's family.

We feel it is essential to note here that the definition of EBP we provide differs somewhat from definitions utilized for evidence-based medicine. One of the most widely accepted, and cited, definitions of evidence-based medicine comes from the Centre for Evidence-based Medicine (CEBM) in Oxford, England: "Evidence-based medicine is the conscientious, explicit and judicious use of current best evidence in making decisions about the care of individual patients."[8]

We could have utilized essentially the same definition for evidence-based practice (replacing the

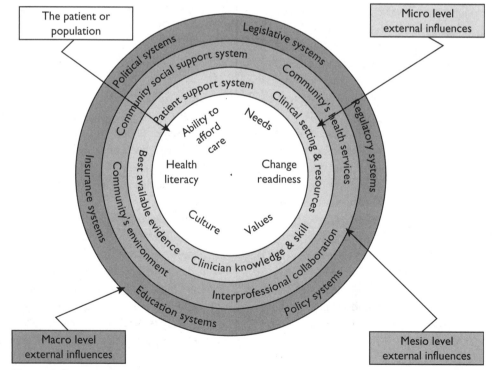

Figure 1–2 Patient-Centered Decision Making

word "medicine" with the word "practice"), but we decided the definition we wanted to use needed to reflect several important characteristics, such as the fact that EBP and EBM are both processes. Clinical decisions tend to be emergent activities, rather than static activities. The definition of EBM describes the, "use of current, best evidence," but does not indicate that decisions might evolve over time and that the activity of using evidence involves a distinct set of procedures.

Additionally, the CEBM definition focuses in making decisions without clarifying who is making them. Because we wanted to emphasize the role of the patient in making clinical decisions, we determined it was crucial to include the concepts of patient-centered and collaborative decision making. In recent years health care has been gradually shifting away from a traditional, paternalistic, and authoritarian relationship between clinicians and patients. This shift not only includes a collaboration with the patient and the patient's family, but also an interprofessional collaboration with other health professionals. We wanted the definition of EBP to reflect this current thinking.

Lastly, the CEBM definition of EBM emphasizes the focus of decisions for individual patients. We believe that the evidence-based process can, and should, be applied to population-based healthcare decisions as well as other group levels, such as families. This also reflects the interprofessional perspective of EBP we utilize. Certain health professions are focused on population-level issues, such as public health. We felt a more inclusive definition was warranted.

We do not, however, believe or wish to convey the message that other definitions of EBP (or EBM) are incorrect. The various definitions available have a common core that allows each to be correct and to reinforce or inform the others. The differences between definitions are generally about nuances, and the meaning is essentially the same from one to the next.

The collaborative process of making decisions following EBP involves multiple influences at multiple levels. A systems approach to decision making best describes the EBP patient-centered decision making process. Figure 1–2 displays the various sources and levels of information to be considered. The patient is at the center and is the focus of the model. There are three rings surrounding the patient, representing external influences at different levels. The further from the center, the broader the influence.

The outermost circle represents macro-level influences, such as political systems, regulatory systems, and so on. The next circle includes mesio-level influences, including interprofessional collaboration among different healthcare disciplines as well as community influences, such as availability of healthcare services. The next circle, the one closest to the patient, is the micro-influence level. The micro-influence level includes the expertise of the healthcare professional, the best available evidence (including qualitative and quantitative evidence), the patient's support system, and so on.

Again, at the center of the process is the patient or the population being served. The patient/population level in the diagram includes influences such as values, needs, level of health literacy, culture, ability to afford care, and readiness to change. There is an interplay among all of the influences represented in the chart. These influences occur consciously and subconsciously for clinicians, for patients, and for communities. Healthcare professionals need to be mindful of all of these influences as well as the various levels of influence, as opposed to focusing on just one level or just one influence.

History of EBP

Historically, clinical decisions have relied almost solely upon the knowledge and authority of the clinician. A paradigm shift has occurred, however, in recent years. Beginning in 1981, a series of articles was published by clinical epidemiologists from McMaster University in Ontario, Canada. These articles provided guidelines for critical appraisal of medical literature. The McMaster team's goal was to teach medical residents the critical appraisal skills needed to use current medical literature to support their clinical decisions.[9] In 1991, the first use of the term *evidence-based medicine* appeared in the American College of Physicians' Journal Club.[10] The term *evidence-based practice* emerged later when other disciplines began to utilize the concept, and there was a realization that the evidence-based process could be applied to many fields of endeavor, both within and outside of health care.

The team from McMaster University connected with a group of academic physicians in the United States and formed the Evidence-Based Practice Working Group. The group produced a series of 25 articles entitled, "The User's Guide to Medical Literature," which was published in the *Journal of the American Medical Association (JAMA)* from 1993 through 2000. These articles have been referenced in literature countless times, and today there are many courses, centers, and professionals teaching and engaging in evidence-based practice. Over that same period of years, the Internet, as we know it, came into existence.

Before the early 1990s, desktop computers were rare and electronic publication was just a dream. In the span of less than a decade, access to information exploded across the planet and clinicians began to have instant access to more information than they could manage. Evidence-based medicine (as it was called at the time) appeared at the right time in light of the emergence of the Information Age. It also provided solutions for contending with the ever-expanding web of health information.

The rationale that underpins EBP has had great appeal in many professions and areas of study, so much so that the term has been adopted and modified to fit a variety of fields. The term *evidence-based practice* is now commonly accepted to apply to any discipline that employs the model. For example, there is *evidence-based nursing, evidence-based policing, evidence-based management*, and even *evidence-based teaching*.

A central concept to the EBP model that has changed the practice of biomedical research is the type of outcomes of interest to practitioners. Historically, physiologic measures (such as laboratory results) were accepted as sufficient representations of illness. EBP advanced the notion that there

are other outcomes that matter to providers and to patients in addition to physiologic outcomes. Today, biomedical research often considers these other outcomes in addition to traditional laboratory data.

Outcomes of Care

The term **outcomes of care** in the context of health care, refers to the measurable or observable results of illness or treatment. Outcomes provide the objective data points for healthcare research. Weight change might be the outcome measured in studying the effects of an exercise program, for example. Satisfaction with nursing care might be an outcome measured in emergency department research. Reduced triglycerides might be the outcome measured in a medication trial.

In EBP, measures of **mortality** (death), **morbidity** (illness), and clinical signs (symptoms, test results) are utilized to determine the presence and severity of disease. They also are used to determine the patient's level of wellness and functioning, as well as efficacy of treatment. A landmark study called the Medical Outcomes Study[11] (MOS) first offered a framework to measure effectiveness of physician practice. The MOS provided outcomes in categories including clinical end points, signs and symptoms, laboratory values, functional status, general well-being, and satisfaction with care. Similarly, the field of nursing utilizes a set of nursing-sensitive patient outcomes called Nursing Outcomes Classification (NOC).[12]

Outcome measures give us information of different types and of relative importance to us as providers and to our patients. For example, a cholesterol test gives us physiologic information, but it does not tell us if the patient has any symptoms, nor does it confirm if heart disease is present. The outcome of a cholesterol test might not matter as much to a patient as the presence of chest pain. Also, the outcome of high cholesterol might not indicate the presence of disease at all. For this reason, it was recognized by the founders of EBP that researchers must measure *outcomes that matter* whenever possible.

Surrogate Outcomes

A **surrogate outcome** is a process of using one outcome to reflect another. Surrogates are selected based on the association of a physiologic or biologic measure with another known clinical end point. For example, arterial blood gas (ABG) levels act as a surrogate for respiratory acidosis. Respiratory acidosis is a medical condition that results from decreased respiration. It leads to increased carbon dioxide (pCO_2) in the blood and decreased blood pH.[13] This state occurs in a number of disorders, including asthma, COPD, and drug overdose, and it can be immediately life threatening.

Many physiologic measures are utilized as surrogates, such as blood pressure, heart rate, cholesterol levels, and white blood cell count. (It would quite impossible to compile a complete list of surrogate measures used in health care.) There is a problem, however, with surrogate outcome measures. Because the surrogate is not a direct measure of what it represents, it can be inaccurate. For instance, a patient might have heart disease, but might not have elevated blood pressure or high cholesterol. And not all patients with high blood pressure or cholesterol have heart disease. Furthermore, any given surrogate might represent many different clinical end points. High blood pressure can be an indicator of a host of different conditions. By itself, high blood pressure provides little information about the condition of a patient.

From a medical research standpoint, however, it is easier, faster, and less expensive to collect surrogate outcome data. The alternative to surrogate outcomes is clinically relevant outcomes such as death, tissue samples, measures of activities of daily living and levels of pain, and so on. It can take significant amounts of time for a clinically relevant outcome to occur, which can allow disease to progress beyond the point of intervention. Clinically relevant outcomes can be difficult or impossible to measure, and their measurement can be invasive. For example, the only way at present to make a definitive diagnosis of Alzheimer's disease is through autopsy of brain tissue.

Outcomes that Matter

Clinically relevant outcomes that provide direct measures of disease are preferable to surrogate outcomes. The term **outcomes that matter** is often used to describe these direct measures of functioning or disease. This term is used because it encompasses more than clinical data; it also includes other outcomes that patients and providers care about, such as the patient's ability to function or the cost of care. Outcomes that matter include such factors as quality of life as well as mortality.

For example, the Action to Control Cardiovascular Risk in Diabetes (ACCORD) trial[14] utilized *incidence* of cardiovascular events (nonfatal myocardial infarction, nonfatal stroke, or death from cardiovascular causes) as its primary outcome measure. The study focused on type 2 diabetes, which has emerged in recent years as a significant health problem in the U.S. population. Type 2 diabetes increases patients' risk for a variety of health problems, including, cardiovascular disease, premature death, blindness, kidney failure, amputations, fractures, frailty, depression, and cognitive decline.[14(p. 2245)] Severity and frequency of these problems are associated with the degree of *hyperglycemia*, which is measured by plasma glucose or glycated hemoglobin level (a measure of the mean blood glucose level during the previous 2 to 3 months). These two tests are commonly used as surrogates for the many potential disease states that occur in patients with type 2 diabetes.

In the ACCORD trial, the outcome that mattered contradicted the surrogate outcome. The surrogate outcome showed that intensive glucose-lowering therapy was more effective than standard therapy. After 1 year of treatment, patients receiving intensive therapy had greater improvements in glycated hemoglobin levels than patients receiving standard therapy. However, intensive therapy also resulted in increased mortality and did not significantly reduce the incidence of major cardiovascular events.[14(p. 2545)] Although these findings occurred early in the study, intensive treatment was discontinued due to the risk to patients. Had only a surrogate outcome measure (glycated hemoglobin level) been used, intensive therapy might have continued, resulting in disastrous outcomes for some patients.

Another example of the value of using outcomes that matter came from the Cardiac Arrhythmia Suppression Trial (CAST).[15] The study demonstrated that several drugs that were highly effective in treatment of arrhythmia actually increased mortality after myocardial infarction. Prior to the publication of the CAST study, it was common emergency department practice to give patients antiarrhythmic drugs to suppress asymptomatic arrhythmias following an acute myocardial infarction.[16] This practice has been curtailed since the release of this study and others with similar findings.

EBP Skills

The process of EBP involves accessing the best-available evidence when a patient-care question arises and then considering that information in the context of the clinical situation. To engage in this process clinicians must hone three key skills: (1) developing **focused clinical questions**, (2) quickly locating applicable information, and (3) critically appraising that information. The following discussion introduces each of these concepts.

Focused Clinical Questions

Some examples of the kinds of questions that arise during patient care were brought up earlier in the case of Mr. Martinez. He is overweight, smokes cigarettes, and has elevated low-density lipoproteins (LDL) and triglycerides. In addition to these risk factors, his father died of a heart attack at a young age. Mr. Martinez is of Hispanic descent and is 45 years old. Each of these factors contributes to a focused clinical question. For example, which treatment for elevated LDL is most effective in male patients of his age and ethnicity? Focused clinical questions include the following elements:

- A specific condition or outcome (e.g., treatment of high LDL)
- Patient demographics (e.g., age, ethnicity, gender)
- Patient risk factors (e.g., smoking, overweight)

These details are essential in finding answers that fit with the patient individually. They guide and focus your search.

Locating Applicable Information

Once you have a focused question, the next skill you need is the ability to access appropriate resources. With time and experience, you will develop the ability to perform this task quickly. There are two keys to success with locating information. The first is having your own search protocol, which involves knowing the types of information available in the sources to which you have access. The second is developing a search practice that is *prospective*, *concurrent*, and *retrospective*.

Your search protocol should target sources that are most likely to contain the type of information you need. Each source tends to provide specific kinds of information. For example, PubMed and CINAHL are sources that include original scholarly research articles, whereas an evidence-based service such as DynaMed, Nursing Reference Center (for nursing), or PEDro (for physiotherapy) provide synthesized, peer-reviewed evidence summaries on focused clinical topics. A primary care textbook provides basic science information and common practice procedures, whereas journals such as the *American Journal of Nursing* or the *New England Journal of Medicine* provide results of recent developments and research. A textbook's information is likely to be broad in nature but somewhat dated, whereas a journal is narrow in focus but likely to be more current. The more sources you know of, and the more you know about each source, the faster you will be able to locate focused information. We recommend asking other students, faculty, and clinicians what sources they use as well as what advantages and limitations they see in each source.

You need to combine your search protocol with a prospective, concurrent, and retrospective EBP approach. **Prospective EBP** means seeking information in advance, rather than only in response to patient encounters. It means developing your fund of knowledge and being able to draw on that knowledge in clinical situations. It is about making a habit of searching for the latest developments in your areas of interest and practice. This is often referred to as *scanning*.

Generally, you will engage in prospective practice in order to sustain your license, because many professions require a certain amount of continuing education. Beyond certification requirements, prospective searching also means being watchful for new information. This aspect of practice includes subscribing to journals or online news services, participating in specialty organizations, asking pharmaceutical representatives what new drugs their companies are developing, and participating in a journal club in your organization. With prospective EBP, what you learn today will help the patients you see tomorrow.

Concurrent EBP means looking up information in response to clinical questions and using that information to make decisions regarding an individual patient. This practice can occur while the patient is in clinic. Many healthcare organizations provide ready access to information services. Many clinicians also purchase access for themselves on portable devices such as smartphones, PDAs, and laptops. E-Pocrates and DynaMed are current examples of subscription resources that are available for handheld devices. Concurrent practice requires rapid searching and assessment of information. Sources that provide peer-reviewed, focused summaries fit best with concurrent practice. Your ability to engage in concurrent practice will depend greatly on your success with prospective and retrospective practice. With concurrent EBP, what you learn today will help the patients you see today.

Retrospective EBP means looking up information subsequent to a clinical encounter. During a clinical encounter, you might not have time to search for information. Your clinic day might be too busy or your patients' needs too urgent to allow you to perform searches. However, when you have time later you can follow up on a question. In some cases you might be able to hold off making a decision with a patient until you have the information you need. This practice might be preferable to selecting a course of action when you still have an unanswered question. You might choose a treatment and change your plan after learning more subsequently. It takes a certain amount of humility and finesse to engage in retrospective EBP, but it can save lives and improve quality of care. With retrospective EBP, what you learn today could help a patient you saw yesterday.

Critically Appraising Information

Critical appraisal is a process of evaluating the trustworthiness and relevance of a resource within the context of a given clinical situation. Appraisal involves questions such as potential sources of bias, representativeness of a study's sample, consistency of a study's methods, accuracy of the data collected, duration of the research in light of the question explored, and even just the common sense of a study. In appraising a resource, you will determine where it lies within a *hierarchy* of evidence, a concept discussed later in this chapter (see "Assigning Levels of Evidence").

The resources you access might not be strictly empirical research. Much of what is available, in fact, comes in the form of expert opinion. An essential task when appraising a source is to determine if it is opinion. This situation can be more difficult than it seems, or it should be. Often expert opinions are communicated similarly to research, having the tone and organization of an empirical study. Such opinions are often nothing more than well-written reviews of the literature. Many expert opinions are based on the research of others. Sometimes one expert opinion is derived from prior expert opinions, and there is a complete lack of empirical research. Accessing the publications of the original research can help practitioners avoid this layering of opinions.

Original research publications are referred to as **primary literature**, whereas expert opinions typically fall in the category of **secondary literature** or **tertiary literature**. It is important that you can discern *primary* research from *secondary* and *tertiary* publications. All types are useful and serve important roles in informing providers. Your ability to recognize the type of publication will help you determine how to apply the information it contains.

The EBP Process

The EBP process brings together all of the resources just mentioned with your knowledge, skills, and practices into a model for clinical decision making. With time, you will develop your own EBP process. We provide you with an outline you can use to begin (**Figure 1–3**).

Step 1: Recognize the Need for Information

The first, and perhaps most obvious, step is acknowledging that information is needed. It is essential for you to recognize the boundaries of your knowledge and to be able to say, "I don't know." More than likely, you will easily identify a gap in your understanding, but it may not always be obvious when you need information for other reasons, such as recognizing a controversial standard of care. The prescribing of antibiotics for all acute middle ear infections (otitis media) in children is an example of this. It is a practice that was common in family medicine until recently but has been called into question due to antibiotic resistance, side effects, and allergic reactions. Also, uncomplicated ear infections in otherwise healthy children are often viral and self-resolving.

1. Recognize the need for information

2. Establish the purpose

3. Formulate focused question(s)

4. Identify target resources

5. Perform the search

6. Organize findings

7. Appraise trustworthiness

8. Assess relevance

9. Select action

10. Implement and evaluate

Figure I–3 The EBM Process

Viral infections are unresponsive to antibiotics.[17] However, sometimes circumstances call for the use of antibiotics to treat acute otitis media. In this first EBP step, the key is recognizing your need to know if watchful waiting or antibiotics are indicated. You must identify your assumptions and those of patients and other clinicians, and you must be willing to question those assumptions. Experience will greatly improve your ability to accomplish this step.

Step 2: Establish Purpose

Establishing the purpose of your query is about setting a goal, such as providing optimal fluid management in a hospitalized patient, and categorizing your question in terms of the type of information needed. Categories include **etiology**, **risk factors**, diagnosis, treatment, harm, **prognosis**, and patient education. The reason for identifying the category is twofold: first, it helps with selecting sources in which to search, and, second, it provides a search term to help narrow your results. For example, if you were caring for a patient with a fluid-volume deficit, you might be most interested in etiology (cause) and treatment. A search for "fluid-volume deficit" alone would provide many results unrelated to your question. By adding the term "etiology" or "treatment," you would likely find more focused information more rapidly.

An important companion to the purpose of your question is the nature of the information you seek. Is the information basic science, such as anatomy or physiology? Is it about medications or laboratory tests, or do you have questions across several topics? In the case of Mr. Martinez, for instance, you might be faced with choosing between medication or nutrition with exercise to treat his high triglycerides and LDL. This question clearly falls in the category of treatment. But this treatment question might require you to know or find the answer to other questions, such as whether a given treatment choice is as effective for lowering LDL as it is for lowering triglycerides. You might need to know the *physiology* of each of these compounds in the body in order to make the best treatment choice.

Step 3: Formulate Focused Question(s)

Once you have categorized your informational need, the next step is to add patient characteristics such as sex, age, ethnicity, and other health problems. These pieces are then brought together to formulate your question or questions. The more specific you are, the more successful you will be. For example, a broad question you might ask is, "What is the best treatment for lowering LDL and triglycerides?" But, when you consider Mr. Martinez, you can be more specific, "What is the best treatment for lowering LDL and triglycerides in an adult male of Hispanic descent?"

However, this question is still too broad, because it does not specify which treatments you are considering. Many treatments are available, ranging from a variety of nutritional interventions, exercise programs, and drugs, to even surgery. Furthermore, combinations of interventions are possible, such as diet plus exercise or nutrition plus medication. It is exceedingly rare to find studies that compare all of the possible treatments and combinations of treatments for a given condition.

Thus, a focused question regarding the case of Mr. Martinez might be phrased, "Is a nutrition/exercise program as effective as *statin* drugs in lowering LDL and triglycerides in an adult male of Hispanic descent?" Two more elements in this question must be considered: What type of outcome do we want to see, and what level of evidence do we need? Are we concerned with physiologic outcomes (cholesterol) or rather with the outcomes that matter, such as atherosclerosis, coronary heart disease (CHD), heart attack, or stroke? We might still be interested in evidence regarding cholesterol-lowering treatments, but we should also look for evidence that treatment will reduce morbidity or even mortality. Simply because one treatment is better than another for reducing LDL or triglycerides does not necessarily mean that treatment will result in fewer heart attacks. On a related note, you might also be interested in the potential harms of the various treatment options.

The level of evidence might be a matter of simply starting with the highest level, such as a meta-analysis, or it might be a matter of the type of question. In some cases, you might want to know if there has been a meta-analysis, and in other situations you might be seeking a **practice guideline** or an evidence-based review. Perhaps a meta-analysis was published earlier, but more recent randomized control trials have been conducted and you are looking for them. Later in the chapter we discuss the levels of evidence.

In your search, you will break up the components of your focused question, or questions, and use them in different ways. You might start by typing your complete question verbatim into a search field. This will likely produce few results. Instead, it is typically more effective to use the components of your question in a structured search. You will learn more about this strategy in step 5. For now, write out your question, making note of each of the vital components.

Step 4: Identify Target Resources

Different resources have different areas of emphasis or types of information. The objective at this stage in the process is to select the sources that best fit with the type of information you seek. As you gain experience, you will come to have a general knowledge of what is contained in the various information sources, making this step nearly invisible in the process. A number of sources offer focused evidence-based reviews, including DynaMed, Physician's Information and Education Resource (PIER), MD Consult, BMJ Point of Care, and others.

Focused evidence-based resources are convenient, quick, and *likely* to be valid. (We equivocate here with the word *likely* because you should never assume any source is valid, regardless of its reputation.) Other sources of high-quality evidence are more in-depth, such as the Cochrane Collaboration and the Oregon Evidence-Based Practice Center. Focused evidence-based sources often charge access or license fees.

A rule of thumb we recommend is that if you want to find a comparison of the most commonly used treatments for a well-researched disorder, start with the in-depth sources. For example, with Mr. Martinez you might be interested in finding the highest-level research regarding different cholesterol-lowering medications. Because heart disease and stroke are significant causes of morbidity and mortality, many studies related to the treatment of high cholesterol are available. Medications are increasingly relied upon for this purpose, and there are several medications to choose from. Additionally, lifestyle modifications (nutrition and exercise) have received considerable attention in the literature. An in-depth, high-quality source such as the Cochrane Library offers comparative studies that include multiple treatments.

Although there is a great deal of evidence for a topic such as high cholesterol, many topics have received little attention from researchers. High-level sources are unlikely to contain articles related to such topics. For example, we were recently interested in comparing the generic form of levothyroxine sodium with the brand name form of the drug. We wanted to know if the generic form is as effective as the brand name. Levothyroxine sodium is the treatment of choice for hypothyroidism.[18] Hypothyroidism is abnormally low secretion of thyroid hormone. Hypothyroidism is a somewhat common health problem with several widely accepted treatments (depending on the type and cause of the disorder). Hypothyroidism tends to be slow to progress and, if treated, rarely leads to life-threatening complications,[19] unlike high cholesterol.

We searched the Cochrane Library using the term "levothyroxine," and three articles were retrieved. None of the articles, however, addressed our question. One article examined treatment of subclinical hypothyroidism in pregnant patients, one examined the efficacy of treating subclinical hypothyroidism in general, and the third article compared high- verses low-dose initial treatment of congenital hypothyroidism. Levothyroxine sodium is a relatively inexpensive drug that has been available since the 1950s and is generally known to be highly effective. Hence, there is little incentive to perform new research in the treatment of hypothyroidism.

If you have a patient who does not respond well to the standard treatment for hypothyroidism, you might find it challenging to locate high-level research about this disorder. It is still advisable to start with in-depth or focused evidence-based sources, but you will need to have additional sources at your disposal. More than likely you would need to search in PubMed, go through endocrinology journals (hypothyroidism is a disorder of the endocrine system), or look for studies published by a specialty society. In this case, you might try the journals published by the Endocrine Society. Another option would be to search the National Guideline Clearinghouse for a practice guideline. You must keep in mind that as you move away from evidence-based sources such as the Cochrane Library you must be increasingly wary of resources that are based on opinion rather than on research. The objective at this step in the process is to have a search plan that includes sources with the highest-level evidence available in your area of inquiry.

Step 5: Perform the Search

Most college students have used electronic search tools extensively. You most likely already know how to perform a single-field search. You have probably performed thousands of single-field searches on the Internet. You have also probably had the experience of getting many irrelevant hits in an Internet search. A *single-field search*, in case you are wondering, is when you go to a search page that has just one search field on it and you type words into that field and click a button (**Figure 1–4**). This is the most common search procedure.

We recommend making a habit of choosing the "advanced search" option. Typically, the advanced search screen will allow you to add criteria to your search that will produce more focused results. On an advanced search screen, you can select options such as a date range or type of publication. **Figure 1–5** shows some of the many options available in an advanced search. The "exact wording

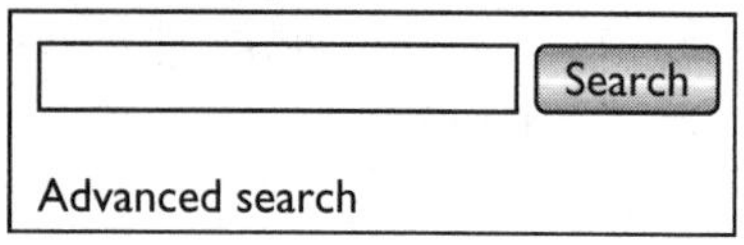

Figure I–4 Single-Field Search Screen

Find pages that have...

all these words:	
this exact wording or phrase:	
one or more of these words:	OR OR

don't show pages that have...

any of these unwanted words:	

more tools

Results per page:	10 results ▾
Language:	any language ▾
File type:	any format ▾
Search within a site or domain:	▾
	(e.g. .com, .edu)
Date: (how recent the page is)	anytime ▾
Numeric range:	..
SafeSearch:	⦿ On ◯ Off

Advanced Search:

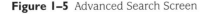

Figure 1–5 Advanced Search Screen

or phrase" field can be particularly useful, as can the "unwanted words" field. The main point we want to convey at present is that for step 5 of the search process you should become familiar with the search options available on the sites you use and to take advantage of them.

While you are searching, be sure to keep track of what terms you have used, in what combinations, and where you have searched. Watch out for different conjugations of words, such as singular versus plural (e.g., *feet* versus *foot*). Do not be afraid to use a basic Internet search engine, such as Google or Yahoo!, or even Wikipedia, to give you ideas and help you identify other places to search. In high school and college, students are often taught not to perform general Internet searches. This is a good rule to follow, because it will help you avoid getting incorrect information. However, a basic Internet search can be useful.

One final message here about step 5: You will have greater success finding valid resources if you are willing to go to the library. Although many resources are available online, many are not. It is common for the current year of a journal, for

example, to be available only in print form. In health care, information evolves rapidly. Often you will need the most recent publication on a topic, but it will only be available in print form. For the sake of your patients, and probably your grade, it is critical that you go into the library to perform your searches. Also, library staff can offer terrific insights when you are digging for information. Their expertise can make your search not only more complete and current, but also more rapid.

The library usually has the ability to order copies of publications that are not in any of its collections. It is not acceptable in the practice of health care for you to miss information simply because your library does not have it. If an item that has information you need is not available through your library, then order it through interlibrary loan or some other means. In fact, your instructor might be able to order it for you without being charged a fee. Do not hesitate to ask. Ultimately, it is your responsibility to get a copy of the resources you need, to read them, and to critically appraise the information contained within them.

Step 6: Organize Findings

As you search, organize your findings into a usable format. This strategy could be as simple as jotting down a few details on a sticky note. It might mean printing patient education materials or using a formal organizational structure, including references. The procedure you use will depend on the complexity of your question, the number of locations you search, and the purpose of your search. For example, imagine that your urgent care clinic is evaluating its standard of care for patients suspected to have pneumonia. You would need to identify the most accurate and affordable diagnostic procedure for community-acquired pneumonia. This is a complex question, because multiple diagnostic tools are available, such as history and physical exam, x-ray, CT, MRI, and blood tests. Clearly CT and MRI are expensive tools, but they might be more accurate than the other options.

In a search for literature related to this question, you would find that there are many studies on each type of diagnostic procedure, but no single study that compares all of them. Because you would have to search in several places, it is important to use an effective organizational strategy to track your findings.

Step 7: Appraise Trustworthiness

In step 7, your goal is to determine if the information provided by a given resource is trustworthy (also referred to as *reliability* and *validity*). How you evaluate trustworthiness depends on the type of resource you are examining. Many different types of resources are available, including textbooks, websites, practice guidelines, case studies, randomized control trials, systematic reviews, and many others. Each type of publication has different traits you will assess. In general terms, you will look for bias, errors, and untested assumptions.

Many of the publications you appraise will be in the form of primary research or summaries of primary research. For these types of resources, you will apply concepts of research design, statistics, and just plain common sense in appraising trustworthiness. You will ask questions such as: Did the

sampling strategy introduce bias? Was an adequate control group utilized? Was the study of sufficient duration? What funding supported the study? Were the correct analytical procedures selected for the type of data? Did the study have an appropriate sample size?

We could go on and on here listing the questions. It is not possible for us to write every question that can be asked during this step. The questions you use when appraising trustworthiness will depend on a number of factors, such as the purpose of your search and the amount of time you have to invest in the search. As with other steps in the EBP process, it takes time and experience to develop the skills needed to perform this step.

We advise you to employ a team approach to EBP. Each member of a clinical team brings different knowledge and experience. When combined, the collective ability of the team to appraise the trustworthiness of a resource is greater than the ability of an individual.

Step 8: Assess Relevance

In step 8, you determine if the information provided in a resource applies to the patient. For example, research on adults might not provide relevant information for a pediatric patient. Or, a study in which the sample was comprised of patients with a previous cardiac event might not provide relevant information to a patient who has not had a cardiac event. The title of the article, if it is well written, will help in making a determination about relevance. Here is an example of an article whose title gives you information on relevance, although not everything you need to know: "Interventions in the management of serum lipids for preventing stroke recurrence."[20] The word *recurrence* in this title is an important clue regarding relevance. It tells you that this study included patients who had already had a stroke.

Consider Mr. Martinez. If you searched the Cochrane Library for articles on "cholesterol," the above article will likely come up in your search results. This study was a systematic review of research involving patients 18 years or older with a history of stroke or TIA (transient ischemic attack). The article is applicable because it involved adults and it related to cholesterol treatment, but it might not be relevant to Mr. Martinez because he has not had a stroke. In this case, it was easy to determine that the article was not relevant because of its title.

Factors to consider regarding relevance include the histories of the patients selected for the study, the age of the patients, the type of intervention (if any), the length of the study, as well as the gender and race or ethnicity of patients. The patients included in a study should resemble the patient you are treating in as many factors as possible. The greater the similarity, the more relevant the results will be for your patient.

Step 9: Select Action

Once you feel you have gathered sufficient information, you will decide what course of action to take. The action chosen depends on the question asked. For example, if the question of your EBP search related to diagnosis, then the action might be to perform the diagnostic procedure. If the question related to the selection of treatment, then the action might be to implement treatment. It might also be that you choose to take no action, other than monitoring, depending on the situation. It could be the action you select is to stop treatment due to discovering potential adverse effects or interactions. The action you select could involve patient education if your question had been related to that topic.

Determining when you have sufficient information on which to act is a matter of the severity of the patient's condition, the status of your knowledge on the topic up to this point, and the patient's needs and preferences. For example, Mr. Martinez has elevated cholesterol, but no urgent health problems. He has risk factors for heart disease, but does not currently have heart disease. His situation gives you time to search for various treatment options, to look for literature on nutrition, exercise, drug therapies, surgical interventions, and so on. At this step in the process, you would need to discuss with Mr. Martinez the types of treatments

available. Patient compliance is essential in whichever treatment is selected, especially if the treatment involves lifestyle change or adherence to a drug regimen. Including the patient in the selection of action is imperative for a patient-centered approach to health care. Together with the patient, you should select the action that fits the health situation, can be achieved with available resources, and matches the patient's values.

You will need to be able to explain to your patient what you found in your review of evidence-based resources. It can help your patient decide which course of action to take, and it can influence the patient's adherence. You will need to communicate with the patient at his or her level of understanding. Effective patient communication is a skill you will be taught in your degree program. Another useful skill at this stage in the EBP process is *motivational interviewing*. It is a practice that incorporates effective patient communication with engagement of the patient in choosing a course of action. The specifics of motivational interviewing are beyond the scope of this text, but we encourage you to learn it and use it in your clinical practice, much as you learn any other clinical skill.

Step 10: Implement and Evaluate

The final step is to implement the action you and your patient have selected and to evaluate its effectiveness. It is important to ensure adequate patient education and to schedule a follow-up visit. Measures of effectiveness can include **objective** and **subjective data;** that is, information you observe or measure (objective) as well as the patient's perceptions (subjective). You must consider several questions at this point. What was the goal of the action taken? Is the outcome what was expected? Is the effect of the action adequate to meet the patient's needs? Are there any adverse effects? Is the patient compliant? Is the patient experiencing an outcome that matters? Is the cost acceptable to the patient?

At this stage in the EBP process, it is advisable to compare your patient's results with the results reported in the literature. The outcome your patient experiences should be communicated to others, whether it matches the stated outcomes in the literature or contradicts them. The growth of knowledge in health care depends on communication of real experiences with patients. Healthcare research is often designed to eliminate the many confounding factors that exist with real patients. This is done in order to ensure that the outcome being measured does not result from some other variable. However, the steps taken in a study to create validity take away the many variables you deal with in everyday clinical practice. The patients you see will usually be more complex than those included in the research you read.

Communication of the results you observe with your patients might simply be tracking within your own clinic and sharing with your colleagues. This process can provide data to support the standard of care your clinic has chosen. Communication of results could mean writing a case review for a journal, participating in a clinical trial, or even performing a study of your own. The anecdotal results of clinicians in day-to-day practice provide the foundation for many discoveries in health care. The EBP process is not complete until some form of communication of results has taken place and you have reflected on how the results apply to future decisions.

Categories of Evidence-Based Practice

We have mentioned that there are several categories in which we group EBP sources, including: epidemiology, prevention, diagnosis, treatment, prognosis, harm, and patient education. The categories we use in this text are commonly used in health profession literature and databases. The purpose of using categories for medical information is twofold: (1) to give you vocabulary to assist with formulating search terms and (2) to make it easier to discuss and explain the EBP process. However, studies often examine more than one of these topics and can be difficult to place squarely into a category. This occurrence does not indicate a flaw in the literature, but rather the nature of categorization systems. We create categories to organize information and to enable communication.

Assigning Levels of Evidence

Another means of categorizing medical information is to assign the level of evidence to a given resource. Several systems have been developed for designating evidence levels. It is common to refer to these systems as **evidence pyramids**.

Recent research has supported the concept of an evidence pyramid, which is a visual representation and system for categorizing healthcare information according to level of evidence. In most systems the top of the pyramid represents the highest level of evidence, those resources that are considered to be the most trustworthy. A team of researchers led by John Ioannidis has conducted meta-analytic studies in which they have examined the frequency with which well-published research findings have been positively refuted. In describing Ioannidis's research, Freedman[21] reported that 80% of nonrandomized studies (which rank low on the evidence pyramid) turn out to be wrong. Moving up the evidence pyramid, randomized control trials are shown to be wrong approximately 25% of the time. Near the top of the pyramid, large, high-quality randomized control trials are shown to be erroneous nearly 10% of the time. The higher a study appears on the pyramid, the less likely it is to be discredited by later research. There is no guarantee, of course, but Ioannidis's research has demonstrated the utility of the evidence pyramid.

The peak of the pyramid includes systematic reviews and meta-analyses that summarize well-designed randomized control trials. A Cochrane Review is this type of resource. The next level includes critically appraised synthesis or synopsis resources, also known as evidence-based reviews, critically appraised topics (CAP), or patient-oriented evidence that matters (**POEMs**). Sources such as DynaMed, Physician's Information and Education Resource (PIER), and BMJ Point of Care generally provide this level of evidence. It is not unusual for medical information providers to offer various levels of evidence.

The next level includes randomized control trials (RCTs). This level is sometimes subdivided by the size of the study and the levels of blinding. Large size, longitudinal, multicenter, double- or triple-blind studies are generally ranked highest in this group. In the next level, beneath RCTs, are cohort studies. These are then followed in the hierarchy by case-control studies, case series, and case reports. The remaining levels of the pyramid include textbooks, literature review articles (which differ from systematic reviews), laboratory research, and expert opinion pieces.

A number of different evidence hierarchy systems are available. We do not claim any one system to be the definitive system. You might find it useful to perform an Internet search on the term "evidence pyramid" and look at several of the results. The utility of this concept is that it gives you another means for appraising a resource. It is less important that you correctly identify the layer into which a given resource should be placed, but more important that you recognize if a resource is near the top, near the middle, or near the bottom of the hierarchy. See **Figure 1–6** for an example evidence hierarchy.

Some medical information providers give a rating scheme with the resources they provide, making it easier for you to ascertain the level of evidence. Often this information is referred to as the *strength* of a recommendation. For example, the USPSTF provides a grading system for its recommendations. The current USPSTF recommendation on screening men for lipid disorders is to screen men older than 35 years.[22] This recommendation is rated as a "Grade A recommendation," which

means that "There is high certainty that the net benefit is substantial." The USPSTF defines high certainty as follows:

> *The available evidence usually includes consistent results from well-designed, well-conducted studies in representative primary care populations. These studies assess the effects of the preventive service on health outcomes. This conclusion is therefore unlikely to be strongly affected by the results of future studies.*[23]

This definition does not clearly indicate if a USPSTF Grade A recommendation comes from a meta-analysis, systematic review, RCT, or so on, but it does help you determine that information assigned this grade belongs in the upper section of the pyramid.

EBP and Your Time

Engaging in EBP can feel time consuming. And, in the beginning, well . . . it is. It takes time to learn the skills of EBP. It takes time to develop your fund of knowledge. It takes time to learn what is contained in various resources. However, eventually EBP becomes a habit. And as it does, it will cease feeling like a cost to your time and more like a natural part of clinical practice. The perspectives we offered earlier about prospective, concurrent, and retrospective EBP will help with the time cost. Another strategy that will help reduce the time cost is collaborating with other clinicians. As we mentioned earlier, a team approach can be of benefit. It might also help if you expect it to take several years of practice until EBP starts to feel natural to you.

CASE STUDY: WRITING FOCUSED CLINICAL QUESTIONS

We return now to Mr. Martinez in order to bring together some of the concepts addressed in this chapter. In this case study, you will write a set of focused clinical questions following the procedure outlined earlier in the chapter. We also will give you several examples of focused clinical questions and explain how we would approach the case.

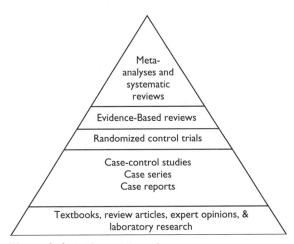

Figure 1–6 Evidence Hierarchy

The Case of Mr. Martinez

Before beginning the case study, we need to explain some of the concepts the case involves. Mr. Martinez has four evident health problems: (1) overweight, (2) dyslipidemia, (3) hypertension, and (4) tobacco abuse. We will give you some information on each of these topics, but this is a good point to have some biology, physiology, and/or pathophysiology textbooks at hand.

Mr. Martinez, a 45-year-old male of Hispanic descent, visits his primary care provider for a routine employment-screening physical. He has been hired as a home construction site manager for a local company that requires a medical release in order for him to start his job. Mr. Martinez appears to be well, although overweight (height: 70 inches, weight: 202 pounds, waist: 38 inches). He has no health complaints. When asked about his family history, he reports that his father died recently at the age of 65 from a heart attack. Further questioning reveals that Mr. Martinez is quite concerned about his own heart health. He has a wife and two teenage sons. He does not want his family to lose him at a young age. Lab tests reveal that he has abnormal lipid levels: total cholesterol = 222 mg/dL, HDL = 30 mg/dL, LDL = 160 mg/dL, triglycerides = 160 mg/dL. He also admits to smoking one pack of cigarettes per day for the last 25 years. On physical exam he is found to have a heartbeat with regular rate and rhythm, without murmurs, rubs, or gallops. His resting heart rate is 78 beats per minute, his blood pressure is 136/88 mm Hg. His lungs are clear to auscultation bilaterally.

Overweight

The term **overweight** is defined by the CDC based on **Body Mass Index** (**BMI**). The calculation of BMI for adults older than 20 years of age uses one of two formulas: weight (kg)/[height (m)]^2 or (weight (lb)/[height (in)]^2) × 703.[24] The first formula uses metric measures and the second one uses standard measures. The calculation for Mr. Martinez's BMI would be as follows:

$$\left(\frac{202}{70^2}\right) \times 703 = 28.98$$

Mr. Martinez's BMI falls within the CDC category of overweight. The BMI categories defined by the CDC are shown in **Table 1–1**.

Dyslipidemia

Dyslipidemia is high levels of total cholesterol and triglycerides in the presence of low levels of HDL (high density lipoproteins). A common generalization is to divide cholesterol into two types: so-called "bad" cholesterol (LDL) and "good" cholesterol (HDL). This is an oversimplification, but it works for our purposes here. According to the Friedwald formula, total cholesterol (TC) is the sum of HDL, LDL, and VLDL (very low density lipoproteins).[25] VLDL can be estimated by taking one-fifth of triglycerides.[26] Mr. Martinez's triglycerides were 160 mg/dL, giving a VLDL number of 32 mg/dL. His LDL value was 160 mg/dL, and his triglyceride value was 160 mg/dL. Thus, his TC calculation is:

$$30_{HDL} + 160_{LDL} + 32_{VLDL} = 222_{TC}$$

Table 1–2 presents the ATP-III (Adult Treatment Panel III)[27] reference ranges for TC, LDL, and triglycerides. Based on this information, his TC is *borderline high*, his LDL level is *high*; and his triglycerides are *borderline high*.

The next factor to consider is Mr. Martinez's HDL, or "good cholesterol," level. The reference ranges

Table 1–1 CDC BMI Categories

BMI	Weight Status
Below 18.5	Underweight
18.5–24.9	Normal
25.0–29.9	Overweight
30.0 and above	Obese

Table 1–2 ATP-III Total Cholesterol, LDL, and Triglyceride Reference Ranges

Total Cholesterol (mg/dL)	LDL (mg/dL)	Triglycerides (mg/dL)
< 200 Desirable	< 100 Optimal	< 150 Normal
200–239 Borderline high	100–129 Near optimal/ above optimal	150–199 Borderline high
240 High	130–159 Borderline high	200–499 High
	160–189 High	500 Very high
	190 Very high	

Table 1–3 ATP-III HDL Reference Ranges

HDL (mg/dL)	
< 40	Low
≥ 60	High

for HDL are shown in **Table 1–3**.[27] With an HDL level of 30 mg/dL, Mr. Martinez falls into the *low* category. In this case, "low" is a bad outcome, because it means he has a low level of good cholesterol.

Hypertension

Hypertension, simply put, is high blood pressure. The Seventh Report of the Joint National Committee (JNC) on Prevention, Detection, Evaluation, and Treatment of High Blood Pressure[28] defines hypertension as a blood pressure greater than or equal to 140 mm Hg systolic or greater than or equal to 90 mm Hg diastolic. Also, by definition, a patient who is currently using antihypertensive medication has hypertension. The JNC's recommended practice for diagnosing a patient with hypertension is to average several blood pressure measures.[28] It is considered hypertension if that average meets the definition. Mr. Martinez's blood pressure was 136 mm Hg systolic and 88 mm Hg diastolic. With only one measure available to us, however, we cannot determine if he has hypertension. More than likely our next step in his case would be to schedule a follow-up appointment and take another blood pressure reading.

Tobacco Abuse

Mr. Martinez reported that he smokes one pack of cigarettes per day. A patient who smokes 20 cigarettes per day for a year is said to have a "1 pack year" history of smoking.[29] With a 25-year history of smoking 20 cigarettes per day (20 is the number contained in a pack of cigarettes), Mr. Martinez has a 25 pack–year history of smoking.

Case Study Steps

1. On your own, complete steps 1 through 3 of the EBP process. Write down the information you need, the purpose of your query, and your focused clinical question(s). You might have more than one purpose and more than one question for each purpose.
2. Next, work with a group of two to three others and repeat what you just did.
3. Check your work. In the case study summary, you will find a list of focused clinical questions that we came up with regarding the case of Mr. Martinez. The list is not all-inclusive, but it does provide examples for you to compare with your own. We also provide our responses to steps one and two in the EBP process.

Case Study Summary

Step 1 in the EBP process is to recognize a need for information. As we considered the case of Mr. Martinez, we recognized that we had several information needs. Perhaps you had some of the same needs. It is likely that you also came up with different needs than ours or from your classmates.

We needed to know more about the common occupational health concerns for home construction sites. We also did not know which smoking cessation and weight loss strategies are most effective. Additionally, we realized that there have recently been conflicting reports regarding cholesterol-reducing medications and that we need to consider which option is best or whether a behavioral treatment option might be better. There are limitless possibilities to the questions we could ask, but for step 1 what is important is identifying the areas in which we need information. The answer will differ, depending on the practitioner's specialty and experience.

Step 2 in the EBP process is determining the purpose of the evidence search. This can be derived from the reason for the visit, the patient's signs and symptoms, or a request made by the patient. Mr. Martinez was seen for an employment-screening physical exam. Thus, the initial question is whether he is able to perform the job of construction site manager without danger to himself or others.

For this reason, we might center our query on this aspect of the case. As responsible primary care providers, with Mr. Martinez's four health problems we might wish to explore other questions, such as smoking cessation treatment or weight loss. Prevention of heart disease is also high on our list, not only because of his presenting signs but also because Mr. Martinez said he is concerned about heart disease.

In the third step of the EBP process, the objective is to write focused clinical questions. A focused clinical question includes the following six elements: Problem, Patient/Population, Action, Alternative Action, Results, and Evidence. Here we will focus on the first two elements of a focused clinical question:

- P (Problem) = a specific condition of interest
- P (Patient/Population) = patient/population risk factors; patient/population demographics

Mr. Martinez has four conditions: (1) overweight, (2) dyslipidemia, (3) hypertension, and (4) tobacco abuse. As a construction site manager, how might any of these conditions affect his safety and the safety of others? These conditions would be a primary concern to his potential employer. We would construct a focused clinical question related to this concept as shown in **Figure 1–7**.

We will not literally search for this question, verbatim, but we will use it to establish search terms. For the time being, we will set aside the issue of search terms, because it takes us into steps 4 and 5. This exercise is designed to go through steps 1, 2, and 3.

Looking at our question, it occurred to us that there might be another important factor—the environment. Does Mr. Martinez work in a place that is cold, wet, dusty, noisy, and so on? When gathering his history, it would be important to ask these questions. The answers to these questions will help narrow the evidence search and improve our chances of identifying his occupational environment risk factors.

We also would have asked him if he had any existing health conditions such as ringing in his ears, blurry vision, asthma, allergies, orthopedic injuries, arthritis, and so on. Mr. Martinez had none of these conditions. In some instances, we might collect information about the work environment from the employer. Some employers provide that information with the screening physical examination form.

In the question formulated in Figure 1–7, overweight was a risk factor for occupational health conditions. It is also a risk factor for heart disease. So, if we had a question about prevention of heart disease, overweight would again appear as a risk factor. However, if we had a question about

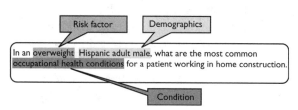

Figure 1–7 Clinical Question

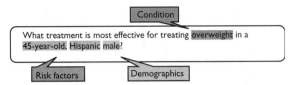

Figure 1-8 Focused Clinical Question

weight loss treatments, overweight becomes the condition. His risk factors for overweight include Hispanic race/ethnicity and age older than 40. **Figure 1-8** shows how we constructed a focused clinical question on weight loss.

One issue remains with this question, however. Which treatments are we considering? At this point, the question is too broad. It would be difficult to locate studies that compare all treatments. This is not always the case, but our prior experience with this area of investigation has already shown this to be the case. There is little research comparing nutritional and exercise interventions, as opposed to something like cholesterol-lowering medications, which have a significant, high-level body of research literature.

Thus, it would be necessary to have a list of treatments we are considering and to include them in the question, or to write several questions. We were interested in nutrition and exercise interventions. Specifically, we wanted to know which nutritional and exercise interventions are effective, whether one is better than the other, and if combining the two is more effective than either one of them individually. This leads to several questions:

- Which nutritional action or intervention is effective for treating overweight in a 45-year-old Hispanic male?
- Which exercise intervention is effective for treating overweight in a 45-year-old Hispanic male?

Then, depending on the answers to the above questions:

- Between [the successful nutritional and exercise interventions], which is most effective for a 45-year-old Hispanic male: nutrition alone, exercise alone, or a combination of the two?

Inside the brackets would be the names of the interventions of interest. It is not unusual to have a single information need lead to multiple focused clinical questions.

Lastly, the process of identifying focused clinical questions is both reflective and iterative. By that, we mean new questions emerge as you reflect on questions you have written. New questions will also emerge as you go through the EBP process. It might take several iterations of the process for you to identify all of your questions. This is one reason it helps to write your questions down. Spending a little time looking at your questions will often cause you to recognize other questions or important additional aspects to your questions, much as we recognized the need to include specific treatments in our focused clinical questions or the need to know about his work environment.

CHAPTER SUMMARY

Historically, decisions in health care have been based on custom or authority. Evidence-based practice (EBP) has begun to change this custom. EBP is the process of combining the best available research evidence with your knowledge and skill to make collaborative, patient- and population-centered decisions within the context of a given healthcare situation. Clinicians today appraise the trustworthiness of information rather than relying strictly on the authority of the information source. Furthermore, clinicians today strive to make choices that result in outcomes that matter, such as reduced morbidity, mortality, and cost.

It takes time and experience to develop the skills to practice EBP effectively. Clinicians practice EBP prospectively, concurrently, and retrospectively. Each clinician develops his or her own EBP process based on the type of practice and patients seen. Clinicians apply EBP to choose diagnostic tools, treatment procedures, and patient education strategies. EBP is needed when a clinic chooses a standard of care, when a pharmaceutical representative offers free samples, or when an insurance company requires a letter from a provider to justify coverage of a requested treatment. Medical information used in the practice of EBP includes not only research on diagnosis and treatment, but also epidemiologic research and studies on harm, prevention, and prognosis.

Meanwhile, the information available to clinicians is expanding at an incredible rate. It is increasingly important that providers can identify valid information. For this reason, information services have emerged that offer pre-appraised evidence-based resources, though often for a fee. The skills of EBP can enable a clinician to differentiate valid information from opinion. They can also improve a clinician's ability to sift through voluminous pages of results and quickly locate relevant information.

The process of EBP begins with your recognition of an information need. It requires self-awareness, humility, and a commitment to lifelong learning. Recognizing a need for information leads you to establishing a purpose for an evidence query and formulation of one or more focused clinical questions. These questions guide the selection of target resources and provide your search terms. As you search, you organize your findings and appraise the trustworthiness and relevance of the information you encounter. Based on this appraisal, you and your patient select and implement a course of action. Then you evaluate the effectiveness of the action you have taken and communicate the outcome.

EBP is more efficient and effective when practiced in teams. Each clinician brings different knowledge, skills, and experiences to the group. This means each clinical team member has different strengths to contribute to the hunt for the best available evidence. Some clinics employ EBP as a part of their operations by holding EBP meetings or running their own journal clubs.

Evidence sources can be categorized according to their level, or strength. Evidence pyramids offer a system for categorizing a source's level of evidence. Some information providers, such as the U.S. Preventive Services Task Force, assign the evidence level of the recommendations they publish. No system for levels of evidence has been identified as the best one. When a resource uses an evidence rating system you will need to read its procedures and definitions.

Lastly, regardless of the source, you will need to regularly appraise information. You will need to consider not only the trustworthiness of the information, but also the limitations of the clinical situation as well as the needs and preferences of the patient and the patient's family. You are not likely to have time, nor a need, to perform an evidence search with every patient. However, you will need to continuously update your knowledge and question your assumptions about health care. Utilizing EBP will help you remain current and make the best choices with your patients.

EXERCISE

Review the following case. Look up any terms or concepts in the case that are unfamiliar and then complete steps 1 through 3 of the EBP process. Write your focused clinical questions. Think about the search terms you might use and where you might begin to look for answers.

Ms. Hooper is a 24-year-old Caucasian woman who presents to the emergency room with acute neck pain following an automobile accident. Her vehicle was struck from behind by another vehicle. She does not know how fast the other vehicle was moving when it struck her car. Her friends drove her to the emergency room. She was able to walk into the hospital and sit upright while waiting to be examined. On physical exam, you find no neurologic deficits. She is alert with a Glasgow Coma Score (GCS) score of 15. She is able to actively rotate her neck 45 degrees to the left and to the right, though it does hurt to do so. However, she does not have midline cervical spine tenderness. A blood test shows no alcohol or other drugs in her system. She has no other serious injuries. She does have a minor contusion above her left eyebrow and bruising across her shoulder and abdomen from the seatbelt. She reports no other health problems. She is taking oral contraceptive pills. Ms. Hooper does not have health insurance and you need to determine if she requires c-spine imaging to rule out a c-spine fracture.

REFERENCES

1. Zimmer C. Answers begin to emerge on how thalidomide caused defects. *New York Times*. March 15, 2010, D3.
2. Long T. Oct. 1, 1957: Thalidomide cures morning sickness, but . . . *Wired*. October 1, 2008. Available at: www.wired.com/science/discoveries/news/2008/09/dayintech_1001. Accessed August 20, 2012.
3. Pergament E, Ormond K, Medlin K. Thalidomide. *ITIS Newsletter*. 1997;6(2). Available at: www.fetal-exposure.org/resources/index.php/1997/12/03/thalidomide/. Accessed June 5, 2010.
4. HistCite (Historiograph Compilation). Available at: www.garfield.library.upenn.edu/histcomp/thalidomide_ti_or/index-py.html. Accessed June 5, 2010.
5. Association of American Colleges. *Liberal learning and the arts and sciences major: The challenge of connecting learning*. Washington DC: AAC; 1991: pp. 16–17.
6. CDC. Defining overweight and obesity. Available at: www.cdc.gov/obesity/defining.html. Accessed July 21, 2010.
7. U.S. Department of Health and Human Services. National Institutes of Health, National Heart, Lung, and Blood Institute. Body mass index table. Available at: www.nhlbi.nih.gov/guidelines/obesity/bmi_tbl.htm. Accessed July 21, 2010.
8. Centre for Evidence Based Medicine. What is EBM? [Webpage]. Updated November 1, 2011. Available at http://www.cebm.net/?o=1014. Accessed September 16, 2012.
9. Guyatt G, Rennie D, Meade MO, Cook DJ. *User's guide to the medical literature: A manual for evidence-based practice*. 2nd ed. New York: McGraw-Hill; 2008.
10. Guyatt G. Evidence-based medicine. *ACP J Club (Ann Intern Med)*. 1991;114(suppl 2):A-16.
11. Tarlov AR, Ware Jr AE, Greenfield S, Nelson EC, Perrin E, Zubkoff M. The medical outcomes study. *JAMA*. 1989;262(7):925–930.
12. Johnson M, Maas M, Moorhead S. *Iowa outcomes project: Nursing outcomes classification (NOC)*. 2nd ed. St. Louis: Mosby; 2000.
13. LeFever Kee J, Paulanka BJ, Polek C. *Handbook of fluid, electrolyte, and acid-base imbalances*. 3rd ed. Clifton Park, NY: Delmar Cengage Learning; 2010.
14. ACCORD Study Group. Effects of intensive glucose lowering in type 2 diabetes. *N Engl J Med*. 2008;358:2545–2559.
15. Connelly SJ. Use and misuse of surrogate outcomes in arrhythmia trials. *Circulation*. 2006;113;764–766.
16. Pratt CM, Moyé LA. The cardiac arrhythmia suppression trial: Casting suppression in a different light. *Circulation*. 1995;91:245–247.
17. U.S. National Library of Medicine and National Institutes of Health. Ear infection: Acute. Medline Plus online encyclopedia. Available at: www.nlm.nih.gov/medlineplus/ency/article/000638.htm. Accessed July 21, 2010.
18. Fitzgerald PA. Endocrine disorders. In: *Current medical diagnosis and treatment*. 49th ed. New York: McGraw-Hill; 2010.
19. Malinowski H. Bioavailability/bioequivalence studies in evaluation of new levothyroxine products. Available at: www.fda.gov/downloads/Drugs/DrugSafety/ostmarketDrugSafetyInformationforPatientsandProviders/UCM186436.pdf. Accessed July 5, 2010.
20. Manktelow BN, Potter JF. Interventions in the management of serum lipids for preventing stroke recurrence. *Cochrane Database Syst Rev* 2009, Issue 3. No.: CD002091. DOI: 10.1002/14651858.CD002091.pub2. Available at: www2.cochrane.org/reviews/. Accessed July 5, 2010.
21. Freedman DH. Lies, damned lies, and medical science. *The Atlantic*. November 2010. Available at: www.theatlantic.com/magazine/archive/2010/11/lies-damned-lies-and-medical-science/308269/. Accessed November 1, 2010.
22. U.S. Preventive Services Task Force. Screening for lipid disorders in adults. Available at: www.ahrq.gov/clinic/uspstf/uspschol.htm. Accessed July 21, 2010.
23. U.S. Preventive Services Task Force. Grade definitions after May 2007. Available at: www.ahrq.gov/clinic/uspstf/gradespost.htm#arec. Accessed July 21, 2010.
24. Centers for Disease Control and Prevention. About BMI for adults. Available at: www.cdc.gov/healthyweight/assessing/bmi/adult_BMI. Accessed July 21, 2010.
25. Friedewald WT, Levy RI, Fredrickson DS. Estimation of the concentration of low-density lipoprotein cholesterol in plasma, without use of the preparative ultracentrifuge. *Clin Chem*. 1972;18:499–502.
26. Beers MH, Porter RS, Jones TV, Kaplan JL, Berkwits (Eds). *Merck manual of diagnosis and therapy*. 18th ed. West Point, PA: Merck & Co.; 2006.
27. National Heart, Lung, and Blood Institute. The seventh report of the Joint National Committee on prevention, detection, evaluation, and treatment of high blood pressure. 2004. Available at: http://www.nhlbi.nih.gov/guidelines/hypertension/jnc7full.pdf. Accessed March 29, 2012.

28. National Heart, Lung, and Blood Institute. National Cholesterol Education Program. Third report of the National Cholesterol Education Program (NCEP) expert panel on detection, evaluation, and treatment of high cholesterol in adults (Adult Treatment Panel III). Available at http://www.nhlbi.nih.gov/guidelines/cholesterol/index.htm. Accessed June 13, 2010.

29. National Cancer Institute. Dictionary of cancer terms (entry for Pack Year). Available at: www.cancer.gov/dictionary/?CdrID = 306510. Accessed July 21, 2010.

Healthcare Research Methods

Bernadette Howlett, PhD

INTRODUCTION

Research methods and statistics are foundational concepts for evidence-based practice (EBP). This chapter was written with the expectation that you have taken courses at the undergraduate level that address both research methods and statistics. We recommend that you have books related to these topics nearby as you read this chapter. Furthermore, we recommend having references regarding statistics and research on your bookshelf throughout your career. We have found two types of books to be particularly useful with this subject matter: a dictionary of statistics/research terminology and a dictionary of epidemiology.

Different degree programs offer varying amounts of instruction on these topics. We have written this text with the assumption that you are taking a course in EBP early in your health professional degree program. If you have had multiple courses in research and statistics, you might be familiar with much of the material in this chapter.

Another piece of advice we have for you is to know people who specialize in research and statistics. It will help you in your professional program and in your career if you know people who have specialized knowledge in these fields. Just as you work with a team of healthcare providers from different disciplines, we recommend that your teams include people with these backgrounds. You might find a classmate or colleague who has worked as a research assistant. Your college, university, or hospital most likely has an office of research. There might even be tutors on your campus who can help you grapple with any concepts you encounter that are new or unfamiliar. We encourage you to identify the resources and people available to you wherever you go as a student and as a clinician.

Research and statistics tend to be areas in which practitioners and students feel hesitant. This is understandable. Each of these domains has numerous degrees and specialties. Full proficiency in these subjects requires advanced education; it would be unrealistic to ask every healthcare provider to also achieve an advanced degree in statistics and another in research. However, avoiding these topics can place you in a dependent position.

If you avoid research and statistics, you will have to rely on the authors of information sources regarding the trustworthiness of the information they provide. One of our goals is to give you the tools to avoid such dependence. In fact, we have already mentioned one of the best tools to use—teaming up with people who have research and statistics knowledge. Furthermore, with time and experience you will become a resource to others. You will be able to share the knowledge and skills you gain from learning EBP with classmates, fellow clinicians, and with your patients.

In this chapter, we focus on the most common research concepts found in healthcare literature. Many of the concepts fall under the category of **biostatistics** (i.e., statistics applied to biological research).[1] Some authorities refer to statistics applied to medical research as **medical statistics**.[2] For the sake of simplicity, we use the term *biostatistics* to refer to medical statistics in this chapter.

By no means can we cover every concept in biostatistics in this chapter. However, as with the rest of health care, biostatistics is an area that requires lifelong learning. Just as you commit to gaining knowledge about health care throughout your career, you will need to continuously grow your knowledge about statistics and research. You will need to commit a little bit of time on a regular basis to these topics.

RESEARCH PARADIGMS

The two major research paradigms are *naturalistic*, also referred to as qualitative, and *positivistic*, which is also known as quantitative. For the purposes of this chapter, the term *qualitative* is used interchangeably with the word *naturalistic*. *Positivistic* and *quantitative* are similarly interchangeable.

The two paradigms of **qualitative** (naturalistic) and **quantitative** (positivistic) research represent different philosophical perspectives regarding knowledge, the design of research, and the types of data collected.

This interchangeability is a matter of much debate among research theorists. In addition to the terminology we have selected, the designation of two research paradigms has been debated. As Pope and Mays explain, "The differences between qualitative and quantitative research [sic] are frequently overstated, and this has helped to perpetuate the misunderstanding of qualitative methods within such fields as health services."[3(p. 5)]

However, these debates are well beyond our purposes here. Because our intended audience is beginning practitioners, we leave the fine points of research philosophy to other courses and texts that prepare you to perform research.

As an aside, we hope someday you do perform research, because there is no better way to learn about a topic than to actively engage in it.

According to the qualitative perspective, knowledge comes from the internal reality of the individual or group, whereas the quantitative perspective views knowledge as coming from an external, measurable reality. Naturalistic researchers usually view reality as fluid and ever-changing, whereas positivistic researchers tend to view reality as fixed and unchanging. Many researchers fall in between these two positions and combine qualitative and quantitative research strategies. Combining qualitative and quantitative perspectives is referred to as **mixed-method research**. **Table 2–1** compares the fundamental distinctions between naturalistic and positivistic research. Few studies fall strictly within one paradigm.

More than likely you are familiar with positivistic research, the type of research that quantifies observations and makes predictions about populations based on samples. The majority of biomedical research falls within the positivistic domain. We will briefly discuss naturalistic research and give some examples of its application in health care. However, this text focuses mainly on research in the positivist domain because of its predominant role in making health decisions. This emphasis on positivism does not diminish the importance of clinicians understanding qualitative research. Qualitative research can expose layers of meaning and significance that cannot be detected by

Table 2–1 Characteristics of Qualitative and Quantitative Research

	Naturalistic/Qualitative	**Positivistic/Quantitative**
Questions	Open-ended	Focused
Focus	Lived experiences of individuals, groups, or cultures that reveal meaning and significance of phenomena	Causal relationships or statistical differences that explain or predict phenomena, measuring effects of interventions
Sampling	Small, purposeful, and sometimes emergent selection or serial selection of participants	Large, preferably random samples blinded to the intervention
Setting	Natural, uncontrolled; studied as part of the research	Laboratory or controlled by design of research
Data	Observation, artifact, textual, visual, field notes, audio recordings, includes data from researchers as well as participants	Numerical, measurable, objective data collected from subjects only
Reasoning	Typically inductive, seeking descriptions	Typically deductive, seeking predictions
Analysis	Thematic, narrative, content-analytic procedures	Descriptive and/or inferential statistics
Role of researcher	Active engagement with participants and phenomenon; researcher is one of many data sources within the study	No or minimal engagement with participants and phenomenon; subjects and instruments are the sources of data, not researchers
Design	Emergent, guided by data as study proceeds, utilizing no intervention	Fixed, predetermined, utilizing one or more interventions

a survey or other instrument.[4] Qualitative research allows us to examine increasingly complex questions and is open to all possible answers to a question, not simply predetermined answers (which are examined in a quantitative study).

It is invaluable for you to understand qualitative research so that you have the skills to assess the quality of a naturalistic study (such as a case report). A foundation in evaluating qualitative research will, for example, give you tools for contending with the marketing tactics of companies that sell health-related products to clinicians and to patients. Perhaps of greater value is the perspective qualitative research can offer regarding the experiences of individuals and groups with health problems and with the healthcare system. Qualitative research has an advantage in this arena due to its holistic focus, which includes the individual and social context, emotions, perceptions, actions, beliefs, values, and interactions of patients with their health.

Naturalistic (Qualitative) Research

Naturalistic research emerged from the social sciences, primarily from anthropology, as researchers recognized the need to understand and describe phenomena experienced by people as well as the nature of the people being studied. Creswell offers the following definition:

> Qualitative research is an inquiry process of understanding based on distinct methodological traditions of inquiry that explore a social or human problem. The researcher builds a complex, holistic picture, analyzes words, reports detailed views of informants, and conducts the study in a natural setting.[5(p. 15)]

In a naturalistic study, the researcher's goal is to gain a deep understanding of the lived experiences of individuals or groups and to develop a rich, thick description of these experiences. Naturalistic researchers attempt to understand the meaning of experiences according to those who live them. Typical data collected during naturalistic studies include field notes, photographs, videos, interview recordings, artifacts, and journals.

Qualitative research can stand alone or complement quantitative research through preliminary or subsequent research. A qualitative study might independently explore a question, such as the criteria family practice physicians use to determine when to refer a patient to a specialist. A qualitative study can be used in advance of a quantitative study to establish the questions and choices used in a survey, for example. Qualitative research can follow positivistic research by helping explain phenomena observed in the quantitative study. For instance, an epidemiologic study found a significant difference in the rate of tonsillectomies across two regions, despite there being no difference in incidence or severity of illness.[3] A subsequent qualitative study found that physicians with high rates of surgical referral had a greater range of clinical signs that they defined as indications for surgery, whereas those with low surgical referral rates had a narrowly defined set of criteria.

Anthropologists are arguably the best known for engaging in qualitative research. They go into the field and immerse themselves into the group that they are studying. They become part of the group, the proverbial fly on the wall. Early anthropologists recognized that "only if one lived with the people who are being studied, and attempted to behave and think like them, could one truly understand a different society."[6(p. 4)] This type of research has come to be known as *ethnography*. Ethnographers diligently collect detailed data on what they observe as well as their own behaviors, assumptions, biases, and reactions. Ethnographic researchers do not perform interventions. The goal of their study is to understand the phenomenon as it occurs naturally.

The amount of qualitative research performed varies by healthcare discipline. Nursing research, for instance, includes more qualitative publications than other healthcare fields. For example, a search of the Internet using the phrase, "Qualitative research in nursing" produced 849,000 hits, whereas a search for "Qualitative research in medicine" resulted in 7,330 hits. Furthermore, the results of the above search led to qualitative nursing research publications that dated back to 1986, whereas those related to medicine dated back to 1999. According to Risjord,[4] qualitative research became popular among nursing researchers in the early 1980s. Risjord explains the appeal of qualitative research in nursing as follows: "The nice fit between qualitative methodology and nursing practice promised a form of nursing theory that would be more congruent with the goals and practices of nursing."[4(p. 190)]

Styles of Naturalistic Research

There are numerous styles of naturalistic research. The most common styles include ethnography, biography, phenomenology, case study, and grounded theory. The definitions of each type are as follows:

- **Ethnography** is a description and interpretation of a cultural or social group or system. The ethnographic researcher examines the group's observable and learned patterns of behavior, customs, and ways of life. Ethnography involves prolonged observation of the group, typically through participant observation in which the researcher is immersed in the day-to-day lives of the people or through one-on-one interviews with members of the group.[5(p. 58)]
- **Biography** is the study of an individual and her or his experiences as told to the researcher or found in documents and archival material.[5(p. 75)]
- **Phenomenology** is the study of the lived experiences of several individuals centered on a single **phenomenon**.[5] A phenomenology is similar to a biography in its procedures,

differing primarily in terms of the examination of a group as opposed to an individual.

- **Case study** is an exploration of a *bounded system* (a case or multiple cases) over time through detailed, in-depth data collection involving multiple sources of information rich in context. The bounded system is bound by time and place such that the case or cases of interest may be an event, an activity, or the individuals themselves.[5]
- **Grounded theory** is the study of abstract problems and their processes.[7(p. 24)] It is a general methodology of analysis linked with data collection that uses a systematically applied set of methods to generate an inductive theory about a substantive area. The research product constitutes a theoretical formulation or integrated set of conceptual hypotheses about the substantive area under study.[(p. 16)]

In medical and nursing research, the **case report** is a commonly used qualitative research strategy. The term *case report* is simply another name for *case study*. A clinical case report explains the course of an illness and often the patient's response to treatment. The clinical case report serves two functions: sharing information and supporting learning in an area of medical or nursing care.[8] In fact, the case report serves a vital function in health research:

> New diseases or unexpected effects of drugs or procedures may all first emerge as case reports. This is particularly true of information related to drugs. Patients selected for clinical trials do not often represent the patients who are offered treatment once the drug is launched and there are many examples where new information on the action of the drugs has emerged after the drug has been licensed for use.[8(p. 97)]

Furthermore, throughout your career as a clinician, you will approach care from the case report perspective as you observe the course of an illness in each patient and critique the patient's response to treatment. On a nearly daily basis you will engage in discussions with colleagues from the viewpoint of a case study.

Applications of Qualitative Research in Health Care

Naturalistic research has many applications in health care, the most obvious being studies related to the impacts of illnesses and treatments. Other uses of qualitative research in health care include sales and marketing, development of classification systems, patient education, patient and provider behavior, law and policy, patient satisfaction, and healthcare ethics. Pharmaceutical sales and marketing, in particular, have immeasurable impact on selection of treatments and patient outcomes.

Marketing researchers frequently use naturalistic studies to learn what motivates consumers and how to influence them to purchase their products. This strategy is of particular interest in health care as it is used by pharmaceutical companies to sell products to healthcare providers and directly to consumers. Each sales strategy is carefully tested on consumers, including patients and healthcare providers as key consumer groups. Pharmaceutical companies conduct studies with target patient populations in order to develop effective direct-to-consumer sales techniques. They also study medical practitioners, pharmacists, and nurses to identify effective methods and channels of communication.

It is important for you to be aware of the motivational techniques employed for purposes of selling healthcare-related products in order to help you and your patients make decisions. Knowledge about motivational research has another helpful purpose. Motivational research can also be useful in helping to identify and overcome barriers to healthy behaviors. One well-documented example of research in this arena is motivational interviewing.

Patient behavior change is an increasingly important aspect of health care in the twenty-first century. The previous century saw astounding advances in curing and preventing acute illnesses and controlling the spread of infectious diseases. Today, "the majority of maladies that now cause people to consult healthcare professionals are largely preventable or remediable through health behavior change."[9(p. 3)] A process called **motivational** interviewing (**MI**) was developed as a treatment modality that identifies and utilizes the intrinsic motivation of individuals with substance-related problems. It has been adapted to many other health areas, such as cancer treatment, smoking cessation, domestic violence, and so on. MI relies on many of the same influencing factors in human behavior as marketing and sales, however with quite different objectives. MI offers a strategy for providers to collaborate with patients to identify their health-related goals and make self-directed changes toward achieving those goals.

Limitations of Qualitative Research

We will begin this discussion of limitations by first mentioning a characteristic of qualitative research that is *not* a limitation. We begin here because some theorists argue that qualitative research is itself of little value because it is not quantitative. Qualitative research is, by nature, designed to explore phenomena in depth. As such, it does not serve the purposes of measuring **differences** or **relationships** between variables (the purview of quantitative research). We liken such declamations of qualitative research as similar to stating that an automobile is limited because it cannot float, whereas a boat is not limited because it can. The two modes of transportation differ in their methods, but each serves a highly useful and worthwhile purpose.

The limitations of qualitative research must, therefore, be judged based on its purposes and intent. Qualitative research is time consuming, for example. A 1-hour interview, including field notes, an audio/video recording, photographs, and transcripts can consume hundreds of pages. These hundreds of pages, as well as the associated audio or video files, require innumerable hours to organize and synthesize into meaningful and digestible chunks of information. The work is laborious and tedious. It must be performed to exacting standards in order to be of high quality. Furthermore, a well-designed qualitative study will include a peer-reviewing researcher as part of the team.

This internal reviewer examines and critiques the data and conclusions generated by the principal investigator. This internal check adds more time and labor to a qualitative study, not to mention expense.

Another limitation of qualitative research is difficulty with sharing data. The size of audio and video files created during interviews or field observations can easily exceed the storage capacity of email attachments or DVDs, USB drives, or other modes of transportable storage. Furthermore, the original data files often include identifying information regarding subjects. Subject identity is information that needs to be carefully protected. It can be exquisitely difficult to de-identify a video recording, for example.

Similarly, anonymity can be a challenge with qualitative research. Procedures for data collection and storage must be rigorously evaluated. Subjects must be carefully informed of the potential risk of inadvertent identification. The use of human subjects in qualitative research can make the approval process more complex and time consuming; yet another reason qualitative research can be slow.

The steps for evaluation of qualitative and quantitative studies are similar and boil down to essentially one question: Is the information provided in the publication trustworthy? The characteristics of trustworthiness differ between the two styles of research, but in the final analysis the quality of the research, and its applicability to your patient, determine the role of a given study in an evidence-based clinical decision.

Positivistic (Quantitative) Research

Positivism displaced the widely accepted philosophy that reality can be known only by God or through God, a belief that held sway in Europe until the Enlightenment.[10] As a general rule, **positivistic research** is thought of as *objective* in its perspective, as opposed to the *subjective* view taken by naturalistic research. A quantitative (or positivistic) study involves the computation of numerical values that represent phenomena. The positivistic perspective emerged from the period in European history referred to as the Enlightenment in the eighteenth century. The term *positivism* was coined by Auguste Comte (1798–1857) to give name to this philosophical perspective.[11] Positivism holds that reality is both external and objective. Reality can be measured using systematic observations of nature, which is a process we refer to today as the scientific method.

A simple definition of the **scientific method** is that it is, "the process of formulating a hypothesis, performing objective experiments, and engaging in sound reasoning supported by the collected data."[10(p. 8)] The term *scientific method* was born from the positivist philosophical paradigm, which can be traced back to some of the earliest authorities in Western civilization, such as Aristotle, Galileo, Francis Bacon, and Descartes.[11] Quantitative research relies on the scientific method as its principal procedural foundation and on positivism for its philosophical underpinning.

One of the earliest published applications of the scientific method in medicine is credited to Dr. John Snow (who is also considered the Father of Epidemiology, as well as the Father of Anesthesiology). Snow, a British physician, lived in London during the mid-nineteenth century.[12] In the 1850s, there had been a series of outbreaks of cholera, leading to significant illness and death. At the time, physicians did not know how cholera spread. There were many beliefs as to how it was spread, but no method of containment had succeeded.

Snow had an insight that the rate of disease appeared to vary with the source of drinking water.[13] Drinking water was supplied to residents by several water companies. He compared the cholera mortality rates for residents who purchased water from two of the major suppliers: Southwark and Vauxhall Water Company and Lambeth Water Company. He visited every house in which a cholera death had occurred and collected information about the family's water supply.

A pattern of illness emerged that was associated with the Southwark and Vauxhall Water Company. The cholera incidence was significantly higher among Southwark and Vauxhall customers. Snow also observed that the Southwark and Vauxhall Water Company used sewage-contaminated water from the Thames River, whereas the Lambeth Water Company obtained its water from a sewage-free source. Based on his discovery, he closed the Southwark and Vauxhall well, and cholera all but disappeared among customers who had received water from that well. This procedure confirmed his hypothesis that water carried the disease.

Through systematic observation, mathematical computations, careful data collection, and reporting of his findings, Snow demonstrated that the cholera outbreak could be traced back to the water supply. His findings also supported the hypothesis that water is the mechanism of transmission of the disease. This important finding led to segregating sewage from the drinking water supply and, thus, perhaps to the first public health intervention based on the use of the scientific method. The story of Dr. Snow exemplifies the scientific method and also represents the founding of the science of epidemiology.

A familiar example of the positivistic research paradigm is the association between cigarette smoking and lung cancer. Cigarette smoking/lung cancer research was positivistic in nature because the outcome and exposure were treated as numbers, and statistical calculations were performed using the numbers. In these studies, researchers were looking for one of two significant findings: relationships between the predictor and response variables or differences between exposure groups. Relationship testing involved counting the numbers of smokers/nonsmokers (predictor variables) and the numbers of lung cancer/non–lung cancer cases (response variables) and then testing the hypothesis that there was a correlation between smoking and lung cancer.

In the tests for differences, researchers calculated rates of lung cancer and compared the rates between groups. They hypothesized that there was a significant difference in lung cancer incidence between smokers and nonsmokers. Tests for relationships and differences are performed in many positivistic (quantitative) studies.

Styles of Quantitative Research

There are many types of quantitative research, which can be grouped into three design categories: observational, quasi-experimental, and experimental. For each type of research discussed in this section, we will describe its location on the evidence pyramid (**Figure 2–1**).

Observational Research

Observational research quantifies phenomena, but it does not involve the use of an intervention. An **intervention**, in the context of biomedical research, is an activity intended to alter an outcome, such as a risk reduction strategy, a pain management procedure, a drug therapy, or a diagnostic tool. In observational research, outcomes are measured without researchers employing any kind of intervention. Observational research can be used to identify trends and variables of interest: "Observations are not just a haphazard collection of facts: in their own way observational studies must apply the same rigor as experimental studies."[2(p.173)] Epidemiologic studies fall in the category of observational research. Case studies can also be categorized as observational. Observational research is low on the evidence pyramid.

Quasi-experimental Research

Quasi-experimental research involves studying a phenomenon in which researchers cannot randomly select subjects or randomly assign subjects

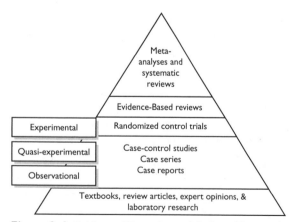

Figure 2–1 Evidence Hierarchy and Styles of Research

to treatment and control groups; however, researchers are able to control some independent variables.[1] An **independent variable** is a **predictor variable** that can affect the **response variable** (also known as a **dependent variable**), such as sex or age being a predictor of heart disease. These studies are often conducted in the same manner as experimental research.[2] For example, in studying lung cancer researchers were unable to randomly assign patients into the treatment (smoking) and control (nonsmoking) groups due to the obvious harm that such random assignments would cause for those in the treatment group. A quasi-experimental design is needed in such situations. There are many instances with interventional research in which a quasi-experimental design is preferable, although the design is inherently limited in terms of generalizing the findings to the entire population of smokers and nonsmokers. For this reason, studies of this type tend to rank in the lower region of the evidence pyramid.

Experimental Research

Experimental research involves dividing patients randomly, selecting subjects from the entire population or randomly assigning participants into intervention and control groups, and measuring differences between them or associations between predictor and response variables. Researchers are able to control variables in this type of study.[1] For example, subjects in a drug trial are randomly assigned to receive the usual treatment (active control) or the experimental treatment (the new drug), and researchers control for explanatory variables such as age, gender, severity of disease, and so on.

Styles of quantitative research also can be grouped according to their time orientation (i.e., **temporal style**) into the categories of *retrospective*, *cross-sectional*, and *prospective*. Not all studies can be easily categorized into just one of these types, but the concepts are helpful in understanding the various quantitative research strategies.

Retrospective Research

Retrospective research examines an outcome or exposure that has already occurred and utilizes numerical data to test for relationships between variables or differences between groups that can be associated with the phenomenon. This type of research is also referred to as a **case-control study**. For example, case-control studies were repeatedly performed when researchers were looking for a relationship between smoking cigarettes and lung cancer. Data were collected from patients with lung cancer, or from their charts, and exposure to cigarette smoking was calculated according to the amount and duration of exposure. This research can be categorized as both observational and retrospective. The research was retrospective because lung cancer had already occurred in the patients and the data were collected after the outcome. The research was observational because no intervention was employed.

Incidentally, cigarette smoking research was conducted because healthcare providers observed a significant difference in incidence of lung cancer among patients who smoked cigarettes compared to those who did not. The striking difference between groups sparked many studies examining the relationship between the outcome (lung cancer) and the exposure (cigarette smoking). Through the early 1960s, as many as 7,000 scientific articles had been published on the topic of smoking and lung cancer.[14] The results of these studies were disputed for decades by tobacco companies.

Clinicians are interested in retrospective research in that it helps identify risk factors associated with disease, or behaviors associated with good health, for that matter. Retrospective studies, however, are generally placed fairly low on the evidence pyramid because they can more readily fall prey to several types of bias. Selection of subjects can be especially problematic. It can be challenging to identify subjects without a given exposure or subjects who will not later develop an outcome that would place them in a different group in a study. Furthermore, patient charts, which are a common data source in retrospective research, can be fraught with errors and omissions.

In addition to data integrity problems in charts and subject-selection bias, there is also a problem with patient-recall bias. When patients with an outcome are asked to remember exposures or behaviors in their past, they are much more likely to respond positively than patients who do not have the outcome. Porta[2] gives the following example of recall bias: "A mother whose child died of leukemia may be more likely than the mother of a healthy living child to remember details of such past experiences as use of x-ray services when the child was in utero."[(p. 208)]

Cross-sectional Research

Cross-sectional research includes studies that collect data at a single fixed point in time. Studies of prevalence are perhaps the most commonly conducted cross-sectional research. **Prevalence** is the proportion of a population with a given disease at a single point in time. The Centers for Disease Control and Prevention (CDC) are best known for this type of research. Surveys are another commonly used cross-sectional strategy. Quality-of-life studies, clinically oriented questionnaires, and satisfaction with hospital stays are other common examples.[15]

Cross-sectional studies are affected by limitations similar to those of retrospective research, with risks including selection bias, recall bias, nonresponse bias, instrument bias, confounding and covarying factors, and reciprocal influences (to name a few). Due to the risk of bias, cross-sectional studies are low on the evidence pyramid. Nonetheless, cross-sectional studies can provide invaluable data about the status of disease and the risk factors or exposures associated with disease. Neither cross-sectional nor retrospective studies are used to make predictions about the outcome of a given intervention. Research of this type is *prospective* in nature, whereas retrospective and cross-sectional research is considered *observational*.

Prospective Research

Prospective research involves the formulation of a hypothesis, followed by the collection of data and subsequent analysis of findings. Data are collected over a defined period of time, of sufficient duration to draw reliable inferences based on the sample. It is possible for prospective research to be observational, quasi-experimental, or experimental in design. The defining characteristic is its forward orientation in time. An outcome is predicted based on a predetermined set of characteristics, a specified experience, or a chosen intervention. The following are commonly used prospective biomedical research strategies.

Control Trial In research, the term *control* has several meanings. It can refer to a group or to a research procedure. In this instance, it refers to the use of a specific group in the design of a study. The **control group** serves as a basis of comparison to ascertain the magnitude of the effect of an intervention. Results in the treatment group are compared to the control group. A control group makes it possible for researchers to determine if the effect of treatment is greater or less than nontreatment. It also allows them to determine if the experimental treatment has a greater or lesser effect than the existing standard of care (which is also referred to as the *usual treatment*). It is possible for researchers to perform studies without control groups; such studies are referred to as **pre/post** designs because the outcomes are measured prior to treatment and again subsequent to treatment. Pre/post studies are greatly limited because it is difficult to determine if the effect is clinically meaningful or if the effect differs from the current standard of care.

A **control trial** (also referred to as *controlled trial*) is a study in which there is at least one treatment group and one control group. In a control trial, group allocation is not random and often cannot be concealed. For example, a study on rotator cuff injuries might compare a surgical intervention with a physical therapy intervention. In this case, it is not possible to conceal from patients and providers what type of intervention the patient receives. Also, in this study patients might be involved in the selection of their treatment modality, which is why random assignment would not be possible.

The distinguishing characteristics of this type of study are the presence of the control group and the lack of random group allocation. The control group might receive no treatment, a placebo, or the usual care given for the condition of interest.

There might be more than one type of control group. Patients also might act as their own controls, or they might be crossed over from the control group to the treatment group (which is referred to as a *cross-over study*). Control trials are relatively low on the evidence pyramid.

Cohort Study **Cohort studies** are large in size and longitudinal in duration. The groups in the study are determined by a given exposure, characteristic, or risk factor rather than subjects being randomly assigned to groups (as occurs in a **randomized control trial**). Patients are followed forward in time to monitor for the development of a given outcome. These studies can include comparisons of various levels of exposures and numerous factors that may influence the frequency of outcomes and their severity.

A well-known cohort study whose results are frequently referenced in healthcare decisions today is the Framingham Heart Study.[16] The study seeks to identify the risk factors (e.g., gender, age, smoking, family history, height/weight, etc.) that predict heart disease and stroke. In 1948, researchers recruited 5,209 men and women between the ages of 30 and 62 to enroll in the study. These patients have been followed ever since, and new cohorts have been enrolled in order to establish representative samples. Based on the findings of this study and others, a set of risk criteria has been established that can be used to help predict the likelihood of a patient having a cardiovascular event within a 10-year period. Cohort studies are relatively low on the evidence pyramid. However, as demonstrated by the Framingham Study, they can produce highly useful information for clinical care decisions and for educating patients.

Randomized Control Trial The **randomized control trial** (RCT) is a study in which the allocation of patients to treatment or control groups is random and concealed. At least one control group must be utilized. Preferably patients, as well as providers, are not informed (blinded) regarding which intervention patients receive. When both the patients and providers are blinded, the study is referred to as a **double-blind RCT**.

Random assignment of patients to treatment and control groups is the defining characteristic of an RCT. Although blinding is important, it is not a requirement in order for a study to be considered an RCT. Nonblinded RCTs are lower on the evidence pyramid than blinded RCTs. Similarly, a double-blind RCT is higher on the pyramid than a single-blind RCT. It is also possible for a study to have additional types of blinding, such as blinding of the data analyst (which would be referred to as a **triple-blind RCT**). Blinding is intended to reduce bias and ensure that the treatment and control groups are representative of the population from which they are drawn.

RCTs are greatly affected by the strategy used for identifying subjects. An RCT is intended to provide data that can be applied to a larger population. Hence, the **sampling strategy** (i.e., procedures for identifying and recruiting subjects) is critical to the validity of findings in an RCT. The degree to which a sample is representative of the population determines the likelihood that the study's results will be generalizable to that population. Well-designed RCTs of sufficient sample size and duration are placed in the upper section of the evidence pyramid. Such studies are considered the gold standard in biomedical research. That is not to say that well-designed RCTs are free from error or bias. Recent research examining the frequency of studies being disproved found that even large, high-quality RCTs are controverted nearly 10% of the time.

Cross-over Trials, Systematic Reviews, Meta-analyses, and Clinical Trials

Several special types of biomedical research do not fit neatly into any of the categories we have discussed in this chapter, including the cross-over trial, the systematic review, the meta-analysis, and the clinical trial.

Cross-over Trial A **cross-over trial** is a prospective study in which patients are moved from one group to another. They are in the control group for a period of time and then are moved to one or more treatment groups. Subjects remain in each group long enough to determine the effect of the

given treatment. Allocation of patients from one group to the next can be randomized. It is not always possible for group allocation to be random, depending on the research circumstances and question. Random allocation makes a cross-over trial stronger, however.

In a cross-over trial, two types of control are possible: the control group in which patients receive the placebo or usual treatment and a within-subject control. This procedure allows researchers to determine if individuals have unique responses to a treatment. A *washout period* is usually required in between the phases of the study in order to reduce the potential for carry-over effects from one treatment to the next.[2] The length of the washout timeframe needs to be of sufficient duration to eliminate the effects of the first intervention before employing the second intervention.

Although it is preferable for a cross-over trial to be performed with random assignment and blinding of treatment, it is not always possible for these studies to be done in this manner. It is important for clinicians to read the study design information carefully in order to determine the level of evidence represented by an individual study. Of course, this consideration is always important, regardless of the type of study. When a cross-over trial is randomized and blinded, it can be considered to be high on the evidence pyramid.

A study performed by Rajaram et al.[18] regarding the effects of walnuts and fatty fish on cholesterol levels is an example of a randomized cross-over trial. In the study, 25 normal to mildly hyperlipidemic (high cholesterol) adults, aged 23 to 65, were randomized into one of three groups: (1) control diet, (2) walnut diet, or (3) fatty fish (salmon) diet. Each subject spent 4 weeks on each of the three diets. Subjects had a weekend break in between diet periods. Subjects were weighed twice weekly, and fasting blood samples were drawn on two alternate days at the end of each study period. Cholesterol levels were compared to baseline levels taken at the beginning of the study and compared to the beginning of each study period.

The cross-over design allowed researchers to compare the three diets with one another and to account for individual patient responses. This design was preferable to having a simple RCT because it helped researchers determine if one diet was particularly effective in individual patients. A criticism of the study design relates to the time of the washout period. Is a weekend enough time to eliminate the effects of one diet? This procedure allows for a smaller sample size while assuring valid results. Without the cross-over, a larger sample and a longer trial period would have been necessary.

Systematic Review and Meta-analysis A **systematic review** is a research procedure in which all prior studies on a given topic are brought together and analyzed collectively. There is a rigorous protocol for performing a systematic review. Systematic reviews are typically deemed to be at the top of the evidence pyramid. An area in which systematic reviews are especially valuable is in comparative effectiveness research. It is costly and time consuming for researchers to perform all available interventions related to the same problem. For example, dozens of interventions have been examined for reducing cholesterol, including psychotherapy, exercise, nutrition, drugs, and even surgery.

Each type of intervention has any number of subtypes. Exercise, for instance, can include various types of activities (walking/jogging, weightlifting, swimming, dancing, etc.) for various amounts of time at various levels of intensity. Researchers generally select a handful of related interventions and compare them to one another. In fact, many studies compare just one intervention with a control. Systematic reviews offer a means for gathering all of the various studies and comparing outcomes across them.

It is critical for readers to carefully ascertain that a publication is in fact a systematic review as opposed to being merely a literature review article. A literature review article is not research, but rather a summary of publications on a given topic. Occasionally, the term *systematic review* is used in the title of a published article that is not in fact a

systematic review. This error has occurred less frequently with time as journals have become more careful in the use of the term.

One way to recognize if a publication is a genuine systematic review is the source of the article. The **Cochrane Collaboration** is considered the leading organization in the world for this type of research, and it sets the standards for design and quality of systematic reviews and meta-analyses. The Cochrane Collaboration explains systematic reviews as studies that "collate all evidence that fits pre-specified eligibility criteria in order to address a specific research question" and "minimize bias by using explicit, systematic methods."[19]

In a systematic review, a research team formulates a question, follows a specified literature search strategy (locating published and unpublished studies), sets strict selection criteria for inclusion of studies in the systematic review, critiques the designs of the studies, summarizes the findings, characterizes the validity of the findings, and provides recommendations about the application of the research to patient care decisions. Systematic review team members perform searches and analyses independently. A separate team member, or group, then evaluates the similarity (homogeneity) of studies identified and the findings reported by the independent reviewers.

A **meta-analysis** is an added step to a systematic review in which a statistical analysis is performed to quantify the findings of the review. Porta describes the meta-analytic process as, "a statistical analysis of results from separate studies, and leading to a quantitative summary of the results if the results are judged sufficiently similar to support such synthesis."[2(p. 154)] A meta-analysis can also include aggregation of pooled data from the original studies, if the data are available. The research question is then retested with the pooled data and results compared to the original separate studies. A systematic review with a meta-analysis is considered the highest level of evidence on the pyramid.

Systematic reviews and meta-analyses might be composed of lower levels of evidence, such as cohort studies, nonrandomized trials, and small RCTs. This does not alter the ranking of systematic reviews and meta-analyses as top-tier evidence, however. They retain their strength because the findings, even when inconclusive, are more reliable than an individual study, even if the individual study is a large RCT. We caution you, however, to look for newer evidence when reading a systematic review or meta-analysis. Even these studies are occasionally found to be incorrect, and new research can refute their findings. Furthermore, new research can fill in missing information or add new information. The Cochrane Collaboration often publishes updates to its studies as new research emerges.

Clinical Trial Another type of study that is difficult to categorize according to the groups discussed in this chapter is the clinical trial. **Clinical trials** take various forms and can combine styles, including case series, surveys, control trials, cohort studies, and RCTs. Clinical trials either directly involve a particular group of people or use materials from humans. Researchers observe subjects and/or collect data to answer a health-related question about the safety or efficacy of an intervention. The National Institutes of Health (NIH) website ClinicalTrials.gov is a repository of federally and privately funded clinical trials conducted in the United States. The NIH divides clinical trials into five types of research questions (treatment, prevention, diagnosis, screening, and quality of life) and into four phases. The phases are defined as follows:[20]

- In **Phase I trials**, researchers test an experimental drug or treatment in a small group of people (20 to 80) for the first time to evaluate its safety, determine a safe dosage range, and identify side effects.
- In **Phase II trials**, the experimental study drug or treatment is given to a larger group of people (100 to 300) to see if it is effective and to further evaluate its safety.
- In **Phase III trials**, the experimental study drug or treatment is given to large groups of people (1,000 to 3,000) to confirm its effectiveness, monitor side effects, compare it to commonly used treatments, and collect information that will allow the experimental drug or treatment to be used safely.
- In **Phase IV trials**, postmarketing studies delineate additional information, including the drug's risks, benefits, and optimal use.

Table 2–2 organizes the various types of quantitative research we have discussed into categories

Table 2–2 Quantitative Styles of Biomedical Research

Style of Research	Temporal Characteristic		
	Retrospective	**Cross-sectional**	**Prospective**
Observational	Case studies Case-control studies	Prevalence studies Surveys	Case studies Control trials Phase IV clinical trials
Quasi-experimental	N/A	Longitudinal cross-sectional studies	Cohort studies Nonblinded RCTs Phase I, II, and III clinical trials
Experimental	N/A	Proof-of-concept experiments*	Blinded RCTs Phase I, II, and III clinical trials

*A **proof-of-concept experiment** is a single-group study in which the plausibility of an underlying principle is tested.

according to the most common style of research and the typical temporal characteristics of the studies. This is not a definitive listing of all types of biomedical research, nor are these categorizations set in stone. This table is merely a tool to visually support the discussion in this chapter. It will always be necessary for you to read the authors' descriptions of their studies to determine the style of research and its temporal characteristics.

Applications of Quantitative Research in Health Care

Quantitative research is predominant in health care. It could even be described as ubiquitous. Observational, quasi-experimental, and experimental studies are utilized to determine the following:

- The prevalence or incidence of disease and associated risk factors
- Survival longevity (with and without treatment)
- Accuracy, harms, or side effects of screening tools and diagnostic procedures
- Effectiveness and complications of treatment modalities
- Interactions between interventions
- Quality of life
- Cost of care
- Patient satisfaction

You will often turn to quantitative research for information to facilitate patient care decisions, but quantitative research has many other applications. For example, quantitative research is used to assess health professional workforce issues such as provider-to-patient ratios, reimbursement levels, salaries, and availability of jobs. Quantitative research is utilized by policymakers, organizational administrators, journalists, patients, and just about everyone else. When hospitals or other organizations decide on the standards of care they will follow, they turn to the quantitative research literature for guidance. You might be involved in a decision of this kind at some point in your career. When laws are being written with regard to

health insurance coverage, quantitative research is referenced. When malpractice lawsuits are filed, quantitative research is brought forth as evidence. You might be called as an expert witness or even (hopefully not) as the respondent in a malpractice lawsuit. A command of quantitative research could even protect your career.

Limitations of Quantitative Research

Time and cost are the two greatest limiting factors for all types of research (qualitative and quantitative). Quantitative studies can be limited in a number of different ways. One important limitation of quantitative research lies in the philosophical perspective on which positivism is based. The fundamental assumption of quantitative research is that an inference can be drawn from a sample of patients that will hold true with the population represented by the sample. This concept is referred to as **generalizability**. In order to perform a quantitative study, researchers must formulate a **hypothesis**, a belief about what is true. This hypothesis is tested with rigorous means. However, the formation of a hypothesis limits the potential outcomes to those answers that were imagined by the researcher in advance. Consider the following example.

A team of researchers is interested in the best treatment for high cholesterol. They set out to conduct a comparative systematic review of all of the treatments that have been published. This includes exercise, nutrition, drugs, and other treatments. They select the treatments that have been previously researched, which immediately limits the answer to the question. Even though this type of study would be deemed as high-level evidence, it would not even consider many other potential answers or alternate perspectives.

By formulating the hypothesis that specific treatments for high cholesterol are better than others, the researchers have excluded any number of other informative views. It might be that an environmental variable is contributing to rising cholesterol levels and that any treatment is inhibited by this variable. It might be that there is a genetic mutation at work. Additionally, it might be that, regardless of the form of treatment, ultimately patients' quality of life and longevity is only minimally affected by any treatment. All of the cost of research and treatment might be wasteful in comparison to other things that might be of greater value to us. Perhaps we would benefit more from having better schools than having 10 points lower cholesterol. We are not saying this is true; we are just using the idea to make a point.

The preliminary formulation of possible answers to a research question, which is essential for quantitative research, by nature precludes a universe of other possible answers and ideas. It becomes necessary, therefore, to research every other possible answer and idea, which then adds time and cost, making the entire endeavor ludicrous. In saying this, we do not by any means discount quantitative research; quantitative research is the best tool for most biomedical questions. Studies that fall within this paradigm are invaluable to healthcare providers and to everyone who receives health care. We criticize it precisely because of the important role it plays in health care and the significant potential for harm.

The research design strategies employed in quantitative studies are intended to overcome their limitations. Quantitative research methods are meant to reduce the potential for errors through sufficient sample sizes, representative samples, adequate duration, and objective analysis. However, mistakes are made. The regularity of drugs being recalled by the FDA evinces the problem (if you are interested visit http://www.fda.gov/drugs /drugsafety/DrugRecalls/default.htm).

Optimally, we would follow patients throughout their lives to determine if a given intervention has had a positive or negative *outcome that matters*. Optimally, we would include samples that represent every subgroup in a population, including those with and without a given disease of both sexes, at every age, from every race and ethnicity, at every income level, with every possible complicating illness. These optimal designs are not possible for practical reasons, not to mention the cost.

As a consumer of research literature, your awareness of the underlying assumptions and limitations of the quantitative research paradigm will help you discern limitations of the studies you encounter. In addition, it could lead you to envisioning the universe of answers and ideas yet to be addressed by researchers, pointing to areas you might choose to investigate yourself. After all, healthcare studies are often inspired by the astute observations of clinicians in their daily practice.

Beyond the general limitations of quantitative research, you should look for several types of limitations in the studies you read as a clinician. In this context, the term **limitations** means aspects of a study that reduce its generalizability. In well-written articles, the authors will describe study limitations. When researchers identify the weaknesses of a study, it indicates two things: first, the conclusions they draw are more likely to be reasonable and, second, there might be further research to be done that can overcome the limitations. This identification helps you as the reader determine if the researchers were rigorous in their methods, and it offers you guidance in your ongoing use of evidence related to the clinical question of interest.

Limitations can lead to **bias** in the outcomes of a study. There are hundreds of types of bias, a full discussion of which is beyond the scope of this chapter. We will describe the most common forms of bias here in order to introduce the concept. All types of bias involve something other than the predictor variable influencing the response variable. It is nearly impossible for studies to completely eliminate bias. For consumers of research information, the key to detecting bias is consideration of all of the possible causes of an outcome reported in a study.

Bias can be divided into three major groups: sampling, measurement, and other sources. *Sampling* is the process of selecting a subset of a population and recruiting members of the subset to participate in the study. *Measurement* includes any procedure used for quantifying information (e.g., counting the number of fall incidents in a hospital ward, weighing patients, and measuring cholesterol levels). Other sources of bias include things that motivate a study to be performed or to be published (or not published, as the case may be). We will finish this chapter with explanations of the more common limitations within each area.

Common sources of **sampling bias** include the sample size, the representativeness of the sample, and selection bias. In order for a statistical test to be accurate, the size of the sample (i.e., the number of subjects) must be adequate in terms of the type of data collected, the nature of the research question, and the desired level of effect. Erroneous conclusions can be drawn from studies that have samples that are too small or too large. We will not go into the complexities of all of the factors involved in determining the correct sample size. However, you can take one simple step as a reader to determine if the sample size in a study is appropriate. Examine the article for a statement regarding a sample size calculation.

A **sample size calculation** is a step researchers take prior to performing the study. In simple terms, a sample size calculation tells researchers how many subjects they need in order to be able to answer their question. This procedure is often included in a section of an article prior to the results. Well-written articles will include a section specifically describing the methods for identifying and enrolling subjects in the study.

If the authors do not mention the results of a sample size calculation, then you cannot be sure if the sample size was appropriate. However, if they did perform a sample size calculation, then the sample size might be considered a strength of the study; that is, if the number of subjects who begin (and complete) the study are greater than the required sample size. If you imagine as you read an article a set of hash marks for strengths of a study and a set for weaknesses of a study, an adequate sample size would mean drawing a hash mark on the strengths side. Also, the number of subjects should not be too much higher than the calculated sample size, because this can also increase the potential for error.

The **representativeness** of a sample is the degree to which subjects in the sample match the population they represent. This aspect of the research is typically described fairly early in an article, usually in the same section as the description of the sampling strategy. The sample should match the population in terms of characteristics such as the distribution of people by sex, age, race/ethnicity, severity of disease, and so on. The characteristics included in an analysis of representativeness are based on the nature of the study itself. Researchers employ **probability (random) sampling** in order to attain a representative sample. This means that all individuals in the population have an equal chance of being selected for a study. When combined with a sample size calculation, the use of probability sampling makes it likely that the sample will be representative of the population.

It is often difficult, however, for researchers to perform a simple random sample (i.e., to include every individual in a population as a member of the pool of subjects from which a sample is drawn). Many factors involved in sampling need to be considered in determining representativeness. In terms of your critique of a publication, you need to decide if you think the subjects in the study are representative of the population the authors intended and if the subjects represent your patient. You will base this decision on the description of the sample and the purpose of the study.

A concept closely related to representativeness is **selection bias**. Selection bias occurs when there is a systematic procedural error in the selection of subjects or when a nonrandom (nonprobability) sample is utilized. It is important to note that random sampling is often not possible or even advisable, depending on the amount of time available for the study as well as financial and labor resources. The population might be spread out geographically such that a true random sample could mean having to conduct the study in thousands of communities.

Nonrandom sampling can be acceptable for certain types of studies, such as proof-of-concept studies. A proof-of-concept study can involve verifying the presence of a condition in a population or it can be used to determine a study's protocol. Several types of nonrandom sampling procedures are possible. The key point for healthcare providers is to recognize when a nonrandom sample has been used. Well-written studies will include a detailed explanation of the sampling procedure and a justification for the use of a nonrandom sample. The authors should avoid making generalizations about the population of interest based on a nonrandom sample.

The second major group of research bias comes from **measurement bias**. Measurement bias can include inaccurate measurement tools, calculation errors, mistakes in recording measurements, participant bias, recall bias, and more. When inaccuracy in measurement occurs, it often leads to incorrect conclusions. There are countless types of measurement errors. Although we cannot describe every type of measurement error, you will have the ability to look for them in the studies you read by considering if there are any ways in which the data collected in the study were inaccurate.

For example, many studies measure BMI (body mass index). BMI is a formula that includes a patient's height and weight. An accurate calculation of BMI requires correct measurement of both variables. Errors in measurement of height can take the form of incorrect positioning of the patient, use of an inconsistent method of measurement, time of day the measurement is taken (patients tend to be taller when they get up in the morning), and so on. It is not unusual for studies to involve patients who are unable to stand, such as those in an ICU or in wheelchairs. For these patients, an estimate of height must be used, rather than a direct measure. Estimates have even greater potential for error than direct measures.

A patient's weight is even more prone to measurement error than height. Factors such as clothing and calibration of the scale can impact the accuracy of a weight measurement. If a consistent and careful protocol is not followed, then errors will occur. Patient weights can vary by several pounds from one standing scale to the next. Thus, the same type of scale must be used every time, in addition to calibrating the scale with every use. Furthermore, the person recording the weight can make mistakes reading the scale or in writing the number into the chart. In many studies, data from the chart are retyped into a computer, which introduces another moment when error can occur. The combination of errors in measurement of height and weight then produces even greater error in the resulting BMI calculation.

Many measurements, like BMI, run the risk of multiple types of measurement errors, including instrumentation error, calculation errors, and data observation errors. When reading studies, consider the ways in which a measurement can be inaccurate and look for careful descriptions from the authors about the procedures they followed. This issue is especially important for the response variable in a study. If BMI were the primary response variable, for instance, then the accuracy of measuring height and weight as well as the calculation of BMI is of great importance. The authors must describe the steps taken to reduce errors in order to demonstrate that their findings are valid. Studies that include this type of detail and demonstrate the validity of their measurement procedures get another hash mark under the strengths heading.

Another type of measurement bias comes from the behavior of the subjects in the study. Patients might alter their behavior for a number of reasons, such as self-consciousness or a desire to please the researchers. For example, a patient might exercise more after enrolling in a study related to nutrition. Or, the patient can simply report a greater level of physical activity than is true. Patients might not be completely honest on a survey, or they might have wildly different perceptions, which can skew the results. On a pain scale, for example, one patient might rate a paper cut as 1 out of 10, whereas another patient might rate it as 5 out of 10. This type of measurement error is referred to as **self-reporting bias**.

A related type of measurement bias caused by the subjects in a study is **recall bias**. Patients might not remember completely or accurately the history of their symptoms, exposures, or behaviors. Furthermore, patients without a disease are less likely to recall prior exposures or behaviors compared to patients with a disease. In fact, recall bias is considered by some experts to be pervasive in case-control studies and to some degree in most observational studies.[21] Even randomized control trials can be limited by recall bias if one of the variables includes information provided by patients. As the user of healthcare literature, your task is to examine each study you read for data sources that might be affected by recall bias.

In addition to the two major categories of bias, there are many other types of bias, such as publication bias, funding bias, extraneous variables, lack of clinical value, and more. **Publication bias** occurs when the determination of whether to publish a study is based on factors other than the quality of the research and the relevance of its findings. Sometimes studies are not published because no statistical significance was found in the research. In other words, if the authors of a study find one medication is not significantly better than another, the study is less likely to get published, even though this information might be of great utility to healthcare providers. Easterbrook et al. found that studies with a statistically significant finding were 2.3 times more likely to be published.[22]

Publication bias also can occur because the editors of a journal disapprove of the research, because the research is considered controversial, or simply because of a journal's tendency to publish the articles written by people who are associated with the journal (a sort of insider's group). Sometimes the authors themselves avoid publishing a study because the findings were contradictory to their expected outcomes.

Funding bias is similar to publication bias in that it can lead to a study not being published for reasons other than the quality and relevance of the research. This type of bias can simply mean the organization funding the study has control over whether the study results are published. If the findings are not a benefit to the funding organization, the study is not released. Furthermore, the researchers themselves might financially benefit from the study by working for the funding organization or by receiving rewards such as travel money or stipends for giving lectures.

Another type of bias is a *lack of clinical or practical significance*. A numerical finding of significance does not indicate that a difference between groups was clinically meaningful. For example, a study comparing cholesterol drugs did find a significant difference in cholesterol levels between two drugs, but this difference might not be related to an outcome that matters (e.g., longer life, fewer heart attacks, or better quality of life). Furthermore, differences between groups might not be meaningful in light of the overall prevalence of the disorder.

For example, in a study comparing medications for insomnia, the researchers found that those who received one of the studied drugs had a higher *incidence* (new cases) of depression than those who received placebo.[23] Two percent of those receiving one of the insomnia medications experienced a new onset of depression, as compared with 0.9% of those who received the placebo. However, according to the CDC, the *prevalence* (rate of existing cases) of depression in the population is 9%. The article did not indicate the prevalence of depression among the research subjects. Nor did the authors account for risk factors, which include geographic location, age, sex, marital status, race/ethnicity, employment status, health insurance status, and other health conditions.[24] The study on depression and insomnia drugs compiled results of other studies that were not designed to measure depression as a primary outcome. Hence, the finding of a difference in depression rates, although statistically significant, might not be associated with the true clinical significance.

Many lists have been created to identify, categorize, and define the types of bias in research. Sackett, for example, developed a list that included 35 types of bias.[25] Other authors offer groupings of three or four categories of bias.[26] Regardless of the labels used, all types of bias have one characteristic in common: Something is influencing the outcome other than the predictor variables. These influences can come in the form of sampling errors, measurement errors, or other kinds of errors, such as publication bias or a lack of clinical significance. The key for healthcare providers is their ability to envision the ways that a study might be influenced by extraneous variables and to look for explanations related to them.

Well-designed articles will include sections related to bias, explaining carefully the sampling strategy, the measurement procedures, sources of funding, the authors' relationships with the funding agency, and limitations of the study. For example, in the study on depression and insomnia medications the authors discussed the limitations of the study as follows:[23]

This is a post-hoc analysis of trials which were not designed primarily to examine depression. The compilation had many limitations which have caused some observers to doubt that causality has been demonstrated. Information limitations included trial details, the length of exposure of many participants (correcting for dropouts), and inadequate specification of the nature and severity of incident depressions. The quality of ascertainment of depression occurring as an adverse event was quite uncertain. It is not evident that a major depressive disorder was always diagnosed by an expert when depression was listed as an adverse event. There are potential statistical pitfalls in compiling results of numerous trials of different design and duration using 4 different hypnotics. Because the FDA online files are a limited source, other methods of ascertainment might have uncovered more trials of these drugs, especially post-marketing trials. The data utilized did not lend themselves to the techniques of formal meta-analysis. Many limitations of this compilation could not be overcome unless new trials with thousands of participants are done, so some uncertainty as to the present conclusions is unavoidable.(p. 2)

Although this excerpt demonstrates several sources of bias in the study, it also exhibits one of the strengths of the study, a clear explanation of the study's limitations. This explanation helps readers determine how to apply the findings of the study to patient care. Although a difference was reported in incidence of depression, it is not clear that providers should avoid treating insomnia with the drugs included in the study. It might indicate that treatment for depression is appropriate, if the insomnia patient has depression.

When you have a patient who receives one of these drugs, because of a study like this one you will be aware to watch for development of depression and to consider withdrawing the insomnia medication if depression occurs. Or, if you are treating a patient who already has depression as well as insomnia, you might monitor the patient carefully (if you decide to prescribe an insomnia medication). It is possible that insomnia is a contributing factor to depression or a complication of it. Hence, you might choose to treat insomnia as part of a depression treatment regimen. We are most assuredly not recommending any specific treatment here, but rather putting the treatment decision into a larger context. Clearly your decision about treatment of insomnia or depression will be based on the specifics of each patient situation and not on the example given here.

CASE STUDY: MR. MARTINEZ HAS INSOMNIA

Mr. Martinez is a 45-year-old adult male of Hispanic descent with high cholesterol and high blood pressure. He is overweight and smokes cigarettes. He works at a construction company. When Mr. Martinez presented to the clinic, he said he was worried about his risk of having a heart attack and dying young like his father.

When taking Mr. Martinez's history, you learn that he suffers from insomnia. You take a general health, sleep, and medication history. You also perform a mental status exam. Based on his history, your examination of him, and his negative history of sedative medications, you decide to explore his insomnia further. You give him a sleep diary to track how long it takes him to fall asleep, how often he wakes, and how long he is awake. Mr. Martinez returns in a month with several nights of his sleep diary completed. He also provides you with information about his sleep hygiene (sleep habits and environment). The data he provides indicate possible chronic insomnia. It is unclear if his apparent insomnia is caused by a separate health condition (secondary insomnia) or if it is its own disorder (primary insomnia).

Following the clinical guideline for the evaluation and management of chronic insomnia in adults,[27] you suggest an overnight sleep assessment (nocturnal polysomnography). You will consider the results of the overnight sleep test in light of his overweight, cigarette smoking, and possible anxiety. It is also possible that he has sleep apnea, which is defined as abnormal pauses in breathing or shallow breathing while sleeping. In some cases, sleep apnea causes insomnia. The overnight sleep assessment will include testing to evaluate him for sleep apnea. Mr. Martinez agrees with the plan and he is comfortable with the expense.

1. What evidence-based practice questions does this case study bring to mind for you in terms of epidemiology and diagnosis? Write a focused clinical question that includes a specific condition or outcome, patient demographics, and patient risk factors.
2. Locate one resource that addresses your focused clinical question.
3. Identify the following information about the resource:
   a. What type of resource is it (review article, qualitative research, randomized-control trial, etc.)?
   b. Identify where the resource would be placed on the evidence pyramid.
4. Share your question and your resource with a partner. Discuss your answers to 3a and 3b with one another. Help one another determine if you have made the correct assessment. Also, discuss the following:
   a. Does the resource apply to the patient?
   b. What are the implications of the resource regarding the question you set out to answer?
   c. What further information would you need, if any, in order to answer your question.

Case Study Summary

A number of different questions might have come to mind regarding Mr. Martinez's possible insomnia. For example:

- What is the incidence of insomnia among adult Hispanic males?
- What are the risk factors for sleep apnea (which is a possible cause of insomnia)?
- How accurate is the overnight sleep assessment for diagnosis of chronic insomnia?

For the sake of this activity, we chose to explore the second question on our list, "What are the risk factors for sleep apnea?" We performed a brief search and found a website provided by the Mayo Clinic.[28] The website describes three types of sleep apnea: obstructive, central, and complex. The most common form is obstructive sleep apnea, which occurs when throat muscles relax. Central sleep apnea occurs when the brain fails to send the proper signals to the muscles to keep breathing. Complex sleep apnea is a combination of both.

The website included a list of risk factors for each type of sleep apnea. For obstructive sleep apnea, the website listed excess weight; neck circumference greater than 17 inches; high blood pressure; a narrow airway; male sex; age older than 65 years; family history of sleep apnea; use of alcohol, sedatives, or tranquillizers; smoking; and prolonged sitting.[28] We already know that Mr. Martinez has several of these risk factors, including being overweight, having high blood pressure, being male, and being a smoker. We have ruled out several other risk factors, including being older than 65 years of age and using sedatives or tranquillizers.

Other risk factors require additional information, such as his family history, his neck circumference, if he drinks alcohol, or if he has a narrow airway. We might also need to ask him about prolonged sitting. His work at a construction company might indicate a certain amount of physical activity, but the only way to be sure is to ask. One implication already evident from the Mayo Clinic's website is our need for additional history from the patient.

Let's return to the questions we gave you to consider for this exercise. Before we go through the questions, you might want to see if you can locate the resource yourself. When we performed this activity the website address was www.mayoclinic.com/health/sleep-apnea/DS00148/DSECTION = risk-factors. Of course it is possible, even likely, that the website address has changed. But if you can locate the Mayo Clinic website, the resource might still be there.

3a. *What type of resource did we use?* The resource is a website provided by the Mayo Clinic. It included a list of medical research references. This resource is an expert review, also known as *opinion*.

3b. *Where would the source be placed on the evidence pyramid?* It would be low on the pyramid because it is opinion. Even though the source has a strong reputation, the evidence itself is still low on the pyramid.

4a. *Does the resource apply to the patient?* Yes, mostly. The resource addresses his age, smoking history, weight, and other risk factors. However, it does not provide information on his race/ethnicity.

4b. *What are the implications for Mr. Martinez's care?* It is more likely that he could have obstructive sleep apnea than the other two types. However, more information is needed to rule out the other forms.

4c. *What further information do we need?* We would like to know if his race/ethnicity might be a risk factor for sleep apnea. Also, how are the other types of sleep apnea ruled out? How accurate is nocturnal polysomnography? What other diseases or disorders cause insomnia? How are they ruled out?

As demonstrated here, many questions can arise as a result of just one focused clinical question. Perhaps more questions come up than there are hours in the day to answer them. However, if we find information we believe to be credible and it fits with our medical knowledge as well as our experience, then we might decide to act on that information even if we have questions as yet unanswered. One of the keys to EBP is the ability to make decisions and choose a course of action. This decision should not be premature, however. It is advisable to work collaboratively with your healthcare team and seek guidance and input. In this case, the expertise of an ear, nose, and throat (ENT) physician might be helpful.

One final consideration is the risk to the patient. This risk can take the form of not getting the insomnia diagnosed and treated, an incorrect diagnosis, and/or the cost of care. In this case, the risks might be less immediate and costly than with other health problems, such as if Mr. Martinez had chest pain. But there are always risks. Your command of the research evidence will help you and your patient, reduce the chances of a bad outcome, and lead to improved quality of life for your patient.

CHAPTER SUMMARY

An understanding of research methods is necessary for healthcare providers as consumers of medical research literature. Your understanding of the foundational concepts of research and statistics will enable you to critically evaluate the studies you read, the information patients bring to you, and the brochures provided by pharmaceutical representatives. The greater your understanding of research design and statistics, the less you will be dependent on information providers about the quality of their information. The scope of topics within research design and statistics is well beyond this text, or any individual text for that matter. As such, practitioners need an arsenal of resources, including books and experts, as well as a practice of engaging in lifelong learning related to research and statistics.

The two major paradigms of research—qualitative and quantitative—offer different perspectives and types of information about health and health care. Each type of research needs to be evaluated on the merits of its design and intent. Qualitative (naturalistic) research focuses on describing experiences with health-related phenomena, but does not focus on making predictions or drawing cause-and-effect conclusions. Quantitative (positivistic) research, in contrast, seeks to predict an outcome in a population based on numerical **data** collected from a representative sample of that population. Quantitative research is more widely published and referenced in healthcare literature. However, qualitative research is growing in importance. Also, it is becoming more common for studies to combine procedures from both paradigms, producing mixed-methods research.

Various styles of research fall under each paradigm. Each style of research has distinct procedures that need to be followed in order to produce trustworthy or valid results. The three major types of quantitative research are observational, quasi-experimental, and experimental. Qualitative research is divided into five types: ethnography, biography, phenomenology, case study, and grounded theory.

When reading studies, one way you can evaluate them is to compare the procedures used in them to the recommended procedures for the given style of research. This is true regardless of the type of research performed. As you deepen your understanding of the styles of research, you will enhance your ability to critically appraise each study you read. For example, in a grounded theory study data from multiple sources need to be triangulated with one another, a **constant comparative** analytical procedure must be used (comparing each datum with every other), and researchers should have **prolonged engagement** in the field with the respondents and with the phenomenon of interest. Researchers need to carefully describe the various procedures used in the study to establish the trustworthiness of their conclusions.

In a randomized control trial, the sample must be randomly selected and representative of the population of interest. Accurate methods of measurement must be used, and the article must carefully describe not only sampling procedures and methods of measurement but also the limitations and risks of bias in the study as well as author affiliations and study funding. The validity of the study must be demonstrated through internal procedures as well as comparison with external information.

Another way to evaluate research is to consider where a study is placed on the evidence pyramid. The pyramid recognizes quantitative research as of greater strength than qualitative research. Observational research is lower on the evidence pyramid than quasi-experimental research, which is, in turn, lower than experimental research. Qualitative studies are by definition observational and could be placed on the lower region of the pyramid if they are rigorous in design and analysis.

Similarly, retrospective and cross-sectional research (which are quantitative styles) are below prospective studies (such as cohort studies and cross-over trials) on the evidence pyramid. Nearer to the top of the pyramid are prospective randomized studies, namely those that use multiple types of blinding. Located at the top of the pyramid are studies that analyze multiple well-designed, blinded, randomized control trials. These top-level studies include systematic reviews and meta-analyses.

The location of a study on the evidence pyramid is just one factor to consider when evaluating the quality of the evidence. As mentioned earlier, the purpose of the study and quality of its design in light of that purpose are essential considerations. Research has many purposes in health care. The most common objectives of health-related research include:

- Determining the prevalence or incidence of disease and associated risk factors
- Survival longevity (with and without treatment)
- Accuracy, harms, or side effects of screening tools and diagnostic procedures
- Effectiveness and complications of treatment modalities
- Interactions between interventions
- Quality of life
- Cost of care
- Patient satisfaction

The most important consideration when evaluating an article is the applicability of the information in the study to the individual patient or population.

REFERENCES

1. Vogt WP. *Dictionary of statistics and methodology: A nontechnical guide for the social sciences*. 3rd ed. Thousand Oaks, CA: Sage; 2005.
2. Porta M. *A dictionary of epidemiology*. 5th ed. Oxford: Oxford University Press; 2008.
3. Pope C, Mays N. *Qualitative research in health care*. 3rd ed. Oxford: Blackwell Publishing; 2006.
4. Risjord M. The rise of qualitative research. In: Risjord M. (ed.). *Nursing knowledge: Science, practice, and philosophy*. Chichester, England: Wiley-Blackwell; 2010: 188–212.
5. Creswell JW. *Qualitative inquiry and research design: Choosing among five traditions*. Thousand Oaks, CA: Sage; 1998.

6. Barrett SR. *Anthropology: A student's guide to theory and methods*. 2nd ed. Toronto: University of Toronto Press; 2009.

7. Glaser BG. *Basics of grounded theory analysis: Emergence vs. forcing*. Mill Valley, CA: Sociology Press; 1992.

8. Dodds L. Medical case reports. In: Stuart MC (ed.). *The complete guide to medical writing*. London: Pharmaceutical Press; 2008: 97–105.

9. Rollnick S, Miller WR, Butler CC. *Motivational interviewing: Helping patients change behavior*. New York: Guilford Press; 2008.

10. Persaud TVN. *A history of anatomy: The post-Vesalian era*. Springfield, IL: Charles C. Thomas Publishing; 1997.

11. Fuller S. *The philosophy of science and technology studies*. New York: Routledge; 2006.

12. Walker-Bone K, Cooper C. Epidemiology and the rheumatic diseases. In: Isenberg DA, Maddison PT, Woo P, Glass D, Breedveld FC (eds.). *Oxford textbook of rheumatology*. 3rd ed. Oxford: Oxford University Press; 2004.

13. Snow J. *On the mode of communication of Cholera*. London: John Churchill; 1860.

14. U.S. National Library of Medicine. The reports of the Surgeon General: The 1964 report on smoking and health. Available at: http://profiles.nlm.nih.gov/NN/Views/Exhibit/narrative/smoking.html. Accessed December, 20, 2010.

15. Lang TA, Secic M. *How to report statistics in medicine: Annotated guidelines for authors, editors, and reviewers*. 2nd ed. Philadelphia: American College of Physicians; 2006.

16. National Heart, Lung, and Blood Institute and Boston University. History of the Framingham Heart Study. Available at: www.framinghamheartstudy.org/about/history.html. Accessed December 22, 2010.

17. Freedman DH. Lies, damned lies, and medical science. *The Atlantic*. November 2010. Available at: www.theatlantic.com/magazine/archive/2010/11/lies-damned-lies-and-medical-science/308269/. Accessed November 1, 2010.

18. Rajaram S, Haddad EH, Mejia A, Sabaté J. Walnuts and fatty fish influence different serum lipid fractions in normal to mildly hyperlipidemic individuals: A randomized controlled study. *Am J Clin Nutr*. 2009;89(suppl):1S–7S.

19. The Cochrane Collaboration. What are Cochrane Reviews? Available at: www.cochrane.org. Accessed December 21, 2010.

20. National Institutes of Health. Understanding clinical trials. Available at: at ClinicalTrials.gov. Accessed December 21, 2010.

21. Grimes DA, Schulz F. Bias and causal associations in observational research. *Lancet* 2002;359:248–252.

22. Easterbrook PJ, Berlin JA, Gopalan R, Matthews DR. Publication bias in clinical research. *Lancet*. 1991 Apr 13;337(8746):867–872.

23. Kripke DF. Greater incidence of depression with hypnotic use than with placebo. *BMC Psychiatry*. 2007 Aug 21;7:42.

24. Centers for Disease Control and Prevention. Depression affects 1 in 10 U.S. adults. Available at: www.cdc.gov/Features/dsDepression/. Accessed February 13, 2011.

25. Sackett DL. Bias in analytical research. *J Chronic Dis*. 1979;32:51–63.

26. University of Medicine & Dentistry of New Jersey. Major sources of bias in research studies. Available at: www.umdnj.edu/idsweb/shared/biases.htm. Accessed March 29, 2012.

27. American Academy of Sleep Medicine. Clinical guideline for the evaluation and management of chronic insomnia in adults. [Online Database]. National Guideline Clearinghouse. Available at: www.guideline.gov. Accessed February 13, 2011.

28. Mayo Foundation for Medical Education. Sleep apnea. Available at: www.mayoclinic.com/health/sleep-apnea/DS00148. Accessed February 13, 2011.

CHAPTER 3

Health Communication

Ellen J. Rogo, PhD

INTRODUCTION

Health communication is essential to health promotion and disease prevention. It has been defined as "the study and use of communication strategies to inform and influence individual and community decisions that affect health. It links the fields of communication and health and is increasingly recognized as a necessary element of efforts to improve personal and public health."[1]

The *Healthy People 2020* topics for the next decade include one for health communication and health information technology. The Healthy People initiative is a federal public health program to improve the health of the nation. It has been in place for more than 30 years. This topic has the potential to benefit patients and the public by developing health knowledge and skills, enhancing health decisions and actions, improving healthcare quality and safety, and facilitating the effectiveness and efficiency of healthcare delivery. Public and private entities are called on to provide patient- and public-centered health care and information in order to improve the health of the nation and reduce health disparities. Within this context, the specific objectives for this topic relate to improving decision making shared between the patient and practitioner, self-management resources based on the patient's individual needs, networks for social support, delivery of tailored health information, health literacy, interaction with vulnerable populations, and access to Web-based health information. Additional objectives include the rapid dissemination of health information to deal with public health emergencies, collaboration among healthcare practitioners and public health professionals, and the development of interventions and programs based on "sound principles."[2]

Effective health communication is based on the interaction of numerous factors related to the source, the message, and the receiver. The source of the health information influences the interaction between the information and the receiver (e.g. patient or public) regardless of whether it is from print media (e.g., newspapers and magazines), broadcast media (e.g., television and radio), websites, schools, community programs, family and friends, or healthcare professionals,. Another factor is the health message being delivered. The content of the message needs to be presented in plain language instead of professional jargon, based on evidence and accurate information, tailored to the patient or community, and articulated clearly and concisely. The receiver of the message is the last factor to consider. Health communication is influenced by the severity of the patient's disease or condition as well as the patient's level of health literacy, educational level, cognitive level, socioeconomic level, and cultural background, to name just a few aspects. When considering all three of these factors, health communication is a complex and dynamic process. This chapter explores and offers strategies to enhance health communication in the context of patient- and public-centered health care.

HEALTH COMMUNICATION DURING THE PROCESS OF PATIENT CARE

A patient-centered approach was recognized by the Institute of Medicine as an essential key element in the provision of quality health care.[3] The traditional healthcare model, the biomedical model, focuses on the healthcare provider as the expert, and the interaction with patients revolves around the disease. The patient is expected to comply with the recommendations made by the provider. In comparison, when using a **patient-centered health care** approach, the patient's role is transformed from a passive observer to an active participant in the decision-making process. The goal of this interaction is to build a relationship on trust and respect where treatment and self-management procedures are negotiated between the two collaborative parties.[4] The clinician's role moves from one of being an expert and making decisions *for* the patient to that of being a facilitator and helping the patient make informed decisions.[4] A healthcare professional who employs a patient-centered approach values the patient's right to autonomy and self-determination.

Research has shown that healthcare providers who use a patient-centered approach to communicate are perceived to be more competent in their interpersonal skills as well as their professional skills.[5] Patients also felt more confident in the healthcare provider, which increases the probability of the patient accepting treatment recommendations.[5]

Another important communication issue is the privacy and portability of protected health information (PHI). Patients have rights to access and control how their health information is used. There is a federal law that mandates patient information privacy and security called the Health Insurance Portability and Accountability Act (HIPAA). This law was enacted in 1996 and governs the use and disclosure of PHI. The law covers electronic exchange, privacy, and security of health information. As practitioners working in interprofessional teams it is important to ensure we share patient information within the boundaries of HIPAA guidelines. Therefore, it behooves healthcare professionals to be cognizant of their communication during the process of care. The process of care includes the phases of assessment, planning, implementation, and evaluation.

The Assessment Phase of Patient Care

Health communication is established during the **assessment** phase of care when the patient's chief complaint is explored by the provider. In addition, data are gathered on the patient's health status after reviewing the patient's health history, interviewing the patient, and examining the body. These data relate to the signs and symptoms of disease, which are used (by the same practitioner or another health practitioner) to render a diagnosis or to recommend additional diagnostic procedures to determine a differential diagnosis.

During this initial phase of contact, it is important for the clinician to ask open-ended questions to help patients disclose understanding of the disease and its progression and to aid the clinician in understanding the patient's cultural perspective.[6] **Table 3–1** presents examples of questions to ask patients in order to assess their understanding of the disease or condition influencing their health.

Another aspect of assessment is to determine the patient's current self-management procedures, along with his or her likes and dislikes of these procedures.[4] Table 3–1 also offers suggestions for wording of questions to assess self-management.

Some clinicians might find it useful to assess the patient's health literacy. According to the National Action Plan to Improve Health Literacy, **health literacy** is:

> . . . the degree to which individuals have the capacity to obtain, process and understand basic health information and services needed to make appropriate health decisions [and] is critical to achieving the objectives set forth in Healthy People 2020 and, more broadly, key to the success of our national health agenda.[7]

Health literacy extends beyond basic reading and writing skills to understanding **numeracy** (i.e., application of numbers and measurement into daily tasks, such as medication dosing), listening, and speaking and is influenced by social and cultural factors and science background knowledge.[8] The U.S. population in general has low health literacy; however, vulnerable populations in lower socioeconomic groups and racial/minority groups exhibit significantly lower skills.[9]

Patients with low health literacy use fewer services for prevention, describe their health as poor, and exhibit less knowledge about self-management of diseases.[8] A recent systematic review confirmed an association between low health literacy and inferior use of the healthcare system (e.g., accessing emergency room care instead of preventive care) and increased health conditions and mortality rates.[10] The lack of sufficient health literacy is a risk factor for poor health outcomes and presents significant barriers to health based on the shame associated with lack of skills.[8]

Therefore, screening a patient's health literacy using a series of simple questions or a readiness ruler can help determine the patient's ability. Clinicians might be hesitant to implement this strategy, fearing alienation of the patient; however, the results of a randomized control trial indicated that patient satisfaction with the overall visit was not impacted by the administration of a health literacy assessment instrument.[11]

Table 3–1   Example Questions to Assess the Patient's Understanding and Self-Management

Assessment	Open-Ended Questions
Patient's understanding of the disease or condition	• When did you first notice a problem with tooth decay? • What do you think caused the cavity in your tooth? • How will the cavity get worse if it is not treated? • How does this tooth decay influence the health of the rest of the body? • What type of treatment have you had for cavities? • What improvement do you want for the health of your teeth?
Self-management procedures	• How many times did you brush your teeth yesterday? • What do you like or not like about brushing? • What type of toothpaste are you using right now? • What do you like or not like about the toothpaste? • How many times did you clean between your teeth (e.g., dental floss or toothpicks) your teeth yesterday? • What do you like or not like about cleaning between your teeth? • Do you use anything else to clean your teeth, such as mouthwash or a Waterpik? • What do you like or not like about using these products?

Source: Adapted from Calley KH, Rogo E, Miller DL, Hess G, Eisenhauer L. A proposed client self-care commitment model. J Dent Hyg. 2000:74(1):24–35.

The easiest manner in which to determine the level of health literacy is to ask the patient a series of questions, such as the following:[12]

1. How often do you find it challenging to fill out health forms by yourself?
2. How often do you have problems learning about your health condition because of difficulty understanding written information?
3. How often do you have someone (such as a family member, friend, caregiver or healthcare worker) help you read health materials?

Responses to the questions are based on a five-point Likert scale of 0 = Always, 1 = Often, 2 = Sometimes, 3 = Occasionally, 4 = Never. Chew and associates[12] reported question 1 as the best determinant of health literacy, with no added benefit as a result of asking the other two questions. Patients reporting a response of "often" were categorized as having marginal health literacy, and those responding "always" were classified as having inadequate health literacy. Other researchers have found that the "sometimes" response is the point at which to define inadequate health literacy.[13] Sakar and associates[14] investigated these screening questions in English or Spanish with a predominantly Hispanic population. The findings confirmed the results established by Chew et al.[12] with regard to the effectiveness of question 1 in determining health literacy; however, they also found that asking all three questions was beneficial.

Another question to assess a person's health literacy level is "How do you rate your reading ability?" with responses of "excellent," "very good," "good," "okay," "poor," "very poor," or "terrible."[15] Any one of the last four responses indicates inadequate or marginal health literacy. Caution should be used with this assessment question, because directly asking patients to "confess" to their inability to read might make them embarrassed and uncomfortable. The benefit of asking the three questions previously discussed is that they indirectly measure a person's health literacy.

A variety of health literacy instruments have been developed that might be helpful for clinicians to use in their assessment. Some of the more popular instruments include the Newest Vital Sign, the Rapid Estimate of Health Literacy in Medicine, and the Short Assessment of Health Literacy for Spanish Adults. The Newest Vital Sign instrument is available in English and Spanish; both require 3 minutes on average for completion.[16,17] Both reading and numeracy skills are evaluated by the responses to six questions based on reading an ice cream food label.[16] Patients who answer at least four questions correctly exhibit an adequate level of health literacy; two to three questions with correct responses indicate the possibility of a limited health literacy level; and one or no correct response implies a strong indication of a marginal or inadequate health literacy level.[16]

In comparison, the Rapid Estimate of Health Literacy in Medicine–Short Form (REALM-SF) is an assessment of reading ability that requires the patient to read seven words aloud (e.g., *exercise, jaundice, behavior, anemia*).[18] Patients are instructed to say "blank" when they are unable to read a word. In situations when the patient is having difficulty reading the words, the clinician should instruct the patient to read only the words that he or she knows. The level of health literacy is determined by the number of words pronounced correctly. The assessment is scored as follows:

- Seven correct answers indicates a high school reading level
- Four to six correct answers suggest a seventh- to eighth-grade reading level
- One to three correct answers indicate a fourth- to sixth-grade reading level
- Zero correct answers suggest a third-grade or lower reading level

The healthcare provider needs to be sensitive to the written materials presented to individuals who are not able to read all of the words correctly. For example, patients who score at the seventh- to eighth-grade level will experience difficulty reading most written patient education materials. Individuals who score at the fourth- to sixth-grade level might have problems reading prescription labels and require patient education materials designed for low-literacy readers. At the lowest level of health literacy, patients will likely struggle with low-literacy materials, and the healthcare provider will need to use alternative strategies.[18]

The Short Assessment of Health Literacy for Spanish Adults (SAHLSA-50) is based on the 66 REALM–Long Form words; however, the number of health words is reduced to 50. The clinician uses flash cards with the Spanish medical term printed on one side and two associated words on the back. The side with the term is shown to the patient, who is asked to correctly pronounce the word. Next, the two associated words are spoken by the clinician, and the patient selects the one closest in meaning. One point is received when the patient reads the correct word and pronounces it correctly and identifies the related word. A score of 38–50 suggests adequate health literacy; 37 and less can indicate low health literacy.[18]

Another type of assessment is to determine a patient's readiness to eliminate unhealthy behaviors or readiness to engage in healthy behaviors. Many times a patient's health behaviors are related to self-management procedures that can be modified to impact positive health outcomes. Health behavior theories provide the foundation for EBP related to health education. Theories inform clinicians' decisions in designing patient-centered education. Patient education is becoming increasingly important as a greater proportion of the general population enters their golden years and has to manage chronic health conditions over their lifetime. It is estimated that almost 50% of the U.S. population experiences at least one chronic disease.[19]

This chapter integrates key health behavior theories and provides communication strategies to be used during patient care. This discussion is not intended to be an exhaustive examination of theories related to patient education. Textbooks, as well as public and private websites, are available that provide detailed information on health education. Through ongoing research, new theories are being tested and old theories are being revised; therefore, the healthcare provider needs to remain current with this content.

The **health belief model** was developed in the 1950s to influence individuals to take action to engage in healthy behaviors.[20] The overall premise of this model is that people who perceive or believe that they are vulnerable to a disease and that their health is threatened will take action to prevent the threat and eliminate their vulnerability. Action toward healthy behaviors happens when patients:

- Believe they are susceptible to a health problem (perceived susceptibility).
- Believe the health problem is serious (perceived severity).
- Believe that taking action by engaging in prevention or treatment will reduce the threat of the health problem (perceived benefits).
- Believe the benefits of taking action outweigh the barriers (perceived barriers).[20]

During patient education, the healthcare professional can address these aspects of the health belief model to help stimulate the patient into action.

Two theories, the transtheoretical model[21] and the precaution adoption process model,[22] are helpful in understanding the stages of change. They promote the idea of change as a process, not a single event, depending on the patient's readiness to change.

The transtheoretical model has five stages: **precontemplation** (patient is not willing or ready to change behavior within the next 6 months), **contemplation** (patient is considering action to change behavior in the next 6 months), **preparation** (patient is preparing for the change within the next month and is partially engaged in changing the behavior), **action** (patient is actively engaged in changing the behavior in less than 6 months), and **maintenance** (patient has sustained the behavior change for more than 6 months).[21] Patients do not necessarily start at the precontemplation level, but can enter the process at any stage. Movement to a higher stage is facilitated by health communication strategies targeted at the current stage exhibited by the patient. Patients can regress to a previous stage; in fact, relapse is part of the behavioral change process.

The precaution adoption process model also identifies stages of change; however, these stages differ from those of the transtheoretical model.[22] The first stage is when the patient is unaware of a health issue. The patient enters the second stage when he or she gains awareness but is not engaged to change. Proponents of this process feel that one cannot regress to either of these stages once a higher level is attained.[22] The third stage is characterized by the patient realizing that he or she has a decision to make as to whether to take action. Stages 4 and 5 result when the patient has made a decision as to whether to take action. Stage 4 is the decision not to take action; stage 5 is the decision to take action. Stages 6 (acting) and 7 (maintenance) are similar to those of the transtheoretical model.[22]

The clinician can assess the level of readiness for change by asking the patient questions based on each stage of change. For example, a dental hygienist who is interested in assessing a patient's willingness to implement a daily flossing routine can ask a series of questions to establish patient readiness. **Table 3–2** integrates the stages of both models and provides example questions to use for assessment.

One quick method of assessing readiness for change is by using a readiness ruler.[23] The **readiness ruler** provides a visual means for patients to assess their willingness to change their behaviors and an opportunity for the clinician to actively engage the patient in the change process. The readiness ruler is a visual analog scale that ranges from 0 to 10; the higher the number the patient selects, the more willing he or she is to make a change (see **Figure 3–1**).

Zimmerman et al.[24] incorporated a readiness ruler and a series of questions to ask patients depending on whether the patient's mark was placed toward the left side, the middle, or the right side of the ruler. The clinician engages the patient to

Table 3–2 Example Questions to Assess Stages of Change

Stage of Change	Assessment Questions
Unaware of Health Issue	Are you aware that you have an infection in your gums resulting in redness and bleeding?
Unengaged by the Health Issue	Are you interested in learning how to reduce the infection and prevent it from coming back?
Contemplation	Are you interested in flossing your teeth once a day?
Decision to Act	Have you decided to floss your teeth once a day in the near future?
Action	Are you flossing several times a week?
Maintenance	Are you consistently flossing on a daily basis?

learn about the motivation for behavioral changes by asking the patient why he or she did not place the mark farther to the left side. Likewise, barriers to behavioral change are elicited when the clinician queries the reasons why the patient did not mark the ruler farther to the right. In this patient-centered communication strategy, the patient is asked for suggestions to overcome the perceived barriers and implement concrete actions for changing behavior.

Beliefs about self-efficacy determine an individual's confidence in his or her ability to make a behavioral change by taking action and overcoming

0	1	2	3	4	5	6	7	8	9	10
I never think about eliminating an unhealthy behavior or engaging in a healthy behavior.		I sometimes think about eliminating an unhealthy behavior or engaging in a healthy behavior.		I have decided to eliminate an unhealthy behavior or engage in a healthy behavior.			I am already eliminating an unhealthy behavior or engaging in a healthy behavior.		My behavior has changed to eliminate an unhealthy behavior or engage in a healthy behavior.	

Figure 3–1 Readiness Ruler
Source: Adapted from LaBrie JW, Quinlan T, Schiffman JE, Earleywine ME. Performance of alcohol and safer sex change rulers when compared to readiness to change questionnaires. *Psychol Addict Behav.* 2005:19(1):112–115.

0	1	2	3	4	5	6	7	8	9	10
Not confident in ability to make the change	Slightly confident in ability to make the change			Confident in ability to make the change			Moderately confident in ability to make the change			Extremely confident in ability to make the change

Figure 3–2 Self-Efficacy Ruler

barriers.[25] Greater self-efficacy is considered important for engaging in healthier behaviors, sustaining these behaviors, and recovering from relapse episodes. A ruler (**self-efficacy ruler**) can be used to determine a patient's self-efficacy with making a behavior change (see **Figure 3–2**). The practitioner can ask probing questions to determine the patient's reasons for not marking a score more to the left or the right.

Self-efficacy is one of the behavioral factors in the **social cognitive theory**.[20] This theory proposes that behavioral factors; cognitive factors (knowledge, expectations, and attitudes); and environmental factors, including social norms and interactions with other individuals, determine human behavior.[20] Family members, caregivers, friends, neighbors, and healthcare professionals are examples of individuals with whom the patient might interact, observe, and imitate others' behavior and gain support to implement the changes to their health behaviors. Social support is another factor to assess during this phase.

Communication during all phases of patient care should focus on strategies based on the models and theories previously discussed. The practitioner should be mindful that communication focused on a higher or lower stage than the patient exhibits does not exemplify patient-centered care. **Table 3–3** outlines the characteristics of each stage and the related health communication strategies and support to facilitate movement to a higher stage and ultimately maintain the behavior change.

Planning Phase of Patient Care

Based on the data and information gathered during the assessment phase, the **planning phase of patient care** ensues. This phase requires healthcare providers to use their knowledge of current practice standards. When providers are unsure of how to proceed, the evidence-based process is followed to determine the most effective care in order to make the best recommendations to the patient. During this phase, the patient shares in the decision-making process when the clinician presents his or her findings during the case presentation and gains informed consent to proceed with care. The goal of patient-centered care during the planning phase is for the patient and provider to be partners and negotiate self-management behaviors, as well as the type of treatment, the length of care, and evaluation decisions.[4] The use of effective communication to resolve differences of opinions between the patient and provider and to negotiate care is paramount during this phase.[4] When a negotiated end point is not gained, the clinician needs to respect the patient's decisions and be mindful of his or her right to autonomy and self-determination as core ethical principles.

The healthcare provider needs to develop a comprehensive treatment (care) plan that includes the following items:

- Self-management strategies to decrease diseases and conditions and strategies to monitor, maintain, or improve health
- Diagnostic tests
- Treatment—interventions, services and alternative care
- Length of care—number of visits, length of visits, time between visits
- Evaluation of care
- Estimated cost for all aspects of care

Once the care plan is developed, the clinician presents the case and begins informed consent procedures. Informed consent should be viewed as a

Table 3–3   Communication Strategies

Stage	Characteristics	Health Communication Strategies
Unaware of Health Issue	Patient is not aware that he or she has a health problem or potential health problem.	• Ask questions to make the patient aware and believe that he or she is susceptible to a health problem.
Unengaged by the Issue	Patient is not willing or ready to change behavior within the next 6 months.	• Ask questions to make the patient believe that the health problem is serious. • Discuss the benefits of taking action to change health behaviors and the risks of not changing.
Contemplation	Patient is considering action to change behavior in the next 6 months.	• Guide patient to understand that the benefits of taking action outweigh the barriers. • Provide positive feedback on the patient's willingness to consider a behavioral change. • Educate the patient on alternatives to change (e.g., various tobacco cessation products). • Encourage and motivate the patient to make an action plan.
Decision to Act	Patient is preparing for the change within the next month and is partially engaged in changing.	• Provide positive feedback on the patient's attempts to make changes to support development of self-efficacy. • Assist patient in making an action plan consisting of goals, actions (using a small-step approach), and target dates (see Figure 3–3 for an example).
Action	Patient is actively engaged in changing behavior in less than 6 months.	• Provide positive feedback on engaging in health behaviors to support the patient's self-efficacy. • Provide an opportunity for the patient to revise the action plan (actions and target dates). • Suggest additional strategies to maintain momentum of change (e.g., social support, reminders on sticky notes).
Maintenance	Patient has sustained the behavior change for more than 6 months.	• Provide positive feedback on the behavior change and completing the action plan. • Suggest additional strategies to sustain the change. • In case of a relapse, the patient develops a new action plan.

process of communication and mutual understanding, not as a one-time event of getting the patient's signature to proceed with care.[26,27] Clinicians can make recommendations to support one treatment; however, they need to be mindful of being coercive during their interaction with the patient.[26,27] For instance, clinicians can overly exaggerate the benefit or harm of one treatment option compared to another without being aware of their bias; therefore, the practitioner needs to be attentive of communicating in an objective manner.

The process of informed consent begins by explaining existing conditions related to the patient's chief complaint; however, it is an ethical responsibility to educate the patient about *all* findings from the assessment. This interaction requires the use of plain language and avoidance of professional jargon. Communication is vital for patient understanding, and the patient should be encouraged to ask questions during the conversation. When it is within the scope of practice, the healthcare provider should provide a diagnosis or recommend testing to render a differential diagnosis.

The next part of the informed consent process is to establish self-management procedures. **Self-management** procedures focus on monitoring an existing disease (e.g., diabetic patients testing their blood glucose levels), taking medications and other interventions to maintain or improve a disease or condition (e.g., dietary considerations and exercise for prediabetic patients), and managing the emotions that accompany the illness.[28] Some readers might find it odd to include self-management procedures in the informed consent process, but this author believes that patients need to understand that they play a key role in preventing illness and improving or maintaining health. Their daily self-management actions are vital; therefore, clinicians need to communicate this important aspect of care to patients and ensure their understanding. The development of an action plan for implementing new behaviors or eliminating unhealthy ones should be negotiated with the patient to encourage

commitment to the specified plan. Small changes are preferred over multiple behavioral modifications to help establish patients' self-efficacy or their belief that they are able to change.[25] **Figure 3–3** provides an illustration of this approach.

The next aspect of the informed consent process is to present to the patient the recommended treatment plan, as well as alternative interventions and the consequences of not receiving care. The number of appointments, including follow-up care and evaluation appointments, is explained. The recommended services and their purposes are explained. The patient is also provided with information on the prognosis, potential benefits, potential risks, and the consequences of nonintervention (e.g., allowing the disease to progress without treatment).[26,27] The estimated cost of the recommended and alternative care also is discussed.

During this segment of informed consent, it is important for the patient to have every opportunity to ask questions in order to ensure understanding and foster commitment. The clinician should schedule adequate time to create an environment conducive to open dialogue. The patient should not feel rushed and should have enough time to

Patient's goal for behavior change: Use dental floss between all teeth on a daily basis.		
Action	**Target date**	**Accomplished (Yes or No)**
Use dental floss once a day on bottom front teeth.	Jan 1–Jan 31	
Use dental floss once a day on bottom and top front teeth.	Feb 1–Feb 28	
Use dental floss once a day on previous front teeth and add bottom right back teeth.	March 1–March 31	
Use dental floss once a day on all previous teeth and add bottom right back teeth.	April 1–April 30	
Use dental floss once a day on all previous teeth and add bottom left back teeth.	May 1–May 30	
Use dental floss once a day on all previous teeth and add top left back teeth.	June 1–June 30	

Figure 3–3 Patient Action Plan Using a Small-Step Approach

ask questions and be thoroughly educated before consenting to care. Options for each aspect of the treatment plan need to be thoroughly explained and based on current evidence in order for patients to select the care they feel best addresses their needs, preferences, and financial situation. In patient-centered care, the individual should feel empowered to adhere to the care plan he or she selects.[4]

The patient makes the decision to accept the recommendations made by the clinician, in full or in part, or to decline treatment altogether. Any decisions made by the patient must be documented within the patient's permanent record. Informed consent is best when the patient's signature is written next to his or her decisions for treatment or nonintervention. Note that the patient's reasons for declining care should also be documented. **Figure 3–4** is an example of a generic informed consent form that can be easily adapted to multiple practice settings. This type of form is useful for clinicians to help them complete all the aspects of informed consent. It also benefits the patient to see all aspects of the consent in writing. This form has two unique features: First, there is a statement at the top explaining the clinician's perspective on what he or she values, and, second, near the bottom, the patient has an opportunity to rate the clinician on various aspects of his or her presentation. Some practitioners might want to develop a separate form for the patient to assess his or her interaction with the clinician. Communication assessment instruments or tools (CATs) can be found by conducting a search in the PubMed database or using a search engine such as Google.

The patient should sign the form to acknowledge the acceptance of care. This form should be part of the patient's record and can be used as evidence to prove that the patient was duly informed and consented to treatment. Inadequate informed consent procedures are one cause of lawsuits against healthcare professionals.[26,27] In the event that the patient does not want to make a decision at the present time or declines care, the clinician needs to be mindful of respecting that decision. Positive communication should be employed to convey the message of being available for future decisions.

Implementation Phase of Patient Care

The **implementation phase of care** encompasses the actions the clinician and patient take to maintain or improve health. Whatever interventions or services are rendered, it is important for the practitioner to continue to be mindful of communication with the patient. Before implementing a treatment, the clinician needs to explain the procedures in an understandable manner to the patient, being cognizant of patient's level of health literacy. The healthcare professional needs to be honest with the patient to gain trust and credibility. For example, I remember the first time I had blood taken as a child. The nurse told me, "This is not going to hurt." Well, it was very painful, and the incident created a feeling of distrust for future interactions with hospital personnel. Therefore, patients should be duly informed when an intervention is going to be painful (and such information should be conveyed during the informed consent procedures).

When a procedure has the potential to be uncomfortable, convey to the patient that you want to know when he or she is experiencing pain in order for you to minimize that experience. This message lets the patient know that you are concerned about his or her feelings. Some patients might not want to bother you with their pain; consequently, it is vital that you be mindful of nonverbal cues of pain, such as tensing of the body, clenching of fists, pursing of lips, increased sweating, or moving away from you. Another consideration for the display of pain is based on culture; some cultures value stoicism, whereas others value being emotional. Culture also plays a role in the meaning and interpretation of facial expressions (e.g., a smile can mean happiness, embarrassment, or sadness), body movements (e.g., hand gestures can be interpreted as being friendly or unfriendly), interpersonal distance (e.g., patients are uncomfortable being in close proximity to the provider), physical contact (e.g., touching an older person is a sign of disrespect), and eye contact (e.g., the lack of eye contact or indirect

---

Informed Consent

Patient Name: **Provider Name:**

As a healthcare provider, I am dedicated to informing you of your health status and recommending care. It is also important for you to be a partner in your care and ask questions in order to make the best decisions for yourself.

Existing conditions or diseases:

Diagnosis (within your practice regulations):

Treatment plan:
- Diagnostic tests
- Self-management procedures (e.g., self-monitoring tests, medications, diet and exercise)

Appointment #1	Appointment #2	Appointment #3	Evaluation
• Services • Length of appt • Estimated cost	• Services • Length of appt • Estimated cost	• Services • Length of appt • Estimated cost	• Services • Length of appt • Estimated cost
Explained ☐ Purpose of services ☐ Prognosis ☐ Potential benefits ☐ Potential risks ☐ Consequence of nonintervention	**Explained** ☐ Purpose of services ☐ Prognosis ☐ Potential benefits ☐ Potential risks ☐ Consequence of nonintervention	**Explained** ☐ Purpose of services ☐ Prognosis ☐ Potential benefits ☐ Potential risks ☐ Consequence of nonintervention	**Explained** ☐ Purpose of services ☐ Prognosis ☐ Potential benefits ☐ Potential risks ☐ Consequence of nonintervention
Alternative Care ☐ Purpose of services ☐ Prognosis ☐ Potential benefits ☐ Potential risks ☐ Estimated cost	**Alternative Care** ☐ Purpose of services ☐ Prognosis ☐ Potential benefits ☐ Potential risks ☐ Estimated cost	**Alternative Care** ☐ Purpose of services ☐ Prognosis ☐ Potential benefits ☐ Potential risks ☐ Estimated cost	**Alternative Care** ☐ Purpose of services ☐ Prognosis ☐ Potential benefits ☐ Potential risks ☐ Estimated cost

Patient: Please tell me how well I did.
- Explaining your condition using words you understood
  1 = Could be better   2 = OK   3 = Good   4 = Great
- Explaining the treatment options using words you understood
  1 = Could be better   2 = OK   3 = Good   4 = Great
- Providing answers to all your questions using words you understood
  1 = Could be better   2 = OK   3 = Good   4 = Great
- Letting you make your own decisions about the care you are going to receive
  1 = Could be better   2 = OK   3 = Good   4 = Great

I consent to the recommended care: ☐ Yes   ☐ No

I consent to the treatment with the following alternatives:

I decline the following treatment:
        Explain your reasons:

Patient Signature: Date:

Provider Signature: Date:

Figure 3–4 Generic Informed Consent Form

eye contact is the accepted manner of interaction). Other cultural differences impact the provision of care, and it is necessary for the healthcare professional to receive education in culturally and linguistically competent care, which is defined by the Office of Minority Health as, "a set of congruent behaviors, attitudes, and policies that come together in a system, agency, or among professionals that enables effective work in cross-cultural situations.[29]

The Office of Minority Health provides an excellent website to consult for links to resources for cultural competency training. One of these resources is the National Standards for Culturally and Linguistically Appropriate Services (CLAS).[29] The purpose of these national standards is to address health disparities experienced in the U.S. population and to make healthcare services more user-friendly to all consumers regardless of race, ethnicity, or language. Standards 1 through 3 address **culturally competent care**. Standards 4 through 7 are *mandates* for language access services for healthcare organizations receiving federal funds. Standards 8 through 14 address the structure and policy of the healthcare organization to support the previous seven standards.

Patient education is an important part of the implementation phase of care. The clinician should educate the patient on the self-management procedures negotiated during informed consent. These procedures need to be thoroughly explained to the patient; however, only 20% of the information heard will be retained.[30] Therefore, supporting materials during the explanation will increase retention to 30%. Visual aids such as pictures, diagrams, drawings, models of body parts, and photographs can enhance learning. Written patient education pamphlets generally have illustrations along with text to explain or demonstrate self-management procedures. When the patient is given a pamphlet, the clinician should review the content to enhance understanding. Retention rates improve to 50% when patients see and hear information.[30] The clinician can demonstrate a technique or procedure while talking about each step. Providing resource materials such as videos or CDs to be sent home with the patient can facilitate the recall of the information conveyed at the patient education session.

Patient–provider communication is enhanced when the practitioner is stationed at the same eye level as the patient. The provider needs to give the patient his or her undivided attention and engage in active listening. Active listening should be followed up with summarizing the information presented by the patient. Phrases such as, "What I hear you saying is . . ." or "Let me see if I understand what you are saying . . ." can be used before summarizing the patient's message.

A useful strategy for educating the patient is to (1) tell the patient what you are going to tell them, (2) tell them, and (3) summarize what you told them. The first step orients and prepares the patient for what he or she is going to hear, and the last step reinforces the information presented during the second step. The practitioner should provide an opportunity for the patient to ask questions.

Confusion about medications is a common phenomenon and the source of numerous incidents relating to patient safety; therefore, it is paramount that the practitioner spend time verifying that the patient comprehends the information. One technique used to verify the patient's understanding of self-management procedures is the **teach-back method**.[31] With this method, the patient is asked to teach the procedure back to the practitioner by demonstrating the use of equipment or explaining medication dosing. The clinician uses active listening to determine whether the patient truly understands the information. This method also provides an opportunity to offer feedback to patients to improve their performance at home. The American Medical Association offers a checklist to use for facilitating patient understanding at each appointment (see **Table 3–4**).

Many factors influence the patient's adherence to self-management procedures that healthcare professionals need to keep in mind as they are educating the patient. Physical factors relate to the patient's impairment of vision, hearing, swallowing, memory, information processing, dexterity, and mobility. Other patient factors that should be considered are emotions such as depression, stress, anxiety, and anger produced by the diagnosis of

Table 3–4 Questions to Enhance Patients' Understanding

Area of Care	Questions
Ask-Me-3	What is my main problem? What do I need to do about the problem? Why is it important for me to do this?
Additional services	Where do I go for tests, medicine, and appointments at other offices?
Medication education	When do I take my medication? What does the medicine do? How will I know when the medication is working? How will I know when I need to call the office about this medication? What number do I call when I have questions?
Teach-back method for self-management care	What is it? Why do I use it? How do I do it? When do I do it?
Follow-up care	When do I have to come to the office again? Do I have another appointment scheduled? What is the date and time of the next appointment? What telephone number do I call if I need to change my appointment?

Source: Adapted from Weiss BD. *Health literacy and patient safety: Help patients understand. Manual for clinicians*. Chicago, IL: American Medical Association; 2007.

the illness, multiple chronic diseases, complexity of self-management procedures, or other reasons not related to health. The clinician needs to be aware of the patient's ability to comprehend the information; when the situation is questionable, a support person, such as a family member, can be included in the discussion, but only after asking the patient's permission to do so.

With or without a support system, the patient might need additional reminders about self-management procedures. The clinician or a staff member can provide support through telephone calls to the patient to check on tasks such as side effects of medications or the ease of using a nebulizer. The patient can employ the use of several reminder strategies. One strategy is to write reminder messages on sticky notes and then strategically place them in the kitchen or bathroom. Another strategy is for the patient to set the alarm on a clock or cell phone as a reminder to take medications.

At the end of the appointment, follow-up care needs to be discussed, as outlined on the treatment plan. The patient needs to understand when the next appointment should be scheduled and the purpose of the appointment.

Evaluation Phase of Patient Care

At the next appointment or after a series of appointments, the intervention is evaluated as part of the **evaluation phase of care**. The healthcare practitioner communicates with the patient to determine his or her progress with the intervention and uses subjective information gained from the patient as well as objective measurements of the outcome based on tests. Self-management procedures are evaluated to determine the patient's perspectives on what he or she likes and dislikes. If an action plan was created at a previous appointment, the clinician assesses whether the patient adhered to the plan.

The patient's successes need to be celebrated; the failures should not be emphasized. For instance, if the patient adhered to the plan for 2 months, instead of 6 months, the patient should be commended on his or her accomplishment for the 2-month period. The clinician can ask what would make the patient stick to the plan for a longer time frame. In patient-centered care, the patient's responses are used to create a new plan of action.

The practitioner should remember that taking action toward healthy behaviors is a process, not a single event. Interaction with the patient at subsequent appointments might be necessary to assist his or her interest in sustaining action to promote health.

PATIENT EDUCATION MATERIALS

Patient education materials can be obtained from a wide variety of resources or developed by the practitioner. Each written and visual material selected or designed for use in the practice should be evaluated using the criteria in **Table 3–5**.

A wealth of patient education materials is available on the Internet. Several websites hosted by the federal government have been designed specifically for consumers. The **MedlinePlus** website is sponsored by the National Library of Medicine and the Institutes of Health (NIH). Use a search engine such as Google to locate the MedlinePlus homepage. The home page has three main tabs for health information. The first tab is titled "Health Topic" and is organized by the name of the disease or condition. The second tab, "Drugs and Supplements," provides information about prescription and over-the-counter medications, herbal therapies, and dietary supplements. The third tab, "Videos and Cool Tools," features interactive tutorials on diseases and conditions and videos on surgeries and human anatomy. The MedlinePlus home page also has links to health topics targeted at women, men, children, and seniors. Patients and clinicians can sign up to receive regular email updates about a particular health topic. Materials in languages other than English are available as well as materials designed for individuals with low health literacy, which are referred to as "easy-to-read" materials. The homepage also has a link to a medical dictionary.

Another useful website is **Healthfinder.gov**, which is sponsored by the National Health Information Center. This site has a searchable database of health topics and also provides access to other databases that consumers can use to locate physicians and other providers and healthcare centers, including long-term care or nursing home facilities, hospitals, community health centers, home health programs, and hospice care. Other databases are available to search for health information from health organizations (e.g., government, nonprofit, and professional) and public libraries. The site also features self-management tools, such as health calculators, online check-ups to determine the risk for certain diseases, planners for physical activity, and menus.

PubMed Health is a relatively new website for consumers to access summaries on clinical effectiveness research published in systematic reviews.[32] This database is maintained by the National Center for Biotechnology Information. Systematic reviews are made possible through partnerships with various entities that conduct systematic reviews, such as the Cochrane Collaboration, the National Cancer Institute, the Oregon Health and Science University's Drug Effectiveness Review Project, and the German Institute for Quality and Efficiency in Health Care. Almost 600 articles are available for consumers on a wide variety of interventions, including medications. Due to the complexity of the information it provides, this website is better suited to patients with a high level of health literacy.

Companies that provide point-of-care products often have patient education materials. **Point-of-care products (or resources)** are tools, usually electronic, that are useful to the practitioner while treating the patient. These products contain synthesized evidence similar to the **Cochrane Library**. Some companies do not require a subscription to the product to have access to these materials, whereas others require a subscription. For example, UpToDate allows access to patient education materials without a subscription. The "basic" educational

Table 3–5   Criteria for Selecting or Designing Patient Education Materials

Selection Criteria	Explanation
Content is specific to a target population.	Material considers the patient's age, gender, role (e.g., parent or caregiver), culture, and language.
Information is relevant to the patient.	Information conveyed is relevant to the patient's disease or condition, or self-management procedures.
Literacy level is appropriate for the patient's level.	Information presented is at the appropriate literacy level, as determined during the assessment phase of patient care. A fourth- to sixth-grade reading level is used for easy-to-read materials.
Plain language is used.	Professional or technical jargon is eliminated and information is written in understandable language using personal pronouns (e.g., *you, I, we*) and everyday conversational words. No abbreviations or acronyms are used. Wording is positive rather than negative.
Information presented is accurate and current.	Concepts presented are based on evidence and current research findings.
Format is conducive to reading or listening.	Short sentences and paragraphs are used. Bullets separate important information. White space is used appropriately (e.g., not too much or too little). Headings are bolded to organize information. The voice is pleasant, and the speaker uses inflection. A question-and-answer format is helpful. Only a few salient points are presented.
Illustrations, pictures, and diagrams are provided to support information presented.	Visual aids are labeled with titles, and arrows are used to label important aspects of the information. Keep in mind that people who are color-blind have difficulty distinguishing red from green. Colors should be appropriate to the population.
Material is accessible to the patient.	Materials can be purchased or downloaded from websites and printed to distribute to patients. Links to written and visual materials can be provided to patients who have access to the Internet.

Source: Adapted from U.S. Library of Medicine. *How to write easy-to-read health materials*. 2012. Available at: www.nlm.nih.gov/medlineplus/etr.html. Accessed August 13, 2012.

materials are written at a lower health literacy level than the "beyond the basics" materials.[33] On the patient home page is a search box where a word or phrase (use quotation marks around a phrase) can be entered to locate relevant information on diseases, conditions, tests for diagnosis and self-management, symptoms, interventions, and medications (using the brand or generic name).

MD Consult is another point-of-care product with free access to patient education materials. On the patient education home page, four tabs are located near the top of the page. The first tab is a searchable database for diseases, conditions, and interventions. The second tab is a database for medications; it can be searched by drug classification as well as by generic or brand names. The third tab lists information by medical specialty. The fourth tab is for patient education materials in Spanish. All materials can be customized with information from the healthcare provider.[34]

Two point-of-care products, the Patient Education Reference Center (PERC)[35] and Essential Evidence

Plus,[36] require a subscription to access patient education materials. More than 10,000 items are available, and PERC has materials in 15 languages besides English. Check with someone in the practice where you are employed or at the institution where you go to school to determine if you have a paid subscription to these products.

Patient education materials are available on university websites that have a medical center or that offer healthcare professional programs. The Harvard Medical School, in partnership with Pri-Med Point-of-Care and the Medical Group Management Association, provides a service called Pri-Med Patient Education Center.[37] The materials can be searched by disease or condition or symptoms, such as back pain or headaches. The information provided for diseases and conditions relates to an explanation of the disease or condition, tests and diagnoses, interventions, medications, a glossary, and resources. Interactive tools to enhance learning are provided in the form of quizzes, games, and risk assessment calculators. The website provides information on more than 500 topics, and the information is updated on a regular basis. Another example of a health professional program that offers patient education materials is the Ohio State Sports Medicine program. It offers patient education materials on injuries to many body parts, pool therapy, and back and neck care.

Professional organizations, societies, and associations are excellent sources for patient education materials. The American Diabetes Association's website has information about diabetes and self-management strategies. The Academy of Nutrition and Dietetics has general food and nutrition resources in addition to topics on managing healthy weight loss and childhood obesity. The American Dental Association has a searchable index for oral health topics for consumers. The American Dental Hygienists' Association has information posted for children called "Kids Stuff" that provides answers to frequently asked questions, access to tooth facts, games, and search-related links.

The KidsHealth website is a great source of information and fun activities related to the health of children, teens, and parents. The children's section has information on topics such as how the body works, feelings, staying safe, and health problems, and also offers a kid's health dictionary. The teen topics include sexual health, drugs and alcohol, diseases and conditions, and food and fitness. Topics for parents include pregnancy and newborns, growth and development, positive parenting, general health, and medications. Each of the three sections has information available in Spanish. Support for the website comes from the Nemours Foundation.[38] The information is reviewed by medical experts, including pediatricians, on a regular basis to make sure that the most current information is provided. Practices and institutions that would like to link to this content or reprint it should consult the permissions guidelines on the website.

There are too many websites to mention; however, almost every disease, condition, age group, and gender is represented by a professional group. Use a search engine such as Google to find the website of a particular group of interest. Once you are on the home page, use the search box to locate patient education materials.

Creating Patient Education Media

The proliferation of technology has made its way into the healthcare arena. Practitioners are no longer confined to creating print media for patient education materials; however, it is the easiest type of media to distribute to individuals who are not computer savvy. Patients are becoming more computer literate, and most have access to the Internet in their homes or in public places. Patient education materials can be created and copied to CDs or DVDs, developed as a podcast or as a smartphone application, placed on YouTube, or uploaded onto a website. These media present the opportunity to develop interactive materials; the practitioner is only limited by his or her creative abilities to design a very informative resource that can spur a patient into action.

Regardless of the type of media used, practitioners will benefit from using a process to assist with the development of a resource that will meet patients' needs. The process consists of assessment, planning, pilot testing, evaluation, and improvement. In the first step, assessment, the target population is assessed to learn about its literacy level, cultural aspects of health, specific health needs, and the type of media used most often. Members of the population can be surveyed or interviewed to assess these characteristics; however, if these procedures are not possible, talk to healthcare professionals who work with this population.[39] Another alternative is to consult the Centers for Disease Control and Prevention website named "Audience Insights." Resources are provided on how to design educational materials that communicate more effectively with populations, such as moms with children at home, tweens, teens, boomers, and Hispanics.[40]

In addition, the practitioner must also assess the time and resources needed to accomplish the project. Helpful questions for assessing time and resources include:

- How much time and effort can I (or the practice) invest in this project?
- How much money can I (or the practice) invest in this project?
- What support from others do I need to complete the project (e.g., webpage designer, information technology specialist, professional speaker)?
- Will the cost of developing and publishing the resource fit into my budget (e.g., salary for support staff or cost of printing, CDs, or DVDs)?

The second step of the process, planning, involves deciding on the desired objectives. The purpose of developing the objectives is for the practitioner to have a clear vision of *why* this material is being created. The objectives are stated in terms of *what* the patient should learn. There are three types of objectives: cognitive, affective, and psychomotor. **Cognitive objectives** address a change in knowledge; **affective objectives** state changes in attitudes or values; and **psychomotor objectives** deal with changes to motor skills (or other skills). All three of these objectives need to address outcomes related to improved health. **Table 3–6** presents examples of each of these objectives related to the topic of weight loss.

Next, practitioners must use an evidence-based approach to planning the content of the resource. The most current scientific information must be used to educate patients. One strategy for developing the content is to make an outline of topics to be included. The objectives can be used as headings on the outline, and the corresponding information, visual aids, and activities can be placed below the heading. Remember to actively engage patients at the affective level to enhance their beliefs and values.

Once the outline is completed, it can be reviewed by a web designer or informational technologist for feedback, if you plan to use technology. When designing written or audio material, write a script and keep in mind the criteria for patient education materials presented in Table 3–5. A draft of the resource is created. Written drafts can be assessed

Table 3–6   Examples of Cognitive, Affective, and Psychomotor Objectives

Type of Objective	Examples
Cognitive	- Understand the impact of being overweight on the health of the entire body. - Plan a regular walking exercise program for a 3-month time frame. - Determine healthy food choices by reading and understanding food labels.
Affective	- Appreciate the benefits of walking and maintaining a healthy diet. - Value the adherence to a regular exercise program. - Engage in planning and eating a healthy diet.
Psychomotor (or other skills)	- Perform stretching movements prior to walking to prevent injury. - Walk for 30 minutes five times a week without causing injury to yourself.

for reading level by applying one of several tools. For example, Microsoft Word has a built-in tool that can be used. Other resources include the MedlinePlus Easy-to-Read website[39] or the *Toolkit for Making Written Materials Clear and Effective*,[41] which is available on the Centers for Medicare and Medicaid Services website.

The third step is pilot testing. Pilot testing involves testing the resource with members of the target population. It can be done through the use of surveys or a focus group after the sample audience has read or viewed the materials. The key points of the questions on the survey or for the focus group should relate to the following:

1. Did you feel *objective #1* was met? (List a separate question for each objective.)
2. Was the information easy to understand?
3. Were there words you did not understand?
4. Were the visual aids easy to understand (specify each visual aid as an illustration, diagram, photograph, etc.)?
5. What can we do to make this information better?

The evaluation step begins when the practitioner carefully scrutinizes the feedback from the pilot testing and plans changes to the resource. The final step is to make improvements to the draft and create the final version.

E-Health

E-health is the use of technology to communicate information to improve health and health services. Examples of e-health resources are online health information, online self-management tools, online support groups, online communication with healthcare professionals, and online access to health records. The benefits to consumers and their support people include the management of chronic diseases, access to information to make informed decisions about their health, and improved communication with healthcare providers and organizations. The vision for e-health is to gain attention to this national initiative, to motivate individuals and organizations into action, and to create partnerships to increase access to e-resources.[42]

Online social media provide opportunities for health communication. Such media include podcasts, widgets, blogs, smartphone applications, Facebook, and Twitter. The CDC have two publications that are useful for healthcare providers who are interested in using these media for health messages: *The Health Communicator's Social Media Toolkit*[43] and the *CDC's Guide to Writing for Social Media*.[44]

Health promotion apps (applications) are available for smartphones and other mobile devices. Other uses of these devices include scanning **Quick Response (QR) codes.** QR codes are barcodes that are scanned with a smartphone. For instance, some pharmacies offer QR codes for patients to refill and manage their prescriptions from their smartphones (in the event a patient does not have a smartphone, notifications can be established via email or text messages). The smartphone then brings up a website, an online video, a telephone number, a map, or other health information. Examples of three QR codes are shown in **Figure 3–5**, **Figure 3–6**, and **Figure 3–7**. The first QR code (Figure 3–5) takes the user to the MedlinePlus website (located at www.medlineplus.gov). The second code (Figure 3–6) takes the user to environmental health e-maps on a National Library of Medicine, NIH website (located at http://www.nlm.nih.gov/pubs/factsheets/toxmap.html). The third code (Figure 3–7) provides resources on AIDS awareness on the AIDS.gov website (located at http://aids.gov/images/mobile-awareness-code.png).

Users must download a free QR code reader application to their smartphone before it can read the code. The application of QR codes to health and health services is potentially endless. Use a search

Figure 3–5 QR Code for MedlinePlus Website

Figure 3–6 QR Code for NIH Website

Figure 3–7 QR Code for AIDS Awareness Resources

engine to locate websites that provide the software needed to develop QR codes.

NATIONAL HEALTH EDUCATION

The **National Health Education Standards** (**NHES**) articulate the framework for promoting health at the personal, family, and community levels for students in pre-kindergarten, elementary school, middle school, and high school. This framework communicates learning outcomes related to health for administrators, teachers, and students. Each of the eight standards is divided into instructional objectives for the following age groups: pre-kindergarten through second grade, third through fifth grade, sixth through eighth grade, and high school.[45]

The standards convey learning outcomes for students, who will then be able to:[45]

1. Comprehend concepts related to health promotion and disease prevention to enhance health.
2. Analyze the influence of family, peers, culture, media, technology, and other factors on health behavior.
3. Demonstrate the ability to access valid information, products, and services to enhance health.
4. Demonstrate the ability to use interpersonal communication skills to enhance health and avoid or reduce health risks.
5. Demonstrate the ability to use decision-making skills to enhance health.
6. Demonstrate the ability to use goal setting skills to enhance health.
7. Demonstrate the ability to practice health enhancing behaviors and avoid or reduce health risks.
8. Demonstrate the ability to advocate for personal, family, and community health.

In some communities, healthcare students and professionals are asked to deliver health presentations related to their discipline. One way to prepare for such a presentation is to become familiar with the National Health Education Standards for the particular grade level on the CDC's website. Another suggestion is to review the content on the NIH Office of Science Education website for educational resources. Some of these NIH resources are targeted to elementary, middle, or high school audiences and provide modules on various health topics. Additionally, the modules are designed to support the National Science Education Standards. Examples of modules targeted at the middle school population include the science of healthy behaviors, mental illness, and energy balance (i.e., calorie intake and physical activity). The NIH modules consist of six lessons to be presented over a 2- to 3-week period. When the healthcare student or professional is unable to commit to this extended period of time, he or she can collaborate with the teacher to implement the entire NIH module, or selectively use sections of the module.

The NIH modules' instructional design follows the **5E model**, which represents five stages of learning: engage, explore, explain, elaborate, and evaluate. The five stages are beneficial for learning because they promote active over passive learning, they enhance collaboration among the participants, and they apply an inquiry approach to discovery (i.e., asking questions, observing, analyzing, explaining, drawing conclusions, and asking new questions).[46] **Table 3–7** highlights the presenter and participant role in the five phases.

Although the activities contained in the modules are designed for students, it might be beneficial for healthcare professionals to read a relevant module to get ideas to use with adult audiences. Other educational resources, such as online exhibits, photos, graphics, posters, slides and presentations, as well as print materials and information about careers in science, are available on the Office of Science Education home page.

The following criteria have been articulated for an effective health education curriculum:[47]

- Clear health goals are articulated, and instructional objectives are developed that relate to the goals.
- Instructional strategies (e.g., learning activities) provide experiences for participants to achieve the objectives and goals.
- Instructional strategies are based on theories (e.g., constructivism, where participants engage in their own learning; social cognitive theory) and are based on evidence of the best practices in health promotion and education.
- Instructional strategies are student-centered, and learning experiences engage students in their own learning by employing group discussions, role playing, cooperative learning, and problem solving.
- Positive health behaviors are supported through a critical examination of personal values, attitudes, and beliefs.
- Positive health attitudes and beliefs are supported through a critical examination of peer norms and pressure, social norms, and the influence of media.
- Opportunities are provided to students for them to assess their own vulnerability to health problems and engagement in risky behaviors. Opportunities are provided to reinforce preventive and protective behaviors.
- Content presented is based on the most current evidence.
- Skills of self-efficacy, personal competence, and social competence are developed.

- Content is relevant to the age, needs, desires, emotions, and developmental stage of the participants.
- Learning strategies and materials are logically sequenced and are culturally inclusive.
- Time for developing positive health behaviors is adequate, and support systems are established to reinforce these behaviors.

The CDC do not recommend a single presentation in one grade level as an effective means to promote healthy behaviors.[47] An alternative is for a school district to develop a health curriculum from elementary school through high school. As a healthcare practitioner, you might be invited to participate in this endeavor. An interprofessional perspective of designing a health curriculum has the potential to result in a comprehensive health promotion and disease prevention program. Once the curriculum is in place, a strong support system is needed to help students engage in healthy behaviors and avoid/reduce risky behaviors. This support can come from parents and other family members, peers, and other significant individuals. Communication strategies with these support systems need to be implemented in order to maximize behavioral changes.

HEALTH COMMUNICATION FOR COMMUNITY OUTREACH

Health communication at the community level focuses on informing and influencing decisions and behaviors of a collective group. When we hear the word **community**, most of us think about a group of individuals who live in the same location, such as a country, state, public health district, county, city, or neighborhood. However, there are other types of communities to consider. A community can extend to a group of individuals who share common interests or experiences.[48] Communities with common interests can relate to business associations, service organizations, advocacy or support groups, and parent–teacher organizations. Examples of communities with common experiences relate to diseases or conditions (e.g., a community of

Table 3–7 Phases of the 5E Instructional Model

Phase	Presenter's Role	Participant's Role

Engage	• Generates participants' curiosity and interest in the topic.
	• Assesses participants' current knowledge and understanding of the topic.
	• Encourages participants to express what they think about the topic.
	• Encourages participants to raise questions about the topic.
		• Becomes curious about the topic.
		• Explains current knowledge and understanding of the topic.
		• Compares their ideas to those expressed by others.
		• Raises questions such as:
		  • What do I want to know?
		  • How can I find relevant information?

Explore	• Encourages participant interaction with each other. • Monitors the interaction. • Enhances exploration by asking probing questions. • Allows participants to work through problems related to their understanding.	• Interacts with learning materials. • Explores topic through investigations to observe, describe, and record data. • Creates alternative solutions to problems or answers to questions. • Gains common experiences to use for comparison among participants.
Explain	• Encourages participants to explain concepts and definitions in their own words. • Formulates questions to help participants verbalize their understanding and explanations. • Asks for evidence to support participants' explanations. • Presents definitions and explanations after participants articulate their ideas.	• Uses own words to explain concepts. • Provides evidence based on previous investigations. • Shares ideas and debates them with other participants. • Records ideas and understanding using scientific terminology. • Evaluates own ideas compared to scientific knowledge.
Elaborate	• Provides opportunities for participants to use new terminology, explanations, and skills. • Advances the participants' understanding through the application of knowledge to new situations. • Reinforces participants' use of scientific terms and explanations. • Poses questions helping participants formulate logical conclusions from evidence.	• Expresses understanding using new terminology, explanations and skills. • Applies scientific terms and explanations to a new situation. • Formulates logical conclusions from evidence. • Articulates their understanding to other participants.
Evaluate	• Observes, gathers evidence and assesses participants' understanding, knowledge and skills. • Allows participants to compare ideas to others and improve their thinking. • Provides participants an opportunity to assess their own learning.	• Exhibits new knowledge and understanding or performance of a skill. • Compares current thinking with that of others and improves ideas when needed. • Assesses own learning by comparing previous understanding with current knowledge.

Source: Adapted from National Institute for Dental and Craniofacial Research. *Open wide and trek inside*. 2000. Available at: http://science.education.nih.gov/Supplements/NIH2/oral-health/guide/pdfs/nih_mouth.pdf.

individuals experiencing diabetes), religious affiliations, or being a member of an ethnic or racial group.

For purposes of this discussion, let us say that the community is a city. Smaller communities or subcommunities of people exist within this larger location. Subcommunities of location (e.g., neighborhoods), interests, and experiences exist within the city. These subcommunities can be viewed as stakeholders in a health initiative to change behavior within the broader community. Stakeholders have a common interest in improving the health of their community, and a collaborative partnership among stakeholders influences a behavioral change in the community.

Effective communication is needed to build partnerships to raise awareness of a health problem, gain the collective community's support, influence the adoption of a health initiative, and then mobilize action. In most cases, a **community health initiative** is spearheaded by a small core of interested individuals. This group's first step is to identify the health problem. Common health problems relate to obesity, diabetes, alcohol or substance abuse, cancer, asthma, teenage pregnancy, or child abuse. Data are collected on the demographics of individuals within the community who are affected by this problem, and statistics are used to support the idea that there is a problem. Health statistics are available from the district or state health department or on the CDC's National Center for Health Statistics website.

Assessment also needs to focus on the physical, social, and economic environment to determine factors supporting and impeding healthy behaviors.[19] Changes to policies (e.g., regulations, laws, rules) and systems (e.g., Medicaid, National School Lunch Program) are assessed as to their influence.[19] A helpful resource for assessing stakeholders in a community is the CDC's *Community Health Assessment and Group Evaluation* (CHANGE).[19] The CDC has two other publications worth investigating: the *CDCynergy*[49] and the *Community Health Promotion Handbook: Action Guides to Improve Community Health*.[50] Five action guides have been developed on diabetes self-management, tobacco use treatment, development of places for physical activity, social support for physical activity, and school-based physical education. All of the action guides were developed from the evidence-based strategies for interventions published in *The Guide to Community Preventive Services*.[51]

The next step for this small group is to raise the awareness of the magnitude of the problem within the community. A town hall meeting can be arranged to discuss the problem with the community at large. Another strategy is for individuals of the spearhead group to meet with the executive boards or entire membership of other subcommunities. Whatever strategy is used, the purpose is to raise consciousness and lead to the next step, which is gaining the collective community's support. The goal of this step is to engage as many individuals and subcommunities as time and money allow. When interacting with individuals and subcommunities , it is important to ascertain (1) whether there is interest in participating in the health initiative, (2) who will be the representative to attend and bring ideas to an organizing meeting, and (3) the resources available (e.g., number of volunteers and funding) to accomplish the change. **Table 3–8** lists ideas for stakeholders in a community. An interprofessional cadre of health professionals should be actively involved with the process of community change to ensure a comprehensive view of health.

Engaging these subcommunities will help establish support from the collective community to initiate a behavioral change. This support is important to establish ownership of the health problem, credibility for the change, and political clout, and to mobilize action to initiate the change.[52]

In order to mobilize action, a committee or coalition with representatives from as many stakeholders as possible is necessary to implement a community-wide change. A meeting is planned to bring all representatives together to establish a vision, mission, and desired outcomes of the health change. The Community Toolbox located at http://ctb.ku.edu/en/default.aspx has many useful resources for planning a community health initiative. One or several people from the spearhead

Table 3–8   Subcommunities

Subcommunities	Examples
People affected by the problem	Decide on a disease, condition, or health behavior. Use the *Healthy People 2020* topics/objectives or the leading health indictors.
Government	Mayor, members of city committees, state and federal legislators, chief of police, parks and recreation department, health department
Schools	District administration, teachers, parent–teacher committees, student organizations, class leaders, coaches and team members
Businesses	Business organizations, local merchants, financial institutions, workplaces, health clubs
Service organizations	Rotary Club, Elks, clubs or organizations for males, females, youth, or children
Religious affiliations	Faith leaders, church members
Ethnic and racial groups	Native American or Alaskan Native leaders, Hispanic, and African American organizations
Media	Newspapers, radio, television
High-profile individuals	Individuals recognized for their support of philanthropic efforts, sports, or entertainment abilities
Support or advocacy groups	Children's health, AAA, AARP
Public and private health and dental insurance companies	Medicaid, Medicare, SCHIPS, Blue Cross Blue Shield, Delta Dental
Interprofessional healthcare practitioners	Public health professionals, family practice physicians, nurses, dieticians, dental hygienists, hospital administrators
Healthcare professional organizations	Public health associations, rural health associations, nursing associations
Higher education	University or college administrators, faculty, students, student organizations, health professional programs

group can be the leaders of this initial meeting. An agenda is developed with topics and time frames for discussion of each topic. The agenda should be available to each person attending the meeting by distributing copies or having them visible on a screen. A volunteer should take minutes of the meeting to record all deliberations.

Ground rules for communication are important to discuss at the beginning of the meeting to ensure that an environment of respect and appreciation

for each representative is established. People attending the meeting need to feel equally important in order to gain a sense of ownership with regard to the development and implementation of an action plan. The action plan is developed from the collective ideas of the group members. **Table 3–9** is a template for an action plan. Action statements begin with a verb and articulate very specific tasks that need to be accomplished. The second column identifies a person responsible for

Table 3–9   Action Plan Components

Action	Person Responsible for Specific Tasks	Partners and Tasks	Target Date and Date Completed	Feedback
Schedule meeting with school personnel.	Hospital Infection Control Director will find time and place that works for all participants.	Community Liaison; School District; Hospital; Public Health District.	September 1.	Meeting was successful. Future planning meetings are scheduled for October and November.

the action and the tasks he or she will complete; this person will be designated as the leader. In the column for partners, list individuals who will help the leader and identify the tasks they are responsible for completing. It is important to establish deadlines for the completion of each task and then to identify the actual date of completion. The last component of the action plan is for feedback from the leader or partners about the impact of the action or additional actions that need to be added to a future planning session. When the action plan is completed, it is distributed to all the stakeholders in order to communicate the collaborative efforts of the group and to make sure the desired actions come to fruition. For instance, the following action plan represents early planning steps for reducing incidence of influenza within elementary schools in a community.

The representatives who have attended the meeting act as liaisons between the committee/coalition and their **subcommunity**. They should report back to their committee/subcummunity in order to gain support of the majority of its members. An interprofessional approach is best to engage a wide variety of health disciplines and public health professionals in the initiative.

Funding for the community health initiative is generally needed to support the work to implement the plan. The city and health department might have resources to contribute, depending on the health initiative. Donations, fundraising events, and grants are other means to raise funds. The amount of money generated for use for health communication has a significant impact on the selection and use of various means to disseminate information to support the community-wide health initiative.

An organized plan for health communication is needed to initiate and sustain the health behavior change. One important action to take is to hold a large event to kick off the health initiative. The purpose of this event is to raise the awareness of all members of the public as to the health problem and the initiative. High-profile individuals and the media are engaged as key players in the event, along with participation of as many subcommunities as possible.

The communication plan also promotes actions to engage the community in the behavioral change. Technology can be used to convey health messages, as discussed in the section on patient education materials and e-health. In addition, billboards can be strategically placed along busy roads to convey health messages. Posters can be used for other high-traffic areas, such as workplaces, health clubs, businesses, hospitals, and healthcare offices.

Fliers can be printed and attached to posters or individually distributed in the same areas.

The print media is useful for disseminating news stories or press releases. Letters to the editor and guest editorials can be used for health messages. Other print media worth considering are articles in the healthy living section of the newspaper or a city newsletter. The most expensive strategy is using a paid advertisement.

Local radio and television stations can be another avenue to pursue for health messages. Both media play public service announcements (PSAs) that can be created to communicate short health messages that are usually 30 to 60 seconds in length). High-profile individuals can be recruited to make the message more enticing. For instance, Michael Douglas, the famous actor, donated his time to developing PSAs on oral cancer for the Oral Cancer Foundation after he was treated for throat cancer. Interviews and news stories are another means of transmitting health messages. For example, a news story can focus on the personal experience of someone with the disease or the condition, or the news story could announce a "kick-off" event or fundraising event.

Health communication at the community level should employ the use of as many different forms of communication as possible to initiate and sustain the health initiative. An evaluation of the success of the community health initiative is based on the outcomes established at the beginning of this process.

HEALTH COMMUNICATION USING WRITTEN COMMUNICATION

On occasion, a health professional might be in a situation requiring the construction of some form of written communication (e.g., letter or email message) to advocate on behalf of a patient for approval of care from an insurance company, or to advocate in support or opposition of new policies being considered by policy makers or new laws being considered by legislators (**Figure 3–8**). Before writing, it is advisable to contact the office

of whomever you wish to contact to determine whether a letter or email message is the most effective means of advocacy. In addition, find out who is the best person to contact, the proper spelling of his or her name, and the correct address.

Most likely, you will present some form of evidence in the written communication to persuade the reader to consider your viewpoint. For instance, when advocating for patient care from an insurance company, evidence from radiographs or clinical examinations should be included to support your request (following HIPAA requirements). Likewise, including evidence in written communication to policy makers and legislators can be a means to gain support for your position. Many times the evidence provided is in the form of statistics related to the prevalence or incidence of diseases or conditions. Whenever possible, use statistics appropriate for the situation. For example, when evidence is being used to support a state policy, it is better to use statistics from the state health department rather than national data, if state statistics are available.

In the first paragraph of the communiqué, convey the purpose of the letter in regards to the patient, policy, or legislative bill. In addition, introduce yourself and your credentials as well an explanation of your relationship to the patient, to the policy, or as a constituent of the legislator's district. The second paragraph should explain the reason and provide a rationale for your request. The Healthy People 2020 objectives and leading health indicators can provide support for the justification of your reasoning.

The third paragraph should contain evidence to support your viewpoint that there is a health problem in your community. In certain cases, the content of the second and third paragraphs can be combined into one paragraph. When you are writing to a legislator, you can sometimes make a connection between the legislator's previous voting record and support for the current legislative bill. The fourth paragraph should restate your request and include a statement of appreciation for the individual's consideration of your request.

Return Address	Your Name Address City, State, Zip Code E-mail Address Telephone Number
Date	Insert date
Heading	The Honorable (insert full name, spell correctly) Address City, State, Zip Code E-mail Address
Salutation	Dear Representative [or Senator] (insert last name, spell correctly):
Introduce self and the purpose of the email message	As a resident of Pocatello and a parent, I am writing to ask for your support of House Bill 1234. [The purpose or intent of this letter is to respectfully request your support of Senate Bill 1234]. This bill supports funding for Child Abuse education for community members to improve the health of our state's children and protect them from unnecessary harm.
Explain the reason for the request and provide a rationale	The physical and mental trauma from child abuse affects the healthy development of children. Through the education of key community individuals, abuse and neglect can be recognized and reported to the authorities. Community members can work together to help children heal from these events.
Present evidence or data to establish there is a health problem	In the past you have voted for legislation to improve children's health. [In our community there have been 3000 cases of suspected child abuse reported last year]. Child abuse is a silent problem and all of us must work together to solve the problem.
Restate your request and thank the individual for his/her time	I urge you to support this important legislation. Investing dollars in the lives of our youngsters saves lives. As a constituent, your time and consideration of the bill is appreciated. [Thank you for your ongoing support of healthcare legislation to improve children's health]
Sign off	Sincerely, Your signature Your name and credentials typed

Figure 3–8 Sample Letter to Legislator

Some general rules for written communications are:

- Keep the message concise and clear; for letters, limit to one page
- Use plain language without discipline–specific words
- Limit the use of the word "I" at the beginning of sentences
- Construct paragraphs with at least two sentences

INTERPROFESSIONAL COMMUNICATION DURING PATIENT AND COMMUNITY-CENTERED ACTIVITIES

Interprofessional collaboration requires effective communication among a team of health disciplines to enhance the health outcomes of a patient or a community. Practitioners need to communicate their roles and responsibilities in patient care or community health programs to other team members.[53] Interaction should support a mutual understanding of information, thereby avoiding wording specific to one discipline; when this situation is unavoidable, time should be spent educating other team members. Each practitioner contributes his/her expertise with the interprofessional team in a confident, clear, and respectful manner. Team members are encouraged to contribute their perspectives to the team's endeavors and actively listen to other's ideas.[39] Situations involving conflict and providing performance feedback to team members require the use of respectful language.[53] Above all, the importance of collaboration and teamwork is constantly communicated.

The essential key to interprofessional collaboration is to focus on the welfare of the patient and community, instead of prolonging the profession-centered behaviors that dominate the independent silo mentality of health care. Effective teamwork requires a mentality of collaboration and a perspective that all health professionals are equally capable of contributing to an improvement in the health of the patient or community. Interprofessional collaboration and effective communication is necessary

to attain the national health objectives articulated in the Healthy People initiative.

CASE STUDY #1

During the assessment phase of patient care, you decide to ask the patient, Mr. Martinez, several questions to determine his level of health literacy.

1. How often do you find it challenging to fill out medical forms by yourself? Mr. Martinez's response is "sometimes."
2. How often do you have problems learning about your medical condition because of difficulty understanding written information? Mr. Martinez's response is "often."
3. How often do you have someone (such as a family member, friend, caregiver, or healthcare worker) help you read healthcare materials? Mr. Martinez's response is "always."

From these responses, does Mr. Martinez indicate low health literacy or adequate health literacy? Based on your knowledge of his level of understanding of health information, how would you explain the following information to him using no medical words? You might consider consulting the CDC's Plain Language Thesaurus to help you identify low health literacy phrases. Use a search engine to locate the most current version of this thesaurus.

- Situation 1: Explain the difference between general anesthesia and local anesthesia to help him make an informed choice for deciding on the type of anesthesia he prefers during treatment. What other information would be included in the informed consent discussion?
- Situation 2: Educate Mr. Martinez on the diagnosis of chronic obstructive pulmonary disease (COPD) and the effects of continuing smoking one pack a day while suffering from this disease.
- Situation 3: Educate him on the antibiotic therapy (twice-a-day [the health record abbreviation for twice-a-day is "bid"], taken with food), including the adverse effects of being allergic to the medication.

CASE STUDY #2

A statewide health initiative to engage adults in healthier eating is being considered for implementation by your state Department of Health. This initiative must gain the support of the state director of the Department of Health before it moves to the planning stages and is allocated funding. As a healthcare professional in the state, you want to show your support by writing an email message to the director. Construct one or two paragraphs to explain the reason for your support of the statewide healthy eating initiative, provide a rationale for your support (consult the Health People 2020 objectives and leading health indicators at http://www.healthypeople.gov/2020/topicsobjectives2020/default.aspx), and provide evidence to establish that there is a health problem related to adults being overweight and obese. Be sure to include state-level health statistics, which can be accessed on the state health department's website.

CASE STUDY SUMMARIES

Case Study #1

From Mr. Martinez's responses to the three questions, it indicates marginal health literacy because the responses of "sometimes," "often," and "always" are indicators of this level. Therefore, the explanations that you create for the following situations need to be constructed using plain language rather than medical words.

Situation 1

Explain the difference between general anesthesia and local anesthesia to help him make an informed choice for deciding on the type of anesthesia he prefers during treatment. What other information would be included in the informed consent discussion?

Your response: You have a choice of two different ways to feel comfortable when we treat you. The first choice is giving you a gas that puts you to sleep. The second choice is a shot of a drug that numbs the area where we will be working and you

will remain awake. Other items to address in an informed consent discussion include:

- All findings from the assessment, including the chief complaint and any other finding
- Diagnosis (when it is within the practitioner's scope of practice) or additional diagnostic tests to provide a differential diagnosis
- Self-management procedures to monitor an existing disease, take medications, or use other interventions at home
- Development of an action plan for self-management using a small step approach
- Treatment, alternative treatment, and consequences of not receiving treatment
- Length of treatments, including the number of visits, length of visits, and time between visits
- Evaluation of outcomes
- Estimated cost of treatment and alternative treatments

Situation 2

Educate Mr. Martinez on the diagnosis of COPD and the effects of continuing smoking one pack a day while suffering from this disease.

Your response: You have an illness called chronic obstructive pulmonary disease (COPD) that makes it hard for you to breathe. Every time you inhale smoke into your lungs the smoke causes damage to your lungs. The longer you smoke, the more your lungs are hurt, making your breathing more difficult. If you do not take steps to make the COPD better, such as stopping smoking, it can lead to heart attack, kidney problems, and even death.

Situation 3

Educate him on the antibiotic therapy (bid, taken with food) for an infection, including the adverse effects of being allergic to the medication.

Your response: Mr Martinez, you have a prescription for an antibiotic that is a drug that will help you fight the illness caused by germs. The pills need to be taken with water, two times a day, one pill in the morning and one pill at night. Make sure you eat before taking the pills because otherwise they can make you sick to your stomach. Sometimes people have a bad reaction to these pills. After you take the pills, notify me if you notice an itchy red rash or itchy red bumps on your skin; if you notice swelling of your eyes, lips, or tongue; if you find it hard to breathe, if you feel dizzy or like you are going to throw up, or if your heart is beating very fast. Call our office immediately if you have any of these signs because you might be having a serious reaction to the pills, and you need to receive care immediately.

Case Study #2

Use a search engine such as Google to locate the Healthy People 2020 home page. Once you are on the homepage, locate the list of 2020 Topics & Objectives to determine which one is the closest fit with the statewide initiative. The topic Nutrition and Weight Status is highly relevant. Go to the Nutrition and Weight Status homepage and read the goal for this topic. The message portrayed in the goal can be used to provide a rationale for the healthy eating program. Next, find the information on the Leading Health Indicators on the Healthy People homepage. The leading indicators represent priority areas for the national health agenda. Locate the indicator that is related to the healthy eating program; the indicator, Nutrition, Physical Activity, Obesity fits the situation. Therefore, the fact that it is a high priority for action should be included in the written communication to the state director.

Next, use a search engine such as Google to locate your state's health department. Use the search box on the homepage to locate "statistics for overweight." Find the data for overweight adults. Let us say that the reported statistics are: 66% of adults are overweight or obese and approximately 35% are obese. If you are unable to locate state statistics, go to the CDC's FastStats website for national statistics. Use these data to support the notion that there is a health problem related to weight status in your state.

The following two paragraphs are what we would write in the email to the state director. You might have written something similar in your response to case. This example is not the only correct response to the case.

The justification for a healthy eating program for adults is that being overweight is a risk factor for multiple health problems such as diabetes, heart disease, and high blood pressure, to name a few. Nutrition and weight status are recognized as a leading health indicator in Healthy People 2020, and as such, need top priority and action to reduce the risk of chronic diseases by eating healthy diets and maintaining a healthy weight.

In our state, 66% of the adult population is overweight and obese. A staggering 35% of the same population is obese; therefore, there is a significant health problem related to weight status. The implementation of a healthy eating program for adults will support the Healthy People 2020 goal and initiate action to combat this health problem.

REFERENCES

1. U.S. Department of Health and Human Services, Office of Disease Prevention and Health Promotion. *Health communication.* Available at: www.health.gov/communication/resources. Accessed July 1, 2012.
2. U.S. Department of Health and Human Services. *Healthy People 2020. Health communication and health information technology.* 2011. Available at: www.healthy people.gov/2020/topicsobjectives/2020/overview. Accessed July 1, 2012.
3. Institute of Medicine. *Crossing the quality chasm: A new health system for the 21st century.* Washington, DC: National Academies Press; 2001.
4. Calley KH, Rogo E, Miller DL, Hess G, Eisenhauer L. A proposed client self-care commitment model. *J Dent Hyg.* 2000:74(1):24–35.
5. Saha S, Beach MC. The impact of patient-centered communication on patients' decision making and evaluations of physicians: a randomized study using video vignettes. *Patient Educ Counc.* 2011:84(3):386–392.
6. Kleinman A. Concepts and a model for the comparison of medical systems as cultural systems. *Soc Sci Med.* 1978:12:85–93.
7. U.S. Department of Health and Human Services. *National action plan to improve health literacy.* 2010. Available at: www.health.gov/communication/hlactionplan/. Accessed July 7, 2012.

8. Institute of Medicine. *Health literacy: A prescription to end confusion*. Washington, DC: National Academies Press; 2004.

9. Kutner M, Greenberg E, Jin Y, Paulsen C. *The health literacy America's adults: Results from the 2003 National Assessment of Adult Literacy* (NCES 2006-483): Washington, DC: U.S. Department of Education; 2006.

10. Berkman ND, Sheridan SL, Donahue KE, Halpern DJ, Crotty K. Low health literacy and health outcomes: an updates systematic review. *Ann Intern Med.* 2011:155(2):97–107.

11. Ryan JG, Leguen F, Weiss BD, Albury S, Jennings T, Velez F, Salibi N. Will patients agree to have their health literacy skills assessed in clinical practice? *Health Educ Res.* 2008:23(4):603–611.

12. Chew LD, Griffin JM, partin MR, Noorbaloochi S, Grill JP, Snyder A, Bradley KA, Nugent SM, Baines AD, VanRyn M. Validation of screening questions for limited health literacy in a large VA outpatient population. *J Gen Intern Med.* 2008:23(5):561–566.

13. Wallace LS, Rogers ES, Rokos SE, Holiday DA, Weiss BD. Brief report: Screening items to identify patients with limited health literacy skills. *J Gen Intern Med.* 2006:21:874–877.

14. Sakar U, Schillinger D, Lopez A, Dusore R. Validation of self-reported health literacy questions among diverse English and Spanish-speaking populations. *J Gen Intern Med.* 2010:26(3):265–271.

15. Powers BJ, Trinh JV, Bosworth HB. Can this patient read and understand written information? *JAMA.* 2010:304(1):76–84.

16. Weiss BD, Mays MZ, Martz W, Castro KM, DeWalt DA, Pignone MP, Mockbee J, Hale FA. Quick assessment of literacy in primary care: the newest vital sign. *Ann Fam Med.* 2005:3(4):514–522.

17. Johnson K, Weiss BD. How long does it take to assess literacy skills in clinical practice? *J Am Board Fam Med.* 2008:21(3):211–214.

18. U.S. Department of Health and Human Services, Agency for Healthcare Research and Quality. *Health literacy measurement tools*. 2009. Available at: www.ahrq.gov/populations/sahlsatool.htm. Accessed July 14, 2012.

19. Centers for Disease Control and Prevention. Community health assessment and group evaluation (change) action guide: building a foundation of knowledge to prioritize community needs. Atlanta: U.S. Department of Health and Human Services; 2010.

20. National Institutes of Health, National Cancer Institute. Theory at a glance. 2005. Available at: www.cancer.gov/cancertopics/cancerlibrary/theory.pdf. Accessed July 14, 2012.

21. Prochaska JO, DiClemente CC, Nocross JC. In search of how people change. *Am Psychol.* 1992:47:1102–1104.

22. Weinstein ND, Sandman PM. A model of the precaution adoption process: evidence from home radon testing. *Health Psych.* 1992:11(3):170–180.

23. LaBrie JW, Quinlan T, Schiffman JE, Earleywine ME. Performance of alcohol and safer sex change rulers when compared to readiness to change questionnaires. *Psychol Addict Behav.* 2005:19(1):112–115.

24. Zimmerman GL, Olsen CG, Michael F. Bosworth MF. A 'Stages of Change' approach to helping patients change behavior. *Am Fam Physician.* 2000:61(5):1409–1416.

25. Bandura A. *Social foundations of thought and action: a social cognitive theory*. Englewood Cliffs, NJ: Prentice Hall; 1985.

26. Jones JW, McCullough LA, Richman BW. A comprehensive primer of surgical informed consent. *Sug Clin N Am.* 2007:87:903–918.

27. Bernat JL, Peterson LM. Patient-centered informed consent in surgical practice. *Arch Surg.* 2006:141:86–92.

28. Corbin J, Strauss A. *Unending work and care: Managing chronic illnesses at home*. San Francisco: Jossey-Bass; 1988.

29. U.S. Department of Health and Human Services, Office of Minority Health. *National standards for culturally and linguistically appropriate services in health care*. 2001. Available at: http://minorityhealth.hhs.gov/assets/pdf/checked/executive.pdf. Accessed July 20, 2012.

30. Dale E. *Audiovisual methods in teaching*. New York: Dryden Press; 1969.

31. Weiss BD. *Health literacy and patient safety: Help patients understand. Manual for clinicians*. Chicago: American Medical Association; 2007.

32. National Institutes of Health, National Library of Medicine. *About PubMed health*. 2012. Available at: www.ncbi.nlm.nih.gov/pubmedhealth/about/. Accessed July 22, 2012.

33. UpToDate. *About UpToDate patient information*. 2012. Available at: www.uptodate.com/online/content/about_patient_info.html. Accessed July 22, 2012.

34. MD Consult. *About patient information*. 2012. Available at: www.mdconsult.com/das/patient/body/341912769-6/33/toc?tab = cond. Accessed July 22, 2012.

35. EBSCO Industries Inc. *Evidence-based point-of-care products*. 2012. Available at: www.ebscohost.com/pointOfCare/. Accessed July 22, 2012.

36. Essential Evidence Plus. *Searching and browsing.* 2012. Available at: www.essentialevidenceplus.com /support/search_db.cfm?section = patient#. Accessed July 22, 2012.

37. Patient Education Center, LLC. *About the Pri-Med patient education center.* 2012. Available at: www .patientedu.org/aspx/AboutUs/Aboutus.aspx. Accessed July 22, 2012.

38. Nemours Foundation. *About KidsHealth.* 2012. Available at: http://kidshealth.org/kid/kh_misc /about.html. Accessed July 22, 2012.

39. National Institutes of Health, National Library of Medicine. *How to write easy-to-read health materials.* 2012. Available at: www.nlm.nih.gov/medlineplus /etr.html. Accessed July 25, 2012

40. Centers for Disease Control and Prevention. *Audience insights.* 2012. Available at: www.cdc.gov /healthcommunication/Audience/. Accessed July 25, 2012.

41. Centers for Medicaid and Medicaid Services. *Toolkit for making written materials clear and effective.* 2012. Available at: www.cms.gov/Outreach-and -Education/Outreach/WrittenMaterialsToolkit/index .html?redirect = /WrittenMaterialsToolkit/. Accessed July 25, 2012.

42. U.S. Department of Health and Human Services, Office of Disease Prevention and Health Promotion. *Expanding the reach and impact of consumer e-health tools. Preface: a vision for e-health benefits for all.* 2006. Available at: www.health.gov/communication/ehealth /ehealthtools/preface.htm. Accessed July 25, 2012.

43. Centers for Disease Control and Prevention. *The health communicator's social media toolkit.* 2011. Available at: www.cdc.gov/socialmedia/Tools/guidelines /pdf/SocialMediaToolkit_BM.pdf. Accessed July 30, 2012.

44. Centers for Disease Control and Prevention. *CDC's guide to writing social media.* 2012. Available at: www.cdc.gov/socialmedia/Tools/guidelines/pdf /GuidetoWritingForSocialMedia.pdf. Accessed July 30, 2012.

45. Centers for Disease Control and Prevention. *National Health Education Standards.* 2011. Available at: www.cdc.gov/healthyyouth/sher/standards/index .htm. Accessed July 30, 2012.

46. National Institute for Dental and Craniofacial Research. *Open wide and trek inside.* 2000. Available at: http://science.education.nih.gov/Supplements /NIH2/oral-health/guide/pdfs/nih_mouth.pdf. Accessed July 20, 2012.

47. Centers for Disease Control and Prevention. *Characteristics of an effective health education curriculum.* 2012. Available at: www.cdc.gov /healthyyouth/sher/characteristics/index.htm. Accessed July 30, 2012.

48. Fawcett SB, Francisco VT, Hyra DS, Paine-Andrews A, Schultz JA, Russos S, Fisher JL, Evensen P. *Our model of practice: building capacity for community and system change.* Community Toolbox, University of Kansas. 2012. Available at: http://ctb.ku.edu/en /tablecontents/sub_section_main_1002.aspx. Accessed July 22, 2012.

49. Centers for Disease Control and Prevention. *CDCynergy.* 2011. Available at: www.cdc.gov /healthcommunication/CDCynergy/. Accessed July 22, 2012.

50. Centers for Disease Control and Prevention. *Community health promotion handbook: action guides to improve community health.* 2008. Available at: www.prevent.org/Action-Guides/The -Community-Health-Promotion-Handbook.aspx. Accessed July 25, 2012.

51. U.S. Department of Health and Human Services, Community Preventive Services Task Force. *The guide to community preventive services.* 2012. Available at: www.thecommunityguide.org/index.html. Accessed July 25, 2012.

52. Rabinowitz P. Gaining public support for addressing community health and development issues. Community Toolbox, University of Kansas. 2012. Available at: http://ctb.ku.edu/en/tablecontents /sub_section_main_1027.aspx. Accessed July 22, 2012.

53. Interprofessional Education Collaborative. Core competencies for interprofessional collaborative practice: Report of an expert panel. [Online publication]. 2011. Available at: https://www.aamc.org /download/186750/data/core_competencies.pdf. Accessed September 25, 2012.

Locating Relevant Evidence

Ellen J. Rogo, PhD

INTRODUCTION

One of the key steps in the evidence-based process is locating relevant evidence to use in making decisions. Not only does the evidence need to be relevant, but it needs to be of the highest quality available to the healthcare professional so that he or she can make the best decision. The focus on evidence-based practice (EBP) is generally related to patient care; however, within this chapter the breadth of content is expanded to include professionals who make decisions related to public or community health and epidemiology as well as those who strive to understand people's experiences or perceptions in any healthcare arena.

This chapter is designed as an introduction to locating evidence from a wide variety of evidence-based resources; some are free, whereas others require a subscription. We will explore the sources utilized by many different health professions. We will also focus on the planning steps of locating relevant evidence, searching for evidence, locating full-text documents, recording search strategies, and, lastly, organizing relevant evidence.

Your success in employing EBP is dependent on personal and institutional or practice factors. The first and foremost personal factors relate to your commitment to lifelong learning and orientation toward seeking current quality evidence to answer questions and make decisions. Your ability to use a computer and search resources, coupled with knowledge of the evidence-based process are paramount to the success of implementing this strategy as a practitioner.

It is recommended that beginning professionals work with faculty, colleagues, and librarians to learn how to effectively and efficiently access evidence-based resources and employ methods for securing copies of evidence. Persistence is needed to learn the skills of locating the best available evidence. Healthcare professionals need to practice these procedures in order to hone their skills and seek assistance when difficulties arise. One significant factor related to students in educational institutions or professionals working in practices is the value the faculty or employer, respectively, places on using EBP. These individuals who recognize the importance of EBP to lifelong learning and the provision of quality care directly influence the development of your skills. Additional factors include (1) access to computers, (2) access to evidence-based resources, (3) access to full-text articles, and (4) technical support for learning to use databases. When a healthcare professional is seeking employment, consideration of these factors impacts the implementation of EBP.

PLANNING STEPS TO LOCATE RELEVANT EVIDENCE

Before accessing evidence-based resources, careful planning of the search strategy is necessary. The first step in planning is to identify the situation that requires you to implement the evidence-based process. It is valuable to use a systematic approach to defining the components of the situation. For example, being overweight has serious consequences on health at any age. A healthcare practitioner might be confronted with a junior high school student who exhibits this condition and wants to lose weight in a healthy manner. A professional working in a public or community health setting might want to design an intervention program in a junior high school to combat this condition. An epidemiologist may wish to understand the rates of overweight individuals within a certain age group or geographic population and the contributing factors to this condition. Other professionals, such as mental health or social scientists, might want to understand a person's experience with being overweight to better assist this person with implementing a healthy intervention. These examples represent four broad situations one might face. In practice, you will find that collaboration among different health professions will improve the outcomes of the patient as well as the population.

A practitioner who is new to the evidence-based process might find it useful to break the situation they face into manageable components before searching for relevant evidence; therefore, the acronym **PPAARE** (pronounced "pare") has been created to assist you in this process (see **Figure 4–1**).

Translating the situation into small pieces makes it easier for the practitioner to identify the vital

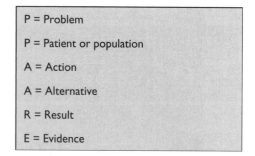

P = Problem

P = Patient or population

A = Action

A = Alternative

R = Result

E = Evidence

Figure 4–1 PPAARE Acronym

elements to use in a search for relevant evidence. These components also are used to write a focused question for the practitioner to use in order to answer the question by gathering evidence.

Problem

The first P in PPAARE represents the *problem*. For a patient care situation, the problem can relate to a disease or condition, such as diabetes, rheumatoid arthritis, pregnancy, or prostate cancer. The problem for a population or community can be applicable to the incidence and prevalence of diseases or conditions, such as the incidence and prevalence of HIV, dental decay, or pregnant teens. An epidemiology problem includes diseases or injuries (e.g., tuberculosis, Lyme disease, traumatic head injuries, sports-related injuries). The qualitative problem relates to the patient's experiences or perceptions of a disease, condition, or access to health services (e.g., cesarean section, cancer, accessing Medicaid services).

Patient or Population

The second P in PPAARE represents the *patient* or *population*. When faced with a patient care circumstance, the need can be related to an individual (patient) or a group (population). For individuals, we are interested in demographic factors, such as age, ethnicity, gender, and education level, and risk factors, including smoking and other unhealthy behaviors.

The population or community aspect of the situation can be applicable to a group's demographics, such as age, ethnicity, and education level, and risk factors, including population density (e.g., urban, rural, frontier), employment opportunities, environmental factors (e.g., quality of water, air, soil), or availability of healthcare providers and health programs.

Epidemiology circumstances include identifying the population's demographics, such as geographic, ethnic, age, and gender characteristics, and the same risk factors as previously mentioned. The qualitative situation requires the identification of the patient's demographics and risk factors, similar to the patient care scenario.

Action

The first A in PPAARE stands for *action* the healthcare provider or patient wants to take. For a clinical situation about patient care, actions can be related to:

- Diagnosis and diagnostic tests
- Etiology
- Prognosis
- Prevention
- Self-management procedures
- Interventions, treatments, or medications
- Follow-up care

An example of a public or community health action is the implementation of a health program and efforts to improve health policy, systems, and practices within a population or community. The action for an epidemiology situation is determining the etiology, distribution (e.g., prevalence and incidence of diseases), and control of diseases and injuries; whereas the action for understanding patients' experiences and perceptions is gaining knowledge to be a more effective healthcare provider.

Alternative

The *alternative* for the action, the second A in PPAARE, is not always identified. There is no need to force an alternative to the action, but when one is available it will help guide the evidence-based process. However, there are situations when an alternative makes sense. For example, a clinician might want to prescribe a newer drug on the market and compare it to one that the practice has used for several years. Likewise, a public health practitioner might compare one type of community health program to another.

Result

The R component represents the *result* of the action. The goal or outcome that the healthcare professional intends to achieve needs to be carefully considered and articulated. The result is directly linked to the P and A components to produce, improve, or reduce the outcome related to the patient, community, population, epidemiology, or understanding of patients' experiences or perceptions. For example, consider the following hypothetical situation for a *problem* related to a diabetic condition. The *patient* is a 32-year-old male Native American. The *action* is a diet restricting carbohydrates combined with an exercise program to reduce BMI, as compared to the *alternative* of consuming oral hyperglycemic medication. The *result* would be a reduction in hemoglobin A1c scores below a 6% level.

Evidence

The last component of PPAARE corresponds to the level of *evidence* you are trying to locate. Consider the hierarchy of evidence shown in **Figure 4–2**.

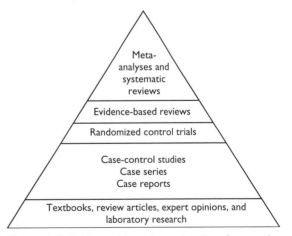

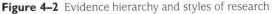

Figure 4–2 Evidence hierarchy and styles of research

Meta-analyses and systematic reviews are the highest level of evidence; evidence-based reviews comprise the next echelon. This level is followed by two additional levels related to specific types of research investigations: randomized controlled trials (RCTs) and case-control studies, case studies, and case reports. The lowest form of evidence is found in textbooks, literature review articles, expert opinion pieces, and laboratory research. Keep in mind that the goal of locating evidence is to find the highest level of evidence available that is relevant to the situation you are facing; however, one can only use the highest level available. For example, a meta-analysis or systematic review might not be in existence on your topic; therefore, lower forms of evidence (e.g., evidence-based reviews or RCTs) have to be used. As you begin to search for evidence, keep in mind the levels of evidence and always search for the highest level available, whatever it might be.

PPAARE Application Examples

In this section, we will apply PPAARE to four different situations, write a question relevant to each situation, and plan the search strategy.

Example: Patient Care

In this example, we will examine the application of PPAARE to a patient care question:

The next patient for the day is a 65-year-old Caucasian male who asks about his risk of prostate cancer. You are wondering if watchful waiting is better than a prostate-specific antigen (PSA) test to reduce the number of unnecessary procedures while resulting in the same progression rate of the disease.

The PPAARE table (**Table 4–1**) can be used to develop the components of a focused clinical question.

Once the PPAARE components are identified, then the practitioner can combine the parts into an answerable question. A patient care question can be formulated using the following template:

Patient care question: *What is the highest level of evidence available to determine whether a patient*

with (P = disease or condition) who is (P = demographics or risk factors) benefits from (A = action) as compared to (A = alternative) to produce, improve, or reduce the (R = result)?

Therefore, the question based on this scenario is:

Example question: *What is the highest level of evidence available to determine whether a patient whose only risk factors for prostate cancer are age and gender, who is a 65-year-old Caucasian male, benefits from watchful waiting as compared to PSA testing to reduce unnecessary procedures and safely monitor the same progression of disease?*

Table 4–1 PPAARE Table for 65-Year-Old Male with Question About Prostate Cancer

PPAARE Component	Case Example
Identify the problem related to the disease or condition (e.g., diabetes, rheumatoid arthritis, pregnancy).	Screening for prostate cancer
Identify the patient related to his or her demographics (e.g., age, ethnicity, gender) and risk factors (e.g., smoking, unhealthy eating practices).	65-year-old Caucasian male
Identify the action related to the patient's diagnosis or diagnostic tests, etiology, prognosis, treatment or therapy, harm, prevention, patient education, or follow-up care.	Watchful waiting
Identify the alternative to the action when there is one (not a required component).	PSA test
Identify the patient's result of the action to produce, improve, or reduce the outcome for the patient.	Reduce unnecessary procedures Monitor same progression of disease
Identify the level of evidence available after searching (use the evidence hierarchy).	Highest available

Table 4–2 PPAARE Table for Prostate Cancer Question

Search Words or Phrases Corresponding to PPAARE Components	Alternative Words or Phrases for Search Words	Search Words or Phrases to be Excluded from Search
Prostate cancer screening	Prostate neoplasm, early detection of cancer, PSA, prostate-specific antigen	
Watchful waiting	Active surveillance	
Prostate biopsy		
Unnecessary procedures		
Rate of progression		

After writing an answerable question to guide the location of relevant evidence, the next step in the planning process is to brainstorm words or phrases to be used in searching evidence-based resources. Search words correspond to the PPAARE components. There are three considerations for planning words or phrases to use in a search for relevant evidence. The first column in **Table 4–2** is where the terms should be recorded. The second column requires a bit of thinking to pinpoint alternative choices for the items in the first column. The practitioner needs to think of additional words, usually synonyms, to locate the best evidence. The purpose of the third column is to identify words or phrases you want to exclude from the search. In some cases words to be excluded from the search might be determined at a later point in time after a database search has been completed. The healthcare practitioner should invest the time in completing this important step before moving ahead to searching for relevant literature.

Example: Public Health or Community Health

The next situation to apply the planning steps is a practitioner faced with a public health or community health problem, such as the one described in the next scenario. A similar process for planning the search strategy can be followed.

Children in Title 1 elementary schools (which are schools in lower socioeconomic areas) exhibit a higher rate of dental decay compared to other schools in the same community. The oral health practitioner wants to know if a fluoride varnish program as opposed to a dental sealant program will reduce the number of teeth with new dental decay in this population.

The public or community health template (**Table 4–3**) can assist you in identifying the PPAARE components.

Once the components have been identified, then a question can be constructed to guide the evidence-based process using the following template:

Public or community health question: *What is the highest level of evidence available to determine whether a community or population with (P = disease or condition) exhibiting (P = demographics or risk factors) benefits from (A = implementation of a health program) as compared to (A = alternative) to produce, improve, or reduce the (R = result)?*

For the dental decay scenario, the following question can be constructed.

Example question: *What is the highest level of evidence available to determine whether a population with a high rate of dental decay exhibiting a low socioeconomic status of elementary school-age children benefits more from a fluoride varnish program as compared to a dental sealant program to improve the prevention of teeth with new dental decay?*

The next step is to identify words or phrases from this scenario to use in the search for relevant evidence (**Table 4–4**).

Table 4–3 PPAARE Table for a Public or Community Health Problem

PPAARE Component	Case Example
Identify the population's problem related to the incidence and prevalence of diseases or conditions (e.g., incidence and prevalence of HIV, dental decay, obesity in children).	High rate of dental decay
Identify the population's demographics (e.g., age, ethnicity, education level) and risk factors (e.g., population density or number of healthcare providers or access to health programs).	Low socioeconomic level Elementary school-age children
Identify the action related to implementation of health programs and efforts to improve health policy, systems, and practices within a population or community.	Fluoride varnish program
Identify the alternative to the action when there is one (not a required component).	Dental sealant program
Identify the result of the action to produce, improve, or reduce results for a community or population.	Reduce dental decay rate
Identify the level of evidence available after searching (based on the evidence hierarchy).	

Table 4–4 PPAARE Table for Public Health Problem with Search Column

Search Words Corresponding to PPAARE Components	Alternative Words or Synonyms for Search Words	Search Words to be Excluded from Search
Children	Child, age 6–12, elementary, school-age	Adult, adults, geriatric
Dental decay	Dental caries	
Title I schools	Low SES, low income	
Fluoride varnish	Topical fluoride	
Dental sealants		
Prevention of dental decay	(Prevention OR control) of dental caries	

Example: Epidemiology

Our next example is an epidemiology situation related to the prevention of skin cancer:

In your practice recently there has been an increase in the number of 45- to 55-year-old patients being diagnosed with cancer on the lips and other areas of the face. You live in a community where people are avid outdoor enthusiasts, and you wonder if the use of sunscreen with a level above SPF 30 is better for preventing skin cancer than no sunscreen or sunscreen below SPF 30.

The PPAARE components can be identified by using the template in **Table 4–5**.

The next step is to construct a question to guide the search for evidence using a template applicable to most epidemiology situations:

Epidemiology question: *What is the highest level of evidence available to determine whether a*

population with (P = disease or injury) exhibiting (P = demographics or risk factors) benefits from (A = control or prevention strategy) as compared to (A = alternative) to produce, improve, or reduce (R = result)?

The template was applied to the scenario for skin cancer, resulting in this question:

Example question: *What is the highest level of evidence available to determine whether a population with skin cancer exhibiting a high level of outdoor activity benefits from sunscreen with an SPF lower than 30 as compared to sunscreen with a SPF above 30 to prevent skin cancer?*

When identifying search words or phrases, it is helpful to think of synonyms for the terms in the first column. The variety of alternative words

Table 4–5 PPAARE Table for Epidemiology Problem

PPAARE Component	Example
Identify the problem related to diseases or injuries.	Skin cancer
Identify the population related to identifying the population demographics (e.g., geographic, ethnic or racial group, age, gender) and risk factors (e.g., population density or environmental factors).	Outdoor activities leading to sun exposure
Identify the action related to determining the etiology, distribution, or control of diseases or injuries.	SPF < 30
Identify the alternative to the action when there is one (not a required component).	SPF ≥ 30
Identify the result of the action to produce, improve the control, or reduce the etiology and distribution of diseases or injuries.	Prevention of skin cancer
Identify the level of evidence available after searching (use the evidence hierarchy).	

Table 4–6 PPAARE Table for Epidemiology Question with Search Column

Search Words Corresponding to PPAARE Components	Alternative Words or Synonyms for Search Words	Search Words to be Excluded from Search
Skin cancer	Skin neoplasms Squamous cell carcinoma Basal cell carcinoma Melanoma	
Outdoor activities	Sun exposure Sunburn	
Sunscreen	Sunscreening agents	Antibiotic
SPF level	Above 30, less than 30	
Prevent skin cancer	Prevention and control of skin neoplasms	

and phrases in the second column (**Table 4–6**) will assist the practitioner in searching for evidence.

Example: Understanding Patient Experiences and Perceptions

The last example relates to the qualitative aspect of patient care and experiences:

You are providing care to pregnant women in a hospital setting. As a staff member in the maternity unit, you routinely come in contact with women who were scheduled for a vaginal birth but who, due to complications that arise during delivery, must undergo a cesarean section. You notice that women who experience this unplanned event seem to be distressed, and you wonder how you can help them before and after the experience to make it less upsetting.

The template in **Table 4–7** is used to identify the PPAARE components related to this example.

Table 4–7 PPAARE Table for Understanding Patient Experiences and Perceptions Question

PPAARE Component	Example
Identify the problem related to experiences and perceptions of a disease, condition, or access to health services (e.g., unplanned cesarean section, cancer, accessing Medicaid services).	Unplanned cesarean section
Identify the patient related to demographics or risk factors.	Mothers
Identify the action related to gaining knowledge to understand patients' experiences or perceptions.	Gain knowledge of these experiences
Identify the alternative to the action when there is one (not a required component).	
Identify the result of the action to produce, improve, or reduce the patients' experiences or perceptions.	Reduce anxiety Improve coping abilities
Identify the level of evidence available after searching (use the evidence hierarchy).	

Writing an answerable question comes next in the planning stage, using a template to produce a relevant question:

> **Understanding patients' experiences or perceptions question:** *What is the highest level of evidence available to determine the experiences or perceptions of (P = disease, condition, or access to care problems) in a (P = demographic or risk factors) patient to (A = gain knowledge) to assist them in producing, improving, or reducing the (R = result)?*

The template was applied to the scenario for women who have had cesarean sections, resulting in this question:

> **Example question:** *What is the highest level of evidence available to determine the experiences or perceptions of an unplanned caesarean section for a pregnant patient to gain knowledge to assist them in reducing anxiety and improving their coping abilities?*

The last step before moving on to conducting a search is to identify words or phrases to employ (**Table 4–8**).

These examples provide you with four broad categories of questions; however, your problem might not fit neatly into one of them. In such situations, use your best judgment to construct a meaningful and answerable question using as many of the PPAARE components as possible.

Table 4–8 PPAARE Table for Understanding Patient Experiences and Perceptions Question with Search Column

Search Words Corresponding to PPAARE Components	Alternative Words or Synonyms for Search Words	Search Words to be Excluded from Search
Pregnant women	Pregnancy Labor	
Unplanned caesarean section	Unplanned caesarean birth Emergency medical services Obstetric labor complications	Vaginal delivery
Anxiety reduction	Stress Postpartum	
Coping abilities	Psychology	
Qualitative research		Clinical trial, RCT

SEARCHING FOR EVIDENCE IN DATABASES

The first set of search strategies we will discuss relates to the most commonly used databases: PubMed, Cochrane Library, and CINAHL. Over the years, these databases have significantly upgraded their features and on-screen appearance. Because of the continuous improvements made to systems like these, it is likely that the screens will have changed from the time we write this text to the time you read it. For this reason, we have not included screenshots, because they would invariably differ from what you will see. Therefore, we recommend that you access the tutorials available on each database to become up-to-date on their features. When you access a database and are confronted with new features and screens, it is in your best interest to seek the assistance of a faculty member, colleague, or librarian who can help you work through the changes.

PubMed is the database discussed first because it is readily available as long as a person has access to the Internet. Searching for evidence can be a challenging experience because of the overwhelming amount of biomedical information available in this database. PubMed currently has more than 5,400 biomedical journals indexed in the database with retrievable journal citations and abstracts. The database is funded by the U.S. National Library of Medicine. Access to citations and abstracts is free; however, access to free articles is limited to those published in PubMed Central. Considering the number of journals indexed in PubMed, a practitioner who is searching for relevant evidence for a patient with diabetes and recommending a physical activity intervention could become overwhelmed when using this database if effective and efficient strategies are not employed to retrieve evidence.

The first screen and search box you encounter after accessing PubMed provides a search of words or phrases within all fields. Phrases entered into the search box, such as "periodontal disease," should have quotation marks around the phrase. The main problem with a subject search is the overwhelming number of citations retrieved on a topic. For example, entering the word "diabetes" into the first search box in PubMed yields more than 380,000 journal citations. Luckily, multiple strategies are available that can be used to find a manageable number of citations.

There are specific reasons for conducting a subject search in the first PubMed screen:

- When searching a brand name of a product
- When searching for information on new diseases (e.g., SARS when it was first identified) for which a Medical Subject Heading (MeSH) has not yet been created
- When searching for evidence before the article is published and/or before it has been indexed using appropriate MeSH

The first strategy to reduce the number of citations retrieved is to access the *controlled vocabulary* used to index journal citations, which in PubMed is called the Medical Subject Heading (**MeSH**). To explain the meaning of controlled vocabulary, think of the yellow pages in a telephone book and the headings used to index businesses. If I am a woman interested in getting a haircut, I go to the yellow pages and look for the heading "Haircut"; however, it is not one of the headings used to index businesses providing this service. Instead, the heading used to index these businesses is named "Beauty Salons & Services." Likewise, if I am a man trying to get a haircut, the heading for these services is "Barbers." In essence, the yellow pages use a controlled vocabulary in a similar fashion as PubMed.

Using MeSH in a search focuses the results on more relevant evidence. The selection of the most appropriate MeSH also is important. PubMed has 41 MeSH related to diabetes, including Diabetes Mellitus; Diabetes Mellitus, Type 1; Diabetes Mellitus, Type 2; and Diabetes, Gestational. For this example, we will use Diabetes Mellitus, Type 2 (DM2). Adding this MeSH to the search box reduces the number of citations to approximately 64,000, which is still an unmanageable number.

The second search strategy to employ is to use the **Boolean operators** AND, OR, and NOT to connect multiple MeSHs (**Figure 4–3**).

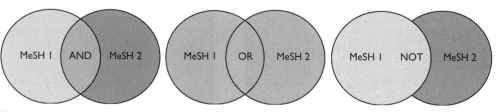

Figure 4–3 Venn diagram of MeSH with Boolean operators

The AND operator links two MeSHs together, limiting citations to those having both headings. The practitioner who is interested in evidence relating to type 2 diabetes mellitus and a physical activity intervention can locate a MeSH for "physical activity intervention" and use the Boolean operator AND to connect the two headings. Two relevant MeSHs for physical activity are "exercise" and "exercise therapy." One search strategy connecting both MeSHs using AND is:

> "Diabetes Mellitus, Type 2"[Mesh] AND "exercise"[Mesh]

Another search strategy is:

> "Diabetes Mellitus, Type 2"[Mesh] AND "exercise therapy"[Mesh]

However, the most efficient strategy would be:

> "Diabetes Mellitus, Type 2"[Mesh] AND "exercise"[Mesh] OR "exercise therapy"[Mesh]

Connecting two MeSHs with the Boolean operator OR expands the search to include citations with both "exercise" and "exercise therapy." Completing this search yields approximately 24,700 citations.

The Boolean operator NOT is helpful to eliminate citations related to articles that are not relevant. For example, if the diabetic client indicates that he will not lift weights as a means of physical activity, eliminate them from the search, as shown below.

With this search, the number of citations was reduced by approximately 300.

> "Diabetes Mellitus, Type 2"[Mesh] AND "exercise"[Mesh] OR "exercise therapy"[Mesh] NOT "Weight Lifting" [Mesh]

The third strategy to further reduce the number of citations to a manageable number is to use the **Limits** feature as a filter in PubMed. Set limits or use **filters** for language to "English" (unless you can read another language fluently) and species to "Human." In addition, limitations to the publication date and publication type are useful. Limiting the search to citations published in the past 5 years and the publication type to meta-analyses yields 12 citations of the highest form of evidence (as of the date we performed this search). **Figure 4–4** recaps the journey from an overwhelming number of citations to a manageable number of best evidence citations.

To provide more detail on using the MeSH as a controlled vocabulary, let us return to the example of the problem of being overweight. A link to the **MeSH Database** is located on the first screen in PubMed. Click the link to search for MeSHs identified in the planning step. When the word "overweight" is entered into the search box, we find that "overweight" is a MeSH and a definition of the MeSH is provided. In addition, 33 subheadings for this MeSH appear (**Figure 4–5**). Subheadings are useful to search for answers to clinical care PPAARE questions related to diagnosis, diet therapy, drug therapy, pathology, physiology, prevention and control, surgery, and therapy. PPAARE questions for epidemiology can use subheadings

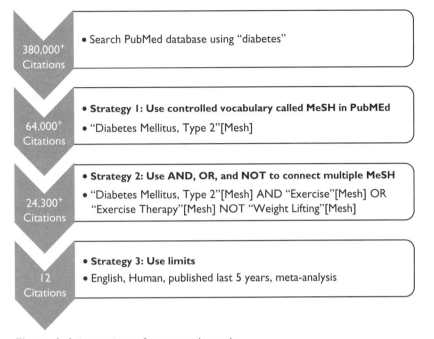

Figure 4–4 Strategies to focus search results

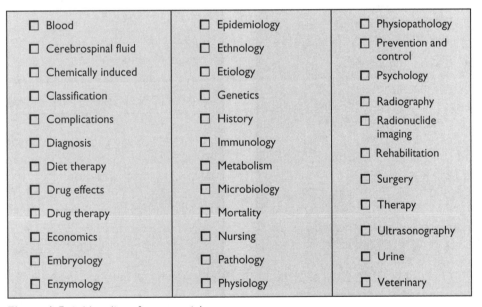

Figure 4–5 Subheadings for overweight

such as epidemiology, etiology, mortality, and ethnology (to determine disease rates in ethnic and racial groups).

At least one MeSH tree is visible (refer to **Figure 4–6** for one example) below the list of subheadings. A **MeSH tree** is useful for determining the hierarchical relationship between headings and selecting the best word or phrase for the search. For example, in the MeSH tree "Overweight" is a broader heading in the hierarchy than is "Obesity."

Another use of the MeSH tree and the hierarchical relationship is to make a decision to include or

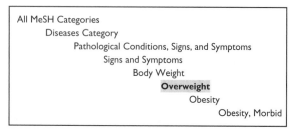

Figure 4–6 MeSH tree for overweight

exclude the headings located below the MeSH. Is the use of "Overweight" or "Obesity" or both the best search strategy? To answer the question, read the definition of each MeSH in the MeSH Database and make that determination. If "overweight" is the best MeSH and you do not want to include "Obesity" and "Obesity Morbid" in the search, you need to check the following check box:

❏ *Do not include MeSH terms found below this term in the MeSH hierarchy.*

The search also can be restricted to MeSH as a major topic as another strategy to focus the results on relevant citations. Placing a check in the box will restrict your search:

❏ *Restrict to MeSH Major Topic.*

For the beginning professional, it is recommended that after you locate a MeSH you add it to the search builder box and conduct a PubMed search on each MeSH separately.

The second strategy for conducting an effective and efficient search is to use AND, OR, and NOT to connect multiple MeSHs by using the search builder feature located in the Advanced Search option. A **history** of your searches also is available in the Advanced Search option, which is a text link (currently) located below the text search box. **Table 4–9** shows a history of PubMed searches.

Notice that each MeSH search has a number in front of it. Also notice that the history feature in PubMed records the number of items retrieved from each MeSH search and the time of the search. Search results are retained for 8 hours after not being active in the database. To conduct a search using the MeSH "Overweight" and the subheading "Diet therapy" and connecting it to the MeSH "Walking," click the word "Add" in the second column before search #5 and #3 and connect them with the Boolean operator AND. The result of this action will place the number of the searches in a search box, and you are ready to click the "Search" button.

```
#3 AND #5
```

When you are unable to locate an appropriate MeSH for use in the PPAARE, you can combine a MeSH search with a subject search. For example, if a practitioner is attempting to understand a teenager's feelings of being overweight, the MeSH "Overweight" and the phrase "Patient experiences," (for which there is no MeSH) can be combined using the AND operator.

```
#2 AND "patient experiences"
```

The third strategy is to use the limits features to further reduce the number of citations. Limits to language, species, publication date, type of article, sex, age, subsets, and text options can help you find relevant evidence of the best quality. One word of caution, however; judiciously use the age, subsets, and text options, because these limits can seriously reduce the number of citations and might create a situation where valuable evidence is missed.

Table 4–9 Search History in PubMed

Search	Add to Builder	Query	Items Found	Time
#5	Add	Search **"Walking"[Mesh]**	14609	19:31:56
#3	Add	Search **"Overweight/diet therapy"[Mesh]**	5060	19:31:27
#2	Add	Search **"Overweight"[Mesh]**	113453	19:30:25

The results are listed as citations; 20 are listed on one screen. **Citations** contain the bibliographic information about the document: title of the document, authors, journal title, volume and issue number, and page numbers. When you click the document title, the **abstract** appears. Read the abstract to determine if the contents are relevant to answering the PPAARE question. When you locate a relevant document, click "Related citations" to locate similar documents. In the PubMed databases, any item in blue is linked to another screen.

Relevant documents can be sent to the **Clipboard**, and this Clipboard can be saved in My NCBI. Using the My NCBI feature requires registering for a free account with a username and password. Once you are logged into your account, you can save your searches for future use and establish an automatic alert to an email account when new documents are added to PubMed that are indexed using the same MeSH as you used in your saved searches. This notification feature helps practitioners remain current on the topic they are searching.

PubMed has a filter called **Clinical Queries** that enables healthcare professionals to conduct specific searches related to the areas of: (1) clinical study categories, (2) systematic reviews, and (3) medical genetics. The link to Clinical Queries is located on the PubMed home page. Once you access the search box in this feature, add the MeSH you want to search and connect multiple MeSHs using Boolean operators. The first filtered search using the Clinical Queries tool relates to the clinical study categories of etiology, diagnosis, therapy, prognosis, or clinical prediction guides. The second filtered search relates to the Systematic Reviews section, which not only includes these types of reviews but also retrieves meta-analyses, reviews of clinical trials, and other types of quality evidence. The third filtered search retrieves citations related to medical genetics.

An example of using Clinical Queries can be related to a previous search strategy using the following MeSHs connected by Boolean operators:

"diabetes mellitus, type 2" AND "exercise therapy" NOT "weight lifting"

Setting the limits to humans, English, and publication date to the past 5 years yields six citations in the Systematic Review section, a manageable number of relevant citations. These citations are at the highest level on the evidence pyramid and include systematic reviews, meta-analyses, evidence-based practice guidelines, and large randomized controlled trials. Results to some searches in the Systematic Reviews can include citations from the Cochrane Database of Systematic Reviews. These systematic reviews are located in the Cochrane Library, a component of the Wiley Online Library.

The Cochrane Library is composed of six databases containing the highest forms of evidence to assist healthcare professionals in making evidence-based decisions: the Cochrane Database of Systematic Reviews, the Cochrane Central Register of Controlled Trials, the Cochrane Methodology Register, the Database of Abstracts of Reviews of Effects (DARE), the Health Technology Assessment Database, and the NHS Economic Evaluation Database.[1] The Database of Systematic Reviews is the most useful for evidence-based practice. The DARE, Health Technology Assessment Database, and NHS Economic Evaluation Database are discussed in a subsequent section of this chapter.

Systematic reviews (and meta-analyses) of interventions and protocols for patient care and public health interventions are found in the Cochrane Database for Systematic Reviews.[2] These components are considered to be the highest level of evidence and the "gold standard" for use in EBP. This high level is designated due to the process and criteria for identifying studies across a wide variety of databases, including unpublished resources; selecting studies to include in the review; evaluating the studies' strengths and weaknesses; collecting data from the studies meeting the inclusion criteria; and then synthesizing and summarizing the data. The goal of these strict protocols and criteria is to produce unbiased publications, resulting from a peer review process, that are reliable resources for healthcare professionals to inform their evidence-based decisions. Currently the Database of Systematic Reviews contains close to 5,000 reviews and more than 2,000 protocols for medical and dental interventions.[1] Because the process for creating a systemic review is a laborious task, relevant systematic reviews or protocols might not be available to answer your PPAARE question. In this case, use the best evidence available to you in Clinical Queries in the PubMed database. Another scenario encountered with the systematic reviews is that conclusive evidence could not be gained from the review. The healthcare professional should use his or her best judgment in this scenario to make a decision.

The Advanced Search feature in the Cochrane Library provides a variety of options for searching. More relevant results are retrieved when MeSHs are used. The Advanced Search page has a link to perform a MeSH search; however, it is less user-friendly than the MeSH Database feature in PubMed. On the advanced search page, multiple MeSHs can be entered into the search boxes and connected with Boolean operators. The default setting is to search all of the six databases, but the advanced feature allows you to select one or several databases to search. Helpful search tips are located on the right side of the screen and provide further help for making a search successful.

In addition to PubMed and the Cochrane Library, another useful database for locating relevant evidence is the Cumulative Index to Nursing and Allied Health Literature (**CINAHL**). There is some overlap of journals indexed in PubMed and CINAHL; therefore, searching both databases is important to retrieve evidence not indexed in both. The focus of CINAHL is on nursing and the allied health literature. The literature from more than 60 nursing specialties can be found in this database.[3] Disciplines in allied health are covered, such as audiology and speech-language pathology, dental hygiene, dietetics and nutrition, occupational and physical therapy, physician assistant, and respiratory therapy. Literature from other specialties, such as alternative medicine, gerodontology, healthcare administration, oncology, and women's health also are referenced in CINAHL.

The CINAHL database uses a controlled vocabulary called *CINAHL headings* or *subject terms*. Some of these subject headings are exactly the same as

the MeSH in PubMed, whereas others are different. To locate controlled vocabulary, go to the Advanced Search feature. Add the word or phrase you want to search and check the box "Suggest Subject Terms." Another option is to click the CINAHL headings tab at the top of the screen. A tutorial is linked to the Advanced Search page that describes how to access the tree hierarchy for the subject heading and subheadings, explode the terms, limit to a major subject heading, and add multiple terms to the search box. The Advanced Search option also allows limits to be set to peer-reviewed articles, publication type, language, and dates of publication. The limit to publication type is beneficial for locating systematic reviews, meta-analyses, RCTs, clinical trials (including RCTs, randomized clinical trials, and clinical trials), and practice guidelines. One word of caution with regard to setting the limit to accessing full-text articles: the search can fail to retrieve important evidence.

Access to CINAHL requires a subscription through EBSCO Industries, Inc. Your institution or employer must pay to have access to this database. Other databases are available through EBSCOhost, including content from disciplines such as sociology, psychology, and education.

EVIDENCE-BASED POINT-OF-CARE RESOURCES

Practitioners employing the use of EBP might be challenged with locating relevant evidence to answer the PPAARE question in a timely fashion. Point-of-care tools contain synthesized evidence, similar to the Cochrane Library, that is useful to the practitioner while treating the patient.[4] These resources continue to grow in number and quality of features available to healthcare professionals. When selecting a point-of-care product, several criteria can be used to determine the currency of evidence, relevancy to the discipline, usefulness of features, amount of time to locate relevant evidence, quality of the review process for synthesizing evidence, and access requirements.

The first criterion, currency of evidence, can be evaluated by determining when the information was last updated. Practitioners need access to synthesized evidence that is updated on a continual basis or at the least on a regular schedule of every 3 to 6 months. Relevancy to the healthcare discipline, the second criterion, is evaluated by determining the value of the evidence in answering PPAARE questions. Some point-of-care products are designed for physicians, nurses, and physician assistants, whereas others target nurses or **rehabilitation** healthcare professionals. Point-of-care tools for dental hygiene and dentistry have not yet been developed. The next criterion, usefulness of features, is evaluated by determining the components available on the website. For example, most point-of-care products have a search feature to locate practice guidelines and recommendations by disease or condition, making access to information easy. Some products have links to take the practitioner to information on related diseases, drugs, and interventions. Additional features the practitioner might want to consider are access to a drug database, patient education materials, images, and regular updates. The amount of time to access relevant evidence is also a consideration for evaluating a point-of-care tool. The searching capabilities should be intuitive versus requiring training to retrieve relevant information. The availability of technical support to answer questions is another consideration.

Another criterion relates to the quality of the review process to synthesize the evidence. This review process can be evaluated by determining the methods used to eliminate bias from the synthesized evidence, the quality of the experts in the healthcare discipline who reviewed the synthesized evidence, and the quality of evidence used in the synthesis. Some tools grade the quality of evidence used in the synthesis of the practice guidelines and recommendations for diseases and conditions. Lastly, access requirements need to be considered. Some products require a paid subscription to access the website; subscriptions are available for institutions and on an individual basis. It is beneficial to take advantage of the free trial offers to apply the aforementioned criteria before making a decision on purchasing one product. Access

to some point-of-care products is free but requires the healthcare professional to register to access additional features on the website. Another access consideration is the availability of the tool via the Internet, smartphones, or other mobile and handheld devices to accommodate the practitioner's access needs.

It is not within the parameters of this chapter to review all of the point-of-care tools available to healthcare professionals. In fact, due to the nature of the changing dynamics of these tools, the information would be outdated in a relatively short time; therefore, the following discussion is based on generalities to provide an overview of the features of several products.

DynaMed is a point-of-care evidence-based resource published by EBSCOhost, providing the interprofessional team with access to high level evidence. According to two independent reviews[5,6], DynaMed is superior in the currency of the evidence available for practitioners to use. This resource uses a "Systematic Surveillance System"[7] to locate new research published in medical journals on a daily basis by teams of experts. When new evidence is found, it is incorporated with existing information. Evidence is reviewed using a seven-step process to ensure the professionals who are responsible for synthesizing new evidence follow a strict protocol. In addition, evidence is classified according to its quality by establishing the level of evidence and grading the recommendations made in the practice guidelines.

The DynaMed database is easy to use[6] to locate information on 3,200 topics related to diseases and conditions. After logging into the database, the homepage contains a search box where words and phrases can be entered and the following categories of information are retrieved on diseases and conditions:

- Related Summaries
- General Information
- Causes and Risk Factors
- Complications and Associated Conditions
- History and Physical
- Diagnosis

- Treatment
- Prognosis
- Prevention and Screening
- Quality Improvement
- Guidelines and Resources
- Patient Information
- ICD-9/ICD-10 Codes
- References

Medications can be searched using the generic and brand names. Listed below are the categories of drug information available in this resource:

- General Information
- Uses and Efficacy
- Dosage and Administration
- Cautions and Adverse Effects
- Mechanism of Action/Pharmacokinetics
- Stability and Compatibility
- Preparations
- Patient Information
- References

Other useful resources are located under the Calculators tab at the top of the web page and the choices include:

- Medical Equations
- Clinical Criteria
- Decision Trees
- Statistics Calculators
- Units & Dose Converters
- Search by Specialty
- Math Calculator
- Glossary

As you can see, the busy clinician has access to a wealth of information in this point-of-care resource. The DynaMed home page contains links to recent updates, or the practitioner can subscribe to receive these updates in a weekly newsletter sent to an email address. Access to DynaMed is available through the Internet and mobile devices and can be integrated with electronic health records. A free trial is offered before purchasing a subscription to this resource.

Another point-of-care resource is MD Consult, which provides access to a variety of features and resources for evidence-based practice. After logging into the website, a search box appears and the clinician is able to search all of the features and resources or limit the search to one. One feature is First Consult, which can be used to search on diseases and their diagnosis and treatment.[8] The disease's name is added to the search box, and the titles of the results are retrieved. Carefully reading the titles will locate the most relevant evidence, which is displayed on one side of the screen as an outline linked to the corresponding section. Links are provided to other resources, such as books, journals, clinical reviews, medications, practice guidelines, images, and patient education information. The content undergoes a thorough peer review before it is added to MD Consult. Medical topics are updated in a continual process and on an as needed basis when new evidence is available.

Resources available to search in MD Consult include medical reference books, journals, and clinical reviews contained in more than 30 clinical journal titles, with access to full text chapters and articles.[8] Another resource, the drug database, can be searched by brand or generic names through Gold Standard and contains FDA approvals and safety notices. The database also includes practice guidelines that are accessible from published journals; information from governmental agencies and professional entities is also available. An images database searches images from the medical reference books on the MD Consult website and can be used to retrieve relevant photographs, tables, and graphs. Clinicians also have access to patient education materials in English and Spanish that can be distributed via customized newsletters.

Essential Evidence Plus is a point-of-care tool published by Wiley-Blackwell. This database contains high-quality evidence from the **Cochrane Systematic Reviews**; patient-oriented evidence that matters (POEM) research summaries; evidence-based guidelines, including those contained in the National Guideline Clearinghouse; evidence summaries; a wide variety of support tools; calculators; and images.[9] POEMs are updated based on a continuous review of more than 100 medical journals coupled with a rigorous editorial process. Most of the information contained in this database relates to clinical medicine; therefore, disciplines such as dentistry, occupational and physical therapy and nutrition are not represented. Information can be accessed via the Internet, smartphone, or other handheld mobile device. Online tutorials and a PDF training manual are available to learn how to use the product. Practitioners can test this product by signing up for a free trial period. Additional features are daily POEM updates, weekly POEM podcasts, and drug safety alerts. Technical support is available on the Web by searching the FAQs for previous problems encountered with the database.

The American College of Physicians (ACP) provides a point-of-care resource known as Physician's Information and Education Resource (PIER) made available through a subscription to Stat!Ref, a medical database. EBP guidelines and recommendations can be accessed by placing the name of a disease in the search box. The results are organized by headings, which include prevention, screening, diagnosis, hospitalization, nondrug therapy (such as lifestyle changes, appliances, surgical interventions, etc.), drug therapy, patient education, management of the disease, and follow-up. Within the text, links are found to resources for additional information, including a drug database. The ACP grades the level of evidence used in developing the guidelines and recommendations.

EBSCOhost Publishing provides evidence-based point-of-care resources through several other products in addition to DynaMed: the Nursing Reference Center, the Rehabilitation Reference Center, the Patient Education Reference Center, and GIDEON (Global Infectious Disease and Epidemiology Network).[10] The Nursing Reference Center provides point-of-care information for nurse clinicians and administrators. Evidence-based resources for physical and occupational therapy and speech and audiology therapy can be accessed in the Rehabilitation Reference Center. The patient education product contains information on topics related to diseases and conditions, medical procedures and lab tests, prevention and wellness, drug information, and discharge instructions in a wide variety of languages. GIDEON is a resource designed for public health practitioners and infectious disease personnel. It features information related to epidemiology on a global level, microbiology of infectious diseases, and therapeutic interventions related to vaccines and drugs.

Other point-of-care products worth investigating are the British Medical Journal's Point-of-Care product, which includes Clinical Evidence; PEDro (physiotherapy evidence database); Medscape Reference; and Mosby's Nursing Consult. The benefits of the point-of-care products are (1) easy access for the practitioner via computer, smartphone, or other handheld device; (2) synthesized evidence to apply during patient care; and (3) access to numerous resources and features simultaneously. A student or practitioner who does not have access to one of these products should compare each product by applying the criteria mentioned in the beginning of this section to determine the product's usefulness to answering PPAARE questions and making decisions.

The primary advantage of point-of-care resources is that they are quick access to information. In some cases this means locating high-level information more rapidly because the information has already been synthesized. However, there are important potential limitations to using point-of-care products. The very characteristic that makes them useful is their major limitation. These products might not provide access to the full array of information on a topic. Also, the information available is determined by the company who is selling the product. It is possible for there to be bias in the selection of available topics. We encourage you to utilize point-of-care products as one tool within a comprehensive information strategy that includes primary resources (such as PubMed and CINAHL).

Meta-Search Engines

SUMSearch2 and Trip Database are two examples of **meta-search engines** that search for evidence-based information in multiple databases at the same time and then generate one list of results. Access to these meta-search engines is free;

however, each provides additional features to practitioners who sign up for an account.

SUMSearch2 accesses PubMed, DARE, and the National Guideline Clearinghouse on the Agency for Healthcare Research and Quality website.[11] Diseases and conditions can be searched using filters to limit results by intervention, diagnosis, age, species, language, and number of results. SUMSearch2 has a unique filter called "iterations," whereby the computer applies different search strategies to access results. For example, when the number of results is too large, the search engine can apply up to six variations of the search to reduce the number of results. Likewise, when the number of relevant results is small, variations to the search are applied to increase the number. The practitioner can view the iterations applied in the search by clicking "Show evidence search details" on the results page. On occasion, the practitioner will get a message "cannot parse the results" from one of the databases. When this happens, a link to the unavailable database is provided to conduct a search within the database.

The list of results contains original research studies, systematic reviews, and practice guidelines; however, each of these three types of evidence can be viewed in a separate list. Original research is retrieved from PubMed, systematic reviews from PubMed and DARE, and practice guidelines from PubMed and the National Guideline Clearinghouse. Results are listed from the most recent publication to the oldest; this feature helps combat the problem of not being able to limit the results to specific publication dates. In order to locate the most relevant evidence and the smallest number of results when using this meta-search engine, use multiple MeSHs connected with the Boolean operators AND and NOT. A convenient link to the PubMed MeSH Database is available on the SUMSearch2 home page.

When numerous results are retrieved, a message is visible suggesting that the practitioner search the Trip database, another meta-search engine for EBP. PubMed plus websites and e-textbooks are simultaneously searched; a complete list of these resources can then be viewed on the database's website.[12] Several features improve the location of relevant evidence, including options for: (1) three types of searches, (2) related articles, and (3) a wide variety of filters to limit the results. The search options include a basic search, advanced search (publication dates can be limited) and a Search Wizard that enables the practitioner to use PPAARE components to conduct a search. The Related Articles option works in a similar fashion as the same feature in PubMed.

The results page contains options to view the items with the following filters: evidence-based synopses, systematic reviews, guidelines by authoring country, core and extended primary research, e-textbooks, patient information and decision aids, and medical images and videos. Results in PubMed are provided in the categories of etiology, diagnosis, therapy, prognosis, and systematic reviews. New features and options are added to this search engine on an ongoing basis to improve its usefulness to practitioners engaged in EBP.

Using Search Engines

Anyone who has been on the Internet has most likely used a search engine to locate information. Common search engines include Google, Yahoo!, Bing, and Ask, to name a few. In this author's experience, the Google search engine features are helpful for locating relevant evidence to answer PPAARE questions; therefore, the discussion will focus on this search engine. Google provides two options for locating evidence: basic search and Google Scholar search. Each of these options has an Advanced Search feature allowing the practitioner to narrow the search to retrieve more focused and relevant results. The main challenge of using a search engine is the number of results retrieved; sometimes results number in the thousands or millions. This discussion presents the most efficient and effective ways of using Google to locate relevant evidence.

The first screen accessed on the Google website (www.google.com) has a search box to conduct a basic search. Words or phrases relevant to the PPAARE question are entered into the box. When searching phrases such as "exercise therapy," place quotation marks around the phrase to tell the computer these words are connected as a phrase. On the results page, the link to an Advanced Search can be found at the top or bottom of the screen. Click the link and you have access to features that will help you focus the search by limiting words and phrases, reading level, results per page, language, and domain. The options for limiting words and phrases in a search include "all of these words," "the exact wording or phrase," and "one or more of these words." The more words you use in each one of these options, the more focused the results. For example, if a practitioner wants the highest level of evidence on diabetes and exercise therapy, the strategy detailed in **Table 4–10** could be used.

The use of quotation marks around phrases is recommended in the first and last search options. Other ways to limit the results is to change the reading level to only advanced results and the language to English. Another useful option in the Advanced Search feature is to limit the search to a specific site or domain. This feature is useful to locate evidence on topics such as the prevalence of diseases. When a public health professional wants to locate statistics on the prevalence of a disease such as diabetes, the domain can be limited to .gov. Results of this search are limited to local, state, and federal governmental agencies, including PubMed. The domain can be further specified to include results from a specific state or federal agency. If I am a healthcare professional interested in diabetes prevalence in Idaho, the domain can be limited to idaho.gov, or if national statistics are needed the domain can be limited to the Centers for Disease

Control and Prevention—cdc.gov. Results can be limited by publication date using the toolbar on the left side of the screen.

When the results are displayed, by clicking the title of the publication the search will lead to access to the document. When relevant results are found, you can use the Related Articles feature to find similar results. The advantage of using Google Scholar is that a filter is applied to the results and only scholarly information is retrieved. Google Scholar also has the Related Articles feature for each result.

Searching Websites

The websites of professional associations and governmental agencies frequently contain useful EBP resources. Each healthcare discipline is represented by one or multiple professional associations. Professional associations can be a resource for evidence, including standards of care, clinical practice guidelines, parameters of care, position statements, and white papers on a variety of topics related to your profession.

Standards of practice are articulated as clinical practices applied to *all* patients and are a benchmark for the provision of care. Standards are formulated based on current evidence and expert opinion. Clinical practice guidelines are recommendations for practice designed to assist the practitioner in decision making on client care; however, deviation from the guidelines is based on the clinical circumstances surrounding the care (e.g., patient's needs and wants, progression of the disease or condition, healthcare setting). Adherence to the guidelines does not guarantee positive patient outcomes. Clinical practice guidelines are developed using current evidence and expert opinion. Parameters of care include both standards of care and clinical practice guidelines. Position papers are written by organizations and associations to provide support or opposition for policies or healthcare interventions. White papers are similar to position papers in that they articulate a philosophy or position on a topic. Current evidence and expert opinion provide the rationale for position and white papers.

Table 4–10 Search Strategy Using Limiters in Google

All of these words	"diabetes mellitus"
This exact wording or phrase	"exercise therapy"
One or more of these words	"meta analysis" OR "systematic review"

In the event that you are not familiar with the associations representing your discipline, a search in Google using a phrase like "nursing associations," for example, can provide you with a list. Once you are on the professional association's website, use the search box usually located at the top of the screen to locate relevant information. Many organizations' websites also have a site map that can be useful in locating evidence. A site map provides a list of the major topics contained on the website.

The **World Health Organization (WHO)** focuses on global health and diseases. Access to guidelines and recommendations for implementing clinical procedures and developing health policies is available on the organization's website. In addition, public health practitioners and epidemiologists will find information on health statistics, health information systems, and disease outbreaks. Practitioners can subscribe to a free weekly epidemiology record to keep abreast of newly emerging and recurrent infection outbreaks.

U.S. government agencies can be accessed as EBP resources, and relevant agencies' websites can be individually searched to locate evidence. The **Agency for Healthcare Research and Quality (AHRQ)**, the **Centers for Disease Control and Prevention (CDC)**, the National Institutes of Health (NIH), and the Department of Veteran Affairs are valuable EBP resources.

AHRQ provides access to information relevant to practice as a healthcare professional through the National Guideline Clearinghouse (NGC). The NGC is a database containing evidence-based clinical practice guidelines for a variety of healthcare disciplines. Guidelines and revised ones are updated on a weekly basis.[13] Guidelines can be searched by using a basic or advanced search or by a listing of topics or organizations. When multiple guidelines exist on a topic, a synthesis of the guidelines comparing key points might be available for review; however, the number of these syntheses is limited. When a synthesis is not available, two or more clinical guidelines can be compared adjacent to each other by accessing the Compare Guidelines feature on the NGC website.[14] Stringent criteria

are established for inclusion of guidelines on this governmental site.[13] Recommendations for prevention developed by the U.S. Preventive Services Task Force are available in the NGC database. These recommendations focus on counseling strategies, screening assessments, and medications and immunizations for prevention of diseases.

The CDC support the National Center for Health Statistics and the Community Preventive Services. The National Center for Health Statistics is a valuable resource to determine the health status of populations, including vulnerable populations; health problems; and trends in the healthcare delivery system. FastStats is a database of A to Z topics related to public health that provides easy access to statistics on a wide variety of health topics. Data also are available for each U.S. state and territory. Another feature is Health Data Interactive, which allows practitioners to customize tables of health information by gender, age, ethnicity, and geographic area for comparison to determine patterns or trends in data. The Community Preventive Services provides access to the Community Guide, a free evidence-based resource containing recommendations for implementing public health interventions and developing health policy. A systematic review process is used to develop recommendations for programs and policies that have been effective in promoting community health.[15] The economic impact of the community intervention also undergoes a systematic review process to understand the program and individual participant cost, economic benefits, and cost-effectiveness.

Another governmental entity, the National Institutes of Health (NIH), consisting of 27 institutes and offices, can be accessed to locate evidence.[16] The entire NIH can be searched simply by using the search box on the home page or each individual institute or center can be searched. The following are examples of just a few of the agencies comprising the NIH:[16]

- National Cancer Institute
- National Institute of Dental and Craniofacial Research
- National Institute of Mental Health

- National Institute on Minority Health and Health Disparities
- National Institute of Nursing Research
- National Center for Complementary and Alternative Medicine

Access to ClinicalTrials.gov also is available on the NIH website. This website provides access to clinical trials funded by the federal government and private organizations.[17] Over 100,000 results from clinical studies can be accessed in the Results database. There are requirements for posting the findings; however, the quality of some might be lacking.[18] ClinicalTrials.gov is another resource for current evidence on health topics.

The **National Library of Medicine** (**NLM**), another NIH entity, supports the National Information Center on Health Services Research and Health Care Technology (NICHSR). This agency has several databases that might be useful for finding evidence. One database, the Health Services Research Projects in Progress (HSRProj) contains citations of studies currently under way.[19] Only studies supported by grants or contracts from state and federal governments, foundations, and organizations are indexed in the database. Details about each study can be viewed, along with an abstract of the planned study. Another database, Health Services Technology Assessment Texts (HSTAT), indexes documents from the ARHQ, the U.S. Preventive Task Force, the Substance Abuse and Mental Health Services Administration, and the NIH Consensus Conference Reports.[20]

The Health Services Research (HSR) database can be accessed on the PubMed home page by clicking the title "Topic-Specific Queries" under the heading "PubMed Tools." A list of specific searches appears; when you locate the one named "Health Services Research (HSR) Queries," click the title. Searches on quality and costs of health care can be limited to one area, such as costs, economics, outcomes assessment, appropriateness, quality improvement, or qualitative research.[21] Another beneficial topic-specific search is for "Comparative Effectiveness Research," which retrieves research indexed in PubMed and

studies in progress. Search boxes are available to search HSRProj and ClinicalTrials.gov. Other specific queries can access information on electronic health records, *Healthy People 2020*, and cancer topics.[21]

The Department of Veteran Affairs is another governmental agency that has clinical practice guidelines on its website. Guidelines related to chronic diseases, mental health, pain, military-related conditions, rehabilitation, and women's health are available. The Substance Abuse and Mental Health Services Administration supports the National Registry of Evidence-Based Programs and Practices.[22] This registry is an online database of more than 200 interventions related to substance abuse and mental health. Interventions can be found by entering a word or phrase in the search box located on the home page.

The Canadian Task Force on Preventive Health Care has developed clinical practice guidelines for a wide variety of primary healthcare providers, public health professionals, and policy makers.[23] The guidelines are based on systematic reviews of evidence developed by the Evidence Review and Synthesis Centre housed in McMaster University.[24] The Task Force rates the quality of evidence, which results in one of two ratings, strong or weak, for the strength of the recommendations made in the guideline.

The National Health Service based in England supports the National Institute for Health and Clinical Excellence (NICE). NICE develops clinical practice guidelines, health technology assessments, and public health recommendations.[25] The database is easily searched by using the search box found under the tab "Find Guidance." Another option is to search for evidence by topic, date, or type of guidance (e.g., cancer, diagnostics, intervention, technology). More than 700 files are available on the NICE website. A more recent feature is NICE Pathways, which provides "interactive topic-based diagrams" of recommendations for healthcare and public health professionals.[25]

Another evidence-based resource supported by the National Health Service is the Centre for Reviews and Dissemination. The Centre maintains the Database of Abstracts and Reviews of Effects (DARE), the Economic Evaluation Database (EED), and the Health Technology Database (HTA). Healthcare professionals have free access to 21,000 systematic reviews, 11,000 economic evaluations, and 10,000 health technology assessments.[26] DARE contains critical abstracts of systematic reviews of health interventions and services that meet specified criteria to ensure quality.[27] Cochrane reviews and protocols also are summarized in the DARE database. Critical abstracts in the EED focus on health intervention costs and the effectiveness of outcomes.[28] The HTA database contains summaries of a wide range of studies on technology assessments, but does not critically analyze these studies.[29]

Evidence-Based Journals

Numerous healthcare disciplines have access to evidence-based journals. There are two types of journals, those that present critical reviews of research and systematic reviews and those that publish original research and systematic reviews. The critical reviews are useful because the evidence is analyzed and evaluated. Main components of the critical reviews vary; however, many contain a summary of the methodology, key study factors, main outcome measures, main results, conclusions, and funding sources. Also included is a commentary written by the review author providing a critical analysis of the validity and reliability of the study or systematic review and relating the findings to previous studies.

The British Medical Journal (BMJ) group publishes evidence-based journals in medicine, nursing, and mental health. Other disciplines, such as dentistry and obstetrics/gynecology, have similar journals available through MD Consult and Elsevier Publishing. Subscriptions to these journals are needed to access the articles, or the healthcare provider can pay for each article available on the publisher's website. Additional information about obtaining documents is discussed in a subsequent section of this chapter.

Open Access Evidence

Due to the ever-increasing costs associated with subscriptions to healthcare and scientific journals, the concept of open access publication of evidence has gained momentum in the last decade. In 2003, the Berlin Declaration supported the Internet as a means to distribute and share scientific evidence with the global community:[30]

Open access contributions must satisfy two conditions:

1. *The author(s) and right holder(s) of such contributions grant(s) to all users a free, irrevocable, worldwide, right of access to, and a license to copy, use, distribute, transmit and display the work publicly and to make and distribute derivative works, in any digital medium for any responsible purpose, subject to proper attribution of authorship (community standards, will continue to provide the mechanism for enforcement of proper attribution and responsible use of the published work, as they do now), as well as the right to make small numbers of printed copies for their personal use.*

2. *A complete version of the work and all supplemental materials, including a copy of the permission as stated above, in an appropriate standard electronic format is deposited (and thus published) in at least one online repository using suitable technical standards (such as the Open Archive definitions) that is supported and maintained by an academic institution, scholarly society, government agency, or other well-established organization that seeks to enable open access, unrestricted distribution, interoperability, and long-term archiving.[30]*

Several open access resources are available for searching to locate evidence. One resource is the Directory of Open Access Journals, which lists all the journals available in which to search for evidence (located at www.doaj.org). Professionals wanting to access theses and dissertations can find them in ProQuest's Open Access Publishing. Another resource for open access and free access to journal articles is PubMed Central. To view the list of journals in the open and free list, go to the PubMed Central home page and view each list. On the home page is a search box to conduct a search in PubMed Central that will result in direct access to articles; however, a search in PubMed retrieves free articles in PubMed Central. More than 2 million articles are archived in PubMed Central.[31]

BioMed Central[32] and the Public Library of Science (PLoS)[33] are open access publishers; the former is a for-profit business and the latter is a nonprofit business. Publication and dissemination time is maximized because of the online publishing environment. Articles are evaluated for quality and must meet standards to be published.[32,33] On both publishers' websites, evidence can be searched in one search box for all disciplines' databases, or each specialty area can be searched individually. BioMed Central publishes research in journals within the disciplines of medicine, biology, genetics, and retrovirology.[32] PLoS publishes research in specialty databases related to medicine, biology, genetics, pathogens, and neglected tropical diseases.[33] A feature available in both open access environments is the ability for researchers from different disciplines to communicate about the study by making comments to the author, thereby promoting scholarly discussion.[32,33]

Open access publishing is an excellent concept to improve retrieval of relevant evidence, and in the future it is likely to have a positive influence on EBP. When documents are not available as open access documents, several strategies are available for obtaining a copy of the document.

Locating Full-Text Documents

When evidence is found in the PubMed, CINAHL, and other EBSCOhost databases or by using a search engine, there are multiple ways to gain access to the **full-text** articles. The most expensive manner to retrieve a full-text article is by going to the publisher's website and using the pay-per-view service.

When citations are located in PubMed, it is best to view each one individually in the Abstract display. The benefit of this method is that links to the full-text article are displayed only when one abstract is viewed. Links to the document are visible as icons, generally in the top-right area on the screen. From within an abstract, links are available to PubMed Central and to publishers who provide either free access or pay-per-view access. Pay-per-view access costs at least $20.00. In addition, your educational or medical institution might have icons notifying you of the availability of the article in print or online access. When icons are not visible, check your institution's library website to locate a list of journal subscriptions available to you.

When you do not have free access to an article, there are two options besides the pay-per-view service from publishers: (1) using an interlibrary loan service or (2) using the National Library of Medicine's Loansome Doc service. Many institutions provide an interlibrary loan service at no charge or assess a minimal charge to provide a copy of a document to you from another library. Consult a librarian to learn how to use this service. Make sure you have a copy of the citation (authors' names, title of article, title of journal, year of publication, volume and issue numbers, page numbers, and the direct object identifier, if available). Some libraries notify you of access to the article via email. A link is provided along with an access code. Generally, your access will be limited, such as viewing the article five times or for 14 days. A good rule of thumb is to access the document as soon as you are notified and download it onto your computer.

If your institution does not have this service, check with a local public library or medical library for your options to secure documents and the associated fees. Another alternative is to use Loansome Doc, which is available on the PubMed website. A free account is required to access this service, which you can establish by using your email address and establishing a password.[34] Once you are logged in, you can check for medical libraries offering this service and then register with the individual library. Fees for retrieving articles can vary between libraries; therefore, check several libraries before ordering an article.

When you find relevant evidence in CINAHL, another EBSCOhost database, or by using a search engine, some institutions have links within the results to notify you of access to the document. When links are not available, the next step is to locate a list of journal subscriptions on your library's website. Interlibrary loan services can be used when the library does not subscribe to the journal.

Online Calculators

Healthcare students and practitioners who are implementing EBP can use **calculators** to assist in making patient care decisions in conjunction with their clinical judgment and the patient's needs and desires. MedCalc 3000 is a resource in Stat!Ref; therefore, a subscription is required to access this online tool. One section of calculators converts units, such as weight from pounds to kilograms, and provides information on dosing of drugs, such as thyroid medications. Another section of calculators provides access to decision trees for diagnosis, risk, treatment, and outcomes of various diseases and conditions. The Clinical Criteria section contains content for assessment of diseases and conditions using tools for screening, risk scores, diagnostic criteria, and scales of measurement. MedCalc can be added to electronic patient records and the various features used with the individual patient data. MedCalc 3000 has more than 500 calculators, decision trees, and clinical criteria available for use during patient care.[35]

Essential Evidence Plus, a point-of-care product discussed earlier, also has diagnostic test calculators, history and physical exam calculators, and decision tools for risk assessment, diagnosis, prognosis, and drug dosing. Drug databases, such as Micromedex, also have a variety of calculators for dosing and antidote dosing and measurement calculators to assist the clinician in making decisions regarding medications. Other point-of-care products, such as DynaMed, have a variety of calculators to enhance EBP.

RECORDING SEARCH STRATEGIES

Table 4–11 provides a way in which to keep a record of your search strategies. Each of the resources for locating evidence are located in the left column. You might not have access to some of the resources requiring subscriptions (e.g., CINAHL and other EBSCOhost databases, point-of-care products) and in that case make a note saying "No Access" or use the acronym "NA." Another significant point that needs to be made is that not every resource has relevant evidence to answer the PPAARE question. For example, when a disease, condition, or intervention is relatively new, there might not be systematic reviews available in PubMed or the Cochrane Library; therefore, the healthcare professional would have to use the "best" available evidence on which to base decisions related to the work setting. Systematically searching each of the evidence resources is necessary to locate the best evidence.

In column 2, indicate the date of the search. In the next column, record the keywords, MeSH, or subject headings used in the search, because you might think of alternative words to use in future searches. In the fourth column, make a note of the limits used in the search. Some of the resources have features allowing you to be notified when new evidence is available on the topic being searched. This feature is important to gather additional evidence for answering the PPAARE question and enhancing future decisions.

ORGANIZING RELEVANT EVIDENCE

The next step in the evidence-based process is organizing the relevant evidence you have located. In column 6 record the title of the evidence. In the next column, indicate the type of access you have to the evidence. When you have a hard copy or have downloaded the file to your computer, indicate "Y" for yes. Hard copies of evidence should be placed in a manila folder with an appropriate title on the tab for easy retrieval. Likewise,

Table 4–11 Organizer Table for Tracking Search Strategies

PPAARE Question:

1. Resource Accessed	2. Date of Search	3. Keywords, MeSH, or Subject Headings Used	4. Limits Set (publication dates or type)	5. Alert Established?	6. Title	7. Access to Evidence? (Y/N, PMID, URL, IL, LD)	8. Level of Evidence	9. Relevance to PPAARE Question (Scale 1–3)
PubMed MeSH								
PubMed Clinical Queries								
Cochrane Library								
CINAHL								
Other EBSCOhost databases								
Point-of-care product								
SUMSearch2								
Trip database								
Google Scholar Search, Advanced Search								
Association websites								
Governmental websites								
Evidence-based journals								
Open access								

when storing evidence on a computer, make a folder with an appropriate title for each topic. Some type of backup system is recommended for the information stored on your personal computer, and the best way is to use an external hard drive or cloud service. If you are using a computer that is not owned by you, download the evidence and email it to yourself or upload it into Google Docs.

Anyone who has a Google email account can use the Google Docs feature, and such an account is easy to establish. Uploading documents into Google Docs has benefits in that as long as you have access to the Internet, you have access to your documents from any computer. The same is true for cloud services.

When you do not have a hard copy of a document downloaded onto your computer, use the "N" and then record the PubMed Identification Number (PMID) if the evidence was found in PubMed Central Identification Number (PMCID), and the Uniform Resource Locator (URL, or web address) when the evidence is located on a website. Also note whether the document was ordered through interlibrary loan (IL) or Loansome Doc (LD). Use bookmarks to record the URLs or web addresses of relevant evidence and organize them by topics into relevant folders to quickly retrieve relevant information.

In column 8, indicate the level of evidence for each title. Lastly, make a notation about its relevancy to answering the PPAARE question. Using a scale of 1 to 3 is an easy manner in which to accomplish this task. A score of 1 indicates that it is "not relevant," a score of 2 would indicate that it is "somewhat relevant," and a score of 3 means that it is "highly relevant." The information in columns 8 and 9 is most useful for determining what evidence will be used to make evidence-based decisions.

CONCLUDING THOUGHTS

Healthcare professionals who are new to EBP might experience information overload with all the choices to locate relevant evidence. The strategies we have discussed in this chapter will reduce the overload of information. By utilizing the procedures we discussed your searches will be more focused, leading to higher level and more relevant results in a more efficient and organized manner. Additionally, a team-based interprofessional approach will reduce the load on you as an individual, not to mention that time and experience will improve your success in conducting information searches. Depending on your discipline in health care, you will find that some resources will be more valuable than others for answering PPAARE questions. In order to make this determination, you have to jump in and learn how to effectively and efficiently use resources to locate the best evidence. Do not be afraid to ask for help from colleagues, faculty, and librarians in this process. Once you have mastered the use of EBP, you can pass it along to others and continue your pursuit of lifelong learning.

CASE STUDY #1: PPAARE QUESTION AND LITERATURE SEARCH ON SMOKING CESSATION PRODUCTS

A 25-year-old female presents to your practice. She recently discovered she was pregnant using an over-the-counter pregnancy test. The purpose of her visit is to be advised of the best way to stop smoking one pack of cigarettes per day in order to prevent harm to her developing baby.

1. Use **Table 4–12** to write one PPAARE question related to the clinical scenario.
2. Brainstorm words or phrases for a database search. Record these words and phrases in Table 4–12.
3. Search databases for controlled vocabulary, such as MeSH or subject headings (**Table 4–13**).
4. Use Boolean operators AND, OR, and NOT to connect multiple MeSH, subject headings, words, or phrases (**Table 4–14**).
5. Set limits (**Table 4–15**).
6. Read the abstracts of evidence found in each database to determine the highest level of evidence available related to the PRAARE components of the question.

Table 4–12

PPAARE	Search Words or Phrases Corresponding to PPAARE Components	Alternative Words or Phrases for Search Words	Words or Phrases to be Excluded from Search
Problem			
Patient or population			
Action			
Alternative			
Result			

Table 4–13

Database Name	Identify Controlled Vocabulary Used in Searches	Identify Words or Phrases Lacking Controlled Vocabulary
PubMed (MeSH)		
CINAHL (Subject Headings)		

Table 4–14

Database Name	MeSH, Subject Headings, Words, or Phrases Connected with AND	MeSH, Subject Headings, Words, or Phrases Connected with OR	MeSH, Subject Headings, Words, or Phrases Connected with NOT
PubMed			
Cochrane Library			
CINAHL			

Table 4–15

Database Name	Identify Limits Used in Search	Identify Type of Evidence Found (e.g., meta-analyses, systematic reviews, RCTs)	Number of Citations
PubMed MeSH			
PubMed Clinical Queries			
Cochrane Library			
CINAHL			

Table 4–16

PPAARE	Search Words or Phrases Corresponding to PPAARE Components	Alternative Words or Phrases for Search Words	Search Words or Phrases to be Excluded from Search
Problem			
Patient or population			
Action			
Alternative			
Result			

CASE STUDY #2: PPAARE QUESTION AND LITERATURE SEARCH ON SLEEP APNEA

A 65-year-old male presents to the practice suspecting he is suffering from sleep apnea. Diagnostic tests are conducted to confirm the condition of obstructive sleep apnea. He is 30 pounds overweight. He said he's heard about the Darth Vader mask available for people to wear at night in bed. He wonders if this mask is the best way to alleviate the symptoms of sleep apnea.

1. Use **Table 4–16** to write a PPAARE question.
2. Brainstorm words or phrases for a database search. Record these words and phrases in Table 4–16.
3. Access the Trip database to locate practice guidelines related to using the CPAP.
4. Determine if you have access to a point-of-care product and log into the website. Locate practice guidelines on CPAP use and weight loss for obstructive sleep apnea.

5. Go to Google and locate the Advanced Search page. Use a combination of words and phrases to locate practice guidelines on the CPAP.

CASE STUDY SUMMARIES

Case Study #1

A 25-year-old female presents to your practice. She recently discovered she was pregnant using an over-the-counter pregnancy test. The purpose of her visit is to be advised of the best way to stop smoking one pack of cigarettes per day in order to prevent harm to her developing baby.

1. Use Table 4–12 to write one PPAARE question related to the clinical scenario.
   What is the highest level of evidence available to determine whether or not a pregnant patient who smokes one pack of cigarettes a day benefits from counseling therapy compared to nicotine replacement therapy to attain a smoke-free lifestyle.
2. Brainstorm words or phrases for a database search.

PPAARE	Search Words or Phrases Corresponding to PPAARE Components	Alternative Words or Phrases for Search Words	Words or Phrases to be Excluded from Search
Problem	Cigarette smoking		Chew tobacco
Patient or population	Pregnant 25-year-old female		
Action	Counseling therapy		
Alternative	Nicotine replacement therapy	Nicotine lozenges, gum, patches	
Result	Smoke free lifestyle	Smoking cessation	

3. Search databases for controlled vocabulary, such as MeSH or subject headings.

    Access PubMed and go to the MeSH Database. Enter the word "smoking" in the search box and you will see that it is a MeSH term. Read the definition to be sure it applies. Click on the word "smoking" so that the subheadings appear. The subheading most appropriate to the PPAARE question is "prevention and control." Next, enter the phrase "smoking cessation" into the search box. Two MeSH terms appear, "smoking cessation" and "tobacco use cessation products." Read the definitions of each MeSH to determine which one is the most appropriate. In this instance, "smoking cessation" fits the bill. Click on the phrase "smoking cessation" and the subheadings will appear. The subheading most appropriate for the PPAARE scenario is "methods." Scroll down to the bottom of the screen and look at the MeSH tree. The MeSH term "smoking cessation" is a narrower search term than "tobacco use cessation."

    Repeat the search in the MeSH Database for "pregnant" and you will find the MeSH is "pregnant women." Search for "counseling therapy" and you will find the MeSH term is "counseling." The subheading most appropriate is "methods." Lastly, search the MeSH database for "nicotine replacement therapy" and you will find there is no MeSH term for this concept because it is subsumed under the "smoking cessation" term.

    Consult your institution to determine if you have access to the CINAHL database. If you have access, log in to the database. This database uses subject headings (or terms) for the controlled vocabulary. Once in the database, click on "Advanced Search" and it will take you to another screen. Near the top, click on the box that says "Suggest Subject Terms." As you type words or phrases into the search box, the database will suggest subject terms that are part of the controlled vocabulary. Type the term "smoking cessation" and you will see it is a subject term. Likewise, type "pregnant women" in the search box and it will suggest the alternative phrase "expectant women" as a subject heading.

Database Name	Identify Controlled Vocabulary Used in Searches	Identify Words or Phrases Lacking Controlled Vocabulary
PubMed (MeSH)	*Smoking/prevention and control* *Smoking cessation/methods* *Pregnant women* *Counseling/methods*	*Nicotine replacement therapy*
CINAHL (Subject Headings)	*Smoking cessation* *Expectant women*	

4. Use Boolean operators AND, OR, and NOT to connect multiple MeSH, subject headings, words, or phrases.

Database Name	MeSH, Subject Headings, Words, or Phrases Connected with **AND**	MeSH, Subject Headings, Words, or Phrases Connected with **OR**	MeSH, Subject Headings, Words, or Phrases Connected with **NOT**
PubMed	*"smoking cessation/methods" [MeSH] AND "pregnant women" [MeSH]*	*"counseling/methods" [MeSH]*	
Cochrane Library	*"smoking cessation" AND "pregnant women"*		
CINAHL	*"Smoking cessation" "Expectant mothers"*		

5. Set limits.

Database Name	Identify Limits Used in Search	Identify Type of Evidence Found (e.g., meta-analyses, systematic reviews, RCTs)	Number of Citations
PubMed MeSH	*Abstract available* *Past 10 years* *Humans* *English*	*RCTs* *Evaluation study* *Review* *Qualitative*	*25*
PubMed Clinical Queries	*Abstract available* *Past 10 years* *Humans* *English*	*Meta-analysis* *Systematic review* *RCTs*	*15*
Cochrane Library	*None*	*Systematic review*	*2*
CINAHL	*Abstract available* *Past 10 years* *English*	*RCT* *Evaluation study* *Case study* *Qualitative* *Descriptive study*	*5*

6. Read the abstracts of the evidence found in each database to determine the highest level of evidence available related to the PPAARE components of the question.
   Systematic reviews and meta-analyses

Case Study #2

A 65-year-old male presents to the practice suspecting he is suffering from sleep apnea. Diagnostic tests are conducted to confirm the condition of obstructive sleep apnea. He is 30 pounds overweight. He said he's heard about the Darth Vader mask that is available for people to wear at night in bed. He wonders if this mask is the best way to alleviate the symptoms of sleep apnea.

1. Use table 4–16 to write a PPAARE question.
   What is the highest level of evidence available to determine whether a patient with obstructive sleep apnea who is middle-aged and overweight benefits from the use of a CPAP compared to weight loss to improve the effects of sleep apnea?
2. Brainstorm words or phrases for a database search.

PPAARE	Search Words or Phrases Corresponding to PPAARE Components	Alternative Words or Phrases for Search Words	Search Words or Phrases to be Excluded from Search
Problem	*Sleep apnea*		
Patient or population	*Adult male*		*Children**
Action	*CPAP*		*Oral appliances**
Alternative	*Weight loss*		
Result	*Reduce symptoms of sleep apnea*		

*These exclusions were determined after conducting initial searches in these various databases and search engines.

Please note: The results of your search will vary because new evidence is added to these databases on a continual basis.

3. Access the Trip database to locate practice guidelines related to using the CPAP.
   The following collection of words and phrases were inserted into the search box to locate evidence in the Trip database: "obstructive sleep apnea" AND "CPAP" NOT children" NOT "oral appliances." This search yielded 10 evidence-based reviews, 39 systematic reviews, and 18 U.S. guidelines. Click on the titles of three pieces of evidence in each category and determine whether or not it is relevant to the PPAARE question.

Next, conduct the same search, but this time replace the word "CPAP" with the phrase "weight loss." This new search located 11 evidence-based summaries, 41 systematic reviews, and 20 U.S. guidelines. Click on at least three pieces of evidence in each category to determine its relevancy to the PPAARE question.

4. Determine if you have access to a point-of-care product and log into the website. Locate practice guidelines on CPAP use and weight loss for obstructive sleep apnea.
   The institution where the author works has a subscription to DynaMed. The phrase "obstructive sleep apnea" was entered into

the search box and results specific to this condition were retrieved. One of the sections for this condition was titled "Treatment." Within this section, mid-level evidence (level 2 evidence) was reported for weight loss, likely reliable evidence (level 1 evidence) for CPAP improving the quality of life, and mid-level evidence for CPAP improving sleepiness symptoms. Another section on the obstructive sleep apnea page is "Guidelines and Resources." Access to this section reports the practice guidelines in bibliographic form with a link that takes you to the website where it is located or to PubMed. Compare the relevance of these evidence-based resources to answer the PPAARE question.

5. Go to Google and locate the Advanced Search page. Use a combination of words and phrases to locate practice guidelines on the CPAP.

Conducting a search using the following strategy yielded 122 results:

- All of these words: "CPAP"
- This exact word or phrase: "obstructive sleep apnea"
- Any of these words: "practice guidelines"
- Language: English
- Site or Domain: nih.gov
- Reading level: Show only advanced results

Check the first two pages of results to determine the type of practice guidelines located using this search strategy and determine how to answer the PPAARE question.

For a second search, replace the word CPAP with the phrase "weight loss" and it will retrieve 136 results. Look at the first two pages of results and determine how to answer the PPAARE question.

REFERENCES

1. Cochrane Collaboration. *About the Cochrane Library*. 2012. Available at: http://www.thecochranelibrary .com.libpublic3.library.isu.edu/view/0/AboutThe CochraneLibrary.html. Accessed February 3, 2012.

2. Cochrane Collaboration. *About Cochrane systematic reviews and protocols*. 2012. Available at: http://www .thecochranelibrary.com.libpublic3.library.isu.edu /view/0/AboutCochraneSystematicReviews.html. Accessed February 3, 2012.

3. EBSCO Industries, Inc. *The CINAHL database*. 2012. Available at: http://www.ebscohost.com/academic /the-cinahl-database. Accessed February 6, 2012.

4. Campbell R. Ash J. An evaluation of five bedside information products using a user-centered, task-oriented approach. *J Med Libr Assoc*. 2006; 435–441.

5. Banzi R, Cinquini MC, Liberati A, Moschetti I, Pecoraro V, Tagliabue L, Moja L. Speed of updating online evidence based on point of care summaries: Prospective cohort analysis. *BMJ*. 2011; 343–350.

6. KLAS Enterprises. *Clinical decision support 2011: Understanding the impact*. Available at: www .KLASresearch.com. Accessed September 20, 2012.

7. EBSCOhost. DynaMed. n.d. Available at: http:// dynamed.ebscohost.com/. Accessed February 6, 2012.

8. MD Consult, Elsevier Health. *MD consult standard*. Available at: http://www.mdconsult.com/php/about /326565934-15/pm_SubOps.html#all. Accessed February 10, 2012.

9. Essential Evidence Plus, Wiley-Blackwell. *Browse databases and tools*. 2012. Available at: http://www .essentialevidenceplus.com/. Accessed February 10, 2012.

10. EBSCO Industries, Inc. *Evidence-based point-of-care products powered by EBSCOhost*. n.d. Available at: http://www.ebscohost.com/uploads/discovery/pdfs /topicFile-273.pdf. Accessed February 6, 2012.

11. University of Kansas School of Medicine. SumSearch2. n.d. Available at: http://sumsearch.org. Accessed February 14, 2012.

12. Trip. *FAQ-Trip Content*. Available at: http://www .tripdatabase.com/faq. Accessed February 14, 2012.

13. Agency for Healthcare Research and Quality. *FAQ*. n.d. Available at: http://www.guideline.gov/faq.aspx. Accessed February 21, 2012.

14. Agency for Healthcare Research and Quality. *Compare guidelines*. n.d. Available at: http://www .guideline.gov/compare/index.aspx. Accessed February 21, 2012.

15. Centers for Disease Control and Prevention. *What is the community guide?* 2012. Available at: http://www .thecommunityguide.org/index.html. Accessed February 21, 2012.

16. National Institutes of Health. *Institutes, centers and offices*. 2012. Available at: http://www.nih.gov/icd/. Accessed February 21, 2012.

17. National Institutes of Health. The ClinicalTrials.gov results database. 2011. Available at: http://www.clinicaltrials.gov/ct2/info/results. Accessed February 21, 2012.

18. Zarin DA, Tse T, Williams RJ, Robert M, Califf RM, Ide NC. The ClinicalTrials.gov results database – update and key issues. *N Engl J Med*. 2011; 364:852–860 March 3, 2011.

19. National Institutes of Health. *Fact sheet HSRPROJ* (Health services research project in progress). 2009. Available at: http://www.nlm.nih.gov/pubs/factsheets/hsrproj.html. Accessed February 26, 2012.

20. National Institutes of Health. *Fact sheet health services technology assessment texts (HSTAT)*. 2004. Available at: http://www.nlm.nih.gov/pubs/factsheets/hstat.html. Accessed March 1, 2012.

21. National Institutes of Health. *PubMed special queries*. 2011. Available at: http://www.nlm.nih.gov.libpublic3.library.isu.edu/bsd/special_queries.html. Accessed February 26, 2012.

22. Substance Abuse and Mental Health Services Administration. *About NREPP*. 2012. Available at: http://nrepp.samhsa.gov/AboutNREPP.aspx. Accessed February 26, 2012.

23. Canadian Task Force on Preventive Health Care. *Canadian task force on preventive health care*. 2012. Available at: www.canadiantaskforce.ca. Accessed February 26, 2012.

24. Canadian Task Force on Preventive Health Care. *Evidence review and synthesis centre*. 2012. Available at: http://www.canadiantaskforce.ca/evidence_review_eng.html. Accessed February 26, 2012.

25. National Health Service. *About NICE pathways*. 2011. Available at: http://pathways.nice.org.uk/about-us. Accessed February 26, 2012.

26. Centre for Reviews and Dissemination. *Welcome to the CRD databases*. 2011. Available at: http://www.crd.york.ac.uk/crdweb/. Accessed February 26, 2012.

27. Centre for Reviews and Dissemination. *About DARE*. 2011. Available at: http://www.crd.york.ac.uk/crdweb/AboutDare.asp. Accessed February 26, 2012.

28. Centre for Reviews and Dissemination. *NHS EED*. 2011. Available at: http://www.crd.york.ac.uk/crdweb/AboutNHSEED.asp. Accessed February 26, 2012.

29. Centre for Reviews and Dissemination. *HTA database*. 2011. Available at: http://www.crd.york.ac.uk/crdweb/AboutHTA.asp. Accessed February 26, 2012.

30. Max Planck Society. *Berlin declaration*. n.d. Available at: http://oa.mpg.de/lang/en-uk/berlin-prozess/berliner-erklarung/. Accessed March 1, 2012.

31. National Library of Medicine. *Open access subset*. 2011. Available at: http://www.ncbi.nlm.nih.gov/pmc/tools/openftlist/. Accessed March 1, 2012.

32. BioMed Central. *About us*. 2011. Available at: http://www.biomedcentral.com/about. Accessed March 1, 2012.

33. Public Library of Science. *Welcome to PLoS*. n.d. Available at: www.plos.org. Accessed March 1, 2012.

34. National Library of Medicine. *Fact sheet loansome doc*. 2011. Available at: http://www.nlm.nih.gov/pubs/factsheets/loansome_doc.html. Accessed March 1, 2012.

35. Foundation Internet Services. *LLC MedCalc 3000 complete edition*. Available at: http://online.statref.com/titleinfo/medcalc.html, 201. Accessed March 1, 2012.

Descriptive Statistics

Bernadette Howlett, PhD

INTRODUCTION

Statistics is the "the theory, procedures, and methodology by which data are summarized."[1(p. 323)] Statistics are employed with quantitative research. As a general rule, statistics fall into two major categories: descriptive and inferential. **Descriptive statistics** serve the function of numerically describing a phenomenon, such as how many patients are diagnosed with lung cancer per year or the average cholesterol levels among patients in the control group and patients in the treatment group. **Inferential statistics** make predictions about a population based on a representative sample. For example, in an inferential study the outcome of the treatment group is assumed to predict how the population will respond. An **inference** is made about the population based on the data collected from the sample. Descriptive research is usually performed in inferential studies to describe the sample and to compare the sample with known population parameters.

Before going into the substance of this chapter, we want you to check what you remember about basic statistics. In the following section, we offer a background knowledge probe that covers the basic statistics concepts you need in order to benefit from the rest of this chapter. If you have a strong understanding of basic statistics, you should score 75% or better on this test. It is set up so that each correct answer is worth one point. So if a matching question calls for three matches (on the left) then the question is worth up to three points, one point per correct match. The answers to Basic Statistics Background Knowledge Probe are included at the end of the chapter.

BASIC STATISTICS BACKGROUND KNOWLEDGE PROBE

1. SAT scores fit into the normal distribution model. The mean score on the SAT is 500

points, with a standard deviation of 100 points. If you scored 600, your score would be better than what percentage of all test takers?

a. 68%

b. 50%

c. 32%

d. 84%

2. Match the standard deviations with the total percentage of values they contain in a normal distribution.

a. 1 (one) standard deviation contains:	i. 100%
	ii. ~99.7%
b. 2 (two) standard deviations contain:	iii. ~95%
	iv. ~68%
c. 3 (three) standard deviations contains:	v. ~50%

3. Where is the mean located on a normal curve?

a. At the center of the *x*-axis, on the same value as the median

b. To the left of the median

c. To the right of the median

d. The mean does not appear on the normal curve

4. In a linear regression test, a result of $r^2 = 0.45$ means that:

a. the treatment group was 45% better than the control group.

b. there is no relationship between the predictor and response variables.

c. 55% of those in the treatment group responded negatively to the treatment.

d. 45% of the variation in the response variable can be accounted for by variation in the predictor variable.

5. In a positive correlation scatter plot, as *x* increases:

a. *y* increases.

b. *y* decreases.

c. *y* does not change.

d. It is not possible to determine the direction of the *y* variable.

6. Match the following terms and definitions.

a. Predicted value	i. An estimate of the response variable based on the linear model.
b. Residual	
c. Observed value	ii. The value of an individual response variable found in a sample.
	iii. The difference between the predicted and observed values.

7. What proportion of values is above the mean?

a. 50%

b. 10%

c. 75%

d. Cannot be determined without knowing if the distribution is normal.

8. In order to use a *t*-test, the sample data need to exhibit which of the following characteristics?

a. A left-skew distribution

b. A right-skew distribution

c. A multimodal distribution

d. A unimodal and symmetric distribution

9. In the following set of data, how many modes are present?

5, 7, 3, 9, 2, 5, 1, 6, 8, 5, 3, 8, 9, 4, 2, 8, 5, 3, 9, 6, 1

a. 0

b. 1

c. 2

d. 3

10. In a scatter plot, when the dots appear to follow a straight (linear) pattern the variables are:

a. unrelated.

b. non-normal in distribution.

c. correlated.

d. outliers.

11. Match the following statistical test with its assumptions.

    a. *t*-test
    b. z-test
    c. ANOVA (F-test)
    d. Chi-square test

    i. A test for differences between more than two groups whose group sizes are nearly equal. The data must be normally distributed and the groups must have similar variance.
    ii. A test for differences between groups, using continuous data, with a known population standard deviation.
    iii. A test which can be used for differences or correlations. Used with categorical data, non-normal distributions, or small sample sizes.
    iv. A test for differences between groups, using continuous data, with an unknown population standard deviation.

12. Match the following terms to their definitions.

    a. Median
    b. Mode
    c. Standard deviation
    d. Correlation
    e. Reliability
    f. Validity
    g. Nominal
    h. Variance
    i. Simple random sample
    j. Stratified random sample

    i. The degree to which a study's data are consistent
    ii. The square root of the sum of squared deviations divided by n − 1
    iii. Categorical data type
    iv. Selecting subjects such that each subject is chosen entirely by chance and every member of the populations had an equal chance of being selected
    v. The average distance of values in a sample from its mean
    vi. The degree to which a study's data are accurate
    vii. The value that splits the distribution in half
    viii. Selecting subjects such that each subject is randomly chosen from categories of participants that meet predetermined criteria
    ix. A type of test which checks for relationships between variables
    x. The most frequently occurring value of values

13. A survey was administered to graduates from medical, nursing, and other health professional colleges/universities. In the survey, respondents were asked to indicate what type of practice they entered for their first job. The following table (**Table 5–1**) represents the fields chosen by those who went into primary care (family practice, internal medicine, pediatrics, OB/Gyn, and urgent care). Of the graphs shown in **Figure 5–1**, which type represents a distorted presentation of the data?

Table 5–1

Family Practice	Internal Medicine	Pediatrics	OB/Gyn	Urgent Care
370	83	26	82	26

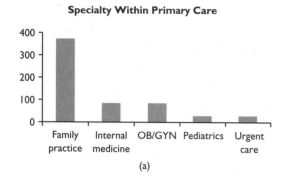

(a)

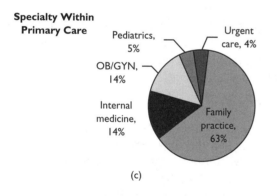

(b)

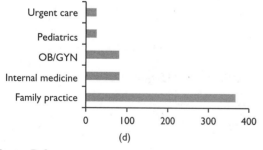

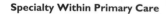

(d)

Figure 5–1

14. What type of distribution is shown in the following histogram (**Figure 5–2**)?

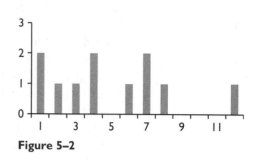

Figure 5–2

a. Normal
b. Symmetrical
c. Binary
d. Multimodal

15. In a skewed distribution like the one shown in **Figure 5–3**, which statistic is the best summary of the center of the distribution (the number at which the distribution is split in half)?

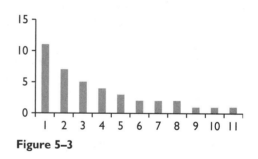

Figure 5–3

a. Mean
b. Mode
c. Median
d. Standard deviation

16. Researchers want to determine whether regular exercise or good nutrition is more effective for weight loss. Which of the following statements is the correct null hypothesis for such a study?

a. Exercise is more effective than good nutrition.
b. Good nutrition is more effective than exercise.

   c. Exercise and nutrition are equally effective.

   d. It is not possible to determine the correct null hypothesis.

17. How many modes does a normal distribution contain?

   a. 2

   b. 1

   c. 0

   d. 3

18. Match the following terms and their definitions.

a. Alpha	i. The probability that the outcome happened by random chance alone
b. Critical value	
c. Test statistic	ii. The proportion of area under the normal curve beyond the test statistic
d. *p*-value	
e. Publication bias	iii. Incorrectly failing to reject the null hypothesis
f. Type I error	iv. When an article is not published for some reason other than the quality of the article or the study
g. Type II error	
h. Alpha halves	v. Incorrectly rejecting the null hypothesis
i. Confidence interval	vi. The numerical value associated with alpha
j. Frequency	vii. A descriptive statistic showing the number of observations or the proportion of observations (if expressed as a percentage)
	viii. The proportion against which a *p*-value is compared in a two-tailed test
	ix. The range of expected values that contains the true population's parameter
	x. The resulting number from a statistical computation

19. The lower quartile in an interquartile range includes the values that fall:

   a. below the 25th percentile.

   b. above the 25th percentile.

   c. between the 25th and 50th percentiles.

   d. below the 50th percentile.

20. A correlation coefficient (r) of 1.0 means that the variables are:

   a. not correlated at all.

   b. 100% positively correlated.

   c. significantly different.

   d. normally distributed.

21. A variable, other than the predictor variable, that influences the response variable is referred to as:

   a. a lurking variable.

   b. a positive association.

   c. a correlation coefficient.

   d. an outlier.

22. What percentage of possible outcomes is contained under the normal curve?

   a. 68%

   b. 90%

   c. 95%

   d. 100%

23. In a two-tailed test, if alpha is less than .05, which of the following *p*-values would be "significant"?

   a. .04

   b. .10

   c. .02

   d. .05

24. In a study on breastfeeding, the authors report differences in the mother's

comfort with different nursing positions on a scale from 1 through 5, with the following options: (1) Very uncomfortable, (2) Somewhat uncomfortable, (3) Neutral, (4) Relatively comfortable, (5) Very comfortable. What type of data were collected in this study?

a. Continuous data
b. Categorical data
c. Ordinal data
d. Ratio data

25. The USDA in 2007 administered a survey to determine if there was a link between the amount of fish in men's diets and their occurrence of prostate cancer. The survey was broken into four categories: (1) Never/seldom, (2) Small part of diet, (3) Moderate part of diet, and (4) Large part of diet. The study found that men who Never/seldom ate fish had a 3.6–4.3% greater incidence of prostate cancer than the men in the other three categories (N = 6,272). In this example, which variable is the independent variable?

a. Number of men
b. Amount of fish in diet
c. Incidence of prostate cancer
d. The year of the study

The answers to this test are included at the end of the chapter immediately prior to the references.

DATA TYPES IN POSITIVISTIC RESEARCH

The words *quantitative* and *qualitative* have more than one meaning to researchers and statisticians. They can refer to the quantitative (positivistic) research paradigm or the qualitative (naturalistic) research paradigm, or they can refer to the type of data used in a positivistic study. In positivistic research, there can be qualitative or quantitative *data types*. This is one reason we prefer the terms *positivistic* and *naturalistic* research to represent the concepts of research paradigms. Alas, the vocabulary of research can be a little muddy sometimes.

The two general types of data in positivistic research are *qualitative data* and *quantitative data*. In positivistic research, the distinction between qualitative and quantitative data is based on the scale of the data. The term *scale* represents a set of attributes of each type of data, such as the distance between points, the presence of an absolute zero, and whether the points on the scale are ordered (fall into a sequential pattern where values next to one another are higher or lower). The types of data scales include: *categorical*, *nominal*, *ordinal*, *interval*, *continuous*, and *ratio*. Data are *categorical* when each **observation** can be assigned to one unique category. Many categories may be possible, such as city of birth (think how many cities there are!), or there may only be two, such as male/female. When there are only two categories, the data are said to be *binary* or *dichotomous*. True/false is a common pair of categories for **binary data.**

Nominal means "name," and it represents data that are unordered and can be grouped into defined categories that are represented by a number. With **nominal data**, the number used is not of any given value; it is only an identifier. Nominal data begin as categorical data. Data become nominal when a numerical code is assigned to each category (e.g., 0 for male and 1 for female). Race, ethnicity, city of birth, and employment status (full time, part time, contract, unemployed) are common examples of **categorical data** that become nominal data when coded into numerical values. Nominal variables are typically used to describe a sample and compare the sample to the population. For example, the proportion of males and females in the sample is usually compared to the proportion of males and females in the population represented.

The practice of converting categorical data to nominal data stems from the need to organize data into the smallest possible space and to perform statistical calculations. It takes less space and is easier to read columns of numbers compared to words. It takes less time to write numbers down as well. Before the advent of computers, everything had to be handwritten, so using nominal shorthand was highly desirable. Additionally, even when statistical software came along, which was fairly recently, it required all variables to be entered as numbers. This has begun to change in recent years, with some applications now being capable of performing statistical calculations with categorical data.

An *ordinal scale* involves variables that have an inherent relative difference in value, but the distance between the points is not definable. An ordinal scale is a series of nominal variables with each point on the scale being higher than the previous one. The responses to Likert survey questions are good examples of **ordinal data.** These scales are ordered (hence the term *ordinal*). You have probably encountered many such scales in which you have indicated your level of agreement, where a higher number was used to indicate a higher level of agreement (**Figure 5–4**). This specific type of ordinal scale is referred to as a **Likert scale.**

Important distinguishing characteristics of an ordinal scale are that the distance from one point to the next is indefinable and the points on the

scale cannot be measured accurately. One person's *Disagree* might be another person's *Strongly Disagree*. Or, an individual might select *Agree* when asked one time and *Strongly Agree* another time, without anything changing in between except perhaps their mood. There is simply no precise way to measure agreement. A pain scale is another common example of an ordinal scale data type (**Figure 5–5**).

One person might describe a paper cut as level 1 (mild), whereas another person might choose level 5 (between moderate and severe). Furthermore, the distance between each level cannot be said to be equal or measurable. We cannot say precisely how much pain is occurring at a given level. We cannot say exactly how much difference in pain there is between level 1 and level 2. We cannot say if the distance from level 1 to level 2 is the same as the distance from level 6 to level 7. In an ordinal scale, we perceive each level to be greater than the previous level, but we cannot give a precise measurement of them.

Interval data have four characteristics:

1. They are ordered, meaning that each successive unit is higher or lower than the next.
2. The distance between each unit is equal, meaning that each unit represents the same magnitude of the variable.
3. The zero point of the scale is arbitrary. It does not represent the absence of the variable, but simply a point we have decided means zero.

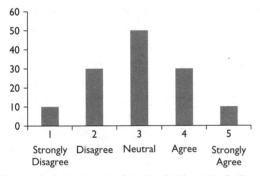

Figure 5–4 Bar Graph of Ordinal (Likert) Scale Data

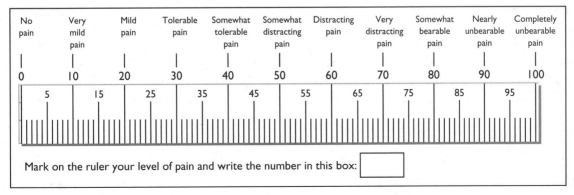

Figure 5–5 Pain Scale (a type of visual analog scale)

4. Values in an interval scale can be added and subtracted, but it does not make sense to multiply or divide them.

Fahrenheit and Celsius temperature scales are good examples of an interval scale. Applying the characteristics of interval scale data, we can say that for temperature scales:

1. The higher the number on the scale, the higher the temperature. The lower the number, the lower the temperature.
2. The distance on the scale from 10 degrees to 20 degrees is equal to the distance from −5 degrees to −15 degrees. The difference is 10 degrees.
3. At zero degrees, temperature is still present. This is because temperature is the presence of kinetic energy. The particles that make up matter at zero degrees Fahrenheit or Celsius still have kinetic energy. Thus, zero on these to scales of measurement is arbitrary. Zero does not indicate the absence of kinetic energy.
4. One can say a patient's temperature has increased by 5 degrees. But it would not make sense to say the patient had a 10% increase in temperature. Similarly, it would be strange to create a ratio of patients' temperatures prior to and subsequent to treatment. We simply add or subtract and report the difference.

Continuous data have all of the characteristics of interval data, but they also can take on any value within the intervals and there is an absolute zero. Continuous data do not have natural categories, as do nominal and ordinal data. A patient may be assigned to only one gender category (male or female), but he or she cannot be readily assigned to only one height category, for example. Continuous data are usually associated with a type of physical measurement. Age, height, weight, distance, volume, and amount of time are usually continuous data. Count data, such as the number correct or incorrect, are also considered continuous. Blood pressure and hip/waist circumference are a couple

more continuous measures you will utilize as a healthcare provider. Kelvin temperature is another example of continuous data, for example:

1. The higher the number on the scale, the higher the temperature. The lower the number, the lower the temperature.
2. The distance on the scale from 10 degrees to 20 degrees is equal to the distance from −5 degrees to −15 degrees. The difference is 10 degrees.
3. At zero degrees Kelvin, the particles of matter have no kinetic energy. Zero is not arbitrary in this measurement scale.

Ratio data, as the name implies, are ratios. Ratios can be calculated on continuous variables. For a ratio to make sense there must be a possibility of a true zero. Ratio data are generally treated the same way as continuous data.

Qualitative Data

All of the above types of data can be grouped into one of two categories: qualitative and quantitative. **Qualitative data** in *positivistic research* include categorical, nominal, and ordinal data scales. Data are considered qualitative when they represent categories rather than measures. **Quantitative data** include interval, continuous, and ratio data scales. The distinction between qualitative and quantitative matters from a statistical testing standpoint. Qualitative data are usually analyzed using *nonparametric statistical tests* (tests that do not require the population to be normally distributed).

A **normal distribution** means that there is a single center point that represents the mean, median, and mode. The values are equally distributed over both sides of the mean, and, when drawn, the **frequency** distribution looks like a bell curve (**Figure 5–6**). Qualitative data, by nature, often cannot satisfy the **assumptions** of normality.

Compare the normal distribution in Figure 5–6 to how a binary distribution such as male/female might look (**Figure 5–7**). The distribution cannot take on the characteristics of normality with only two categories. There is no clear midpoint.

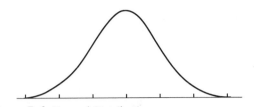

Figure 5–6 Normal Distribution

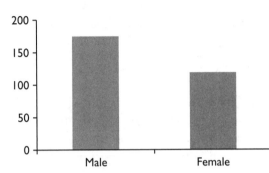

Figure 5–7 Bar Graph of Binary Data

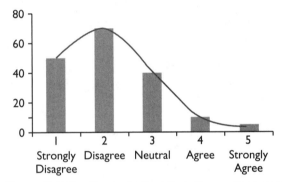

Figure 5–8 Bar Graph of Likert Scale Survey Response Data Appearing Skewed in Shape

Furthermore, the notion of a **mean** (average) or a **median** (the point at which the distribution is split in half) doesn't make sense. Is male the mean or is female? The same problem exists with ordinal data, such as a Likert scale. On the scale shown in **Figure 5–8** non-normality is easy to see because of the lack of a midpoint and the **right skew** (there is a tail going to the right). We have drawn an imaginary line to indicate the shape of this distribution.

Even if the tallest bar was on neutral (in the middle of the distribution), it would not make sense to consider neutral to be the mean. None of the categories can represent the midpoint of the scale in the same way a mean can indicate the midpoint in

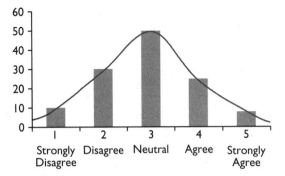

Figure 5–9 Bar Graph of Likert Scale Survey Response Data Appearing Normal in Shape

an interval or continuous scale. **Figure 5–9** shows another Likert scale bar graph with a discernible midpoint and no skew. (Note: This is a **bar graph** by definition because it displays frequencies of qualitative data. A graph that displays frequencies or proportions of quantitative data is called a **histogram.** The two charts have distinct characteristics that we will discuss later in this chapter in the section on visual representations of data.)

Despite the apparent normal shape, the center of this distribution is obscure because the distance between points is indefinable. Although neutral appears to be in the middle from left to right on the x-axis, we cannot say that the distance from agree to neutral is equal to the distance from neutral to disagree.

The shape of the distribution and the nature of the data as qualitative or quantitative determine the type of statistical tests performed on the data. Statistical tests conducted with qualitative data are referred to as **nonparametric statistics.** When reading a study, one quick assessment you can make is whether the authors mentioned using nonparametric statistics. If the scale of the data was categorical, nominal, or ordinal, then nonparametric statistics should be reported, or the data should have been transformed. **Transformation of data** is a procedure that converts data points into another form that has a normal distribution. Data can be transformed in many ways, and a discussion of **data transformation** is beyond the scope of this text. The key for you, as a reader, is to recognize when qualitative data are used in research and to look for the authors mentioning either the use of nonparametric statistics or transformation of the data.

Quantitative Data

Quantitative data come from interval, continuous, or ratio scales. Quantitative data types do not have natural categories within the data into which they can be broken. Quantitative data might come from normally distributed or non-normally distributed populations. In fact, few populations are truly normal in distribution. Age is a quantitative variable. It is precisely measurable with a discernible zero. Age may or may not be normally distributed, depending on the population from which the sample is drawn. There is a tendency for age to be skewed, with a higher number in the lower levels. However, many medical research samples are drawn on age groups, such as 18 to 25 year olds. In many instances the age distribution of a study is nearly normal because of the narrow range of the **sampling frame.**

Figure 5–10 shows a distribution of the ages of patients in a hypothetical study of influenza. In this example, the study involved clinics on college campuses. You can see that the age distribution is skewed, reflecting the age distribution of the college students themselves. The variable is quantitative,

and there is a large sample (363 observations). We can see that the distribution is non-normal, which means nonparametric statistical tests needed to be used.

Scores on a test is another example of a quantitative variable. **Figure 5–11** shows a chart (histogram) of a hypothetical distribution of IQ test scores (shown as a percent score). Three characteristics reveal the data represented here to be quantitative:

1. The data scale in this distribution is continuous.
2. The categories into which the data are divided are not naturally evident in the data. We devised these categories (ranges of 5 percentage points, e.g., 45–49%) in order to create this histogram.
3. The possibility of scoring zero on the IQ test exists, even though that did not happen in this example.

We can make a few other observations about the data based on this chart. The columns in this histogram are shown touching one another. When the columns touch, it indicates that the data are continuous. Notice that the bar charts shown in the qualitative data section had spaces in between the columns. Another observation we can make

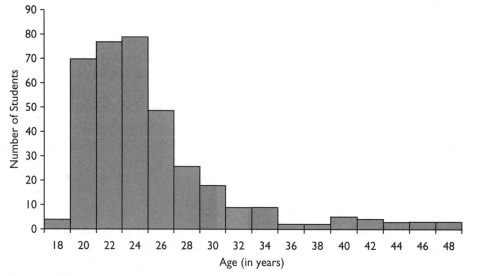

Figure 5–10 Histogram of Patient Age

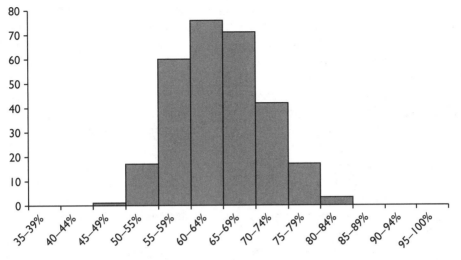

Figure 5–11 Histogram of IQ Test Percent Scores

is that this distribution looks close to normal in shape. However, even if the data were not normally distributed, IQ score would still be considered quantitative.

One final characteristic to consider in this chart of IQ scores is the number of observations in the sample. The number of observations is an important consideration related to normality. Although the data are indeed quantitative and look normally distributed, the sample size needs to be sufficient to make a reliable decision about the shape of the distribution. A sample of more than 100 observations is considered sufficient, as a general rule of thumb, to determine if the population from which the sample was drawn is normally distributed.[2] In this example, it is possible to draw this conclusion because of the size of the sample shown in the graph. You can see by the height of each column how many observations fall into each score range. Approximately 75 scores are in the range of 60–64%. If you add up the number of observations associated with each column, there would clearly be well over 100 observations in the sample. The chart of IQ scores shows a normal distribution of a continuous variable.

Because it has a normal distribution, **parametric** statistical tests can be used. Examples of parametric statistical tests include the one-sample *t*-test, the **paired-samples *t*-test,** one-way ANOVA,

repeated-measures ANOVA, Pearson correlation, simple linear regression, and multiple linear regression. Each of these tests relies upon assumptions about the distribution. If the distribution does not fit with the assumptions, then the results of the statistical test might be inaccurate and could lead to incorrect conclusions.

DESCRIPTIVE STATISTICS

Descriptive Versus Inferential Statistics

Descriptive statistics summarize a data set, but do not make predictions about a population; whereas *inferential statistics* are used to make predictions based on probability. Inferential statistics are all about the probability that the observed outcome happened by random chance. The lower the probability of random chance explaining the outcome, the more likely the outcome was caused by the intervention. For example, let's consider the outcome of a coin toss. If you flipped a coin 75 times and got heads all 75 times, the probability that this happened randomly is very small. Most of us would most likely look at the coin to see if it was heads on both sides. We would make an inference about the coin based on the low probability that one would get 75 heads in a row.

Descriptive statistics will give you the basic values of a sample, such as how many subjects were in a study, their age groups, severity of illness, geographic locations, and so on. Descriptive statistics are discrete numbers about the sample subjects. They are considered accurate and can be verified. (At least they are as accurate as the methods used to measure them.) Examples of descriptive statistics include the sample size (often referred to as **n**), the *mean* (i.e., the average), the **mode** (the most frequent value or values), the **minimum** (lowest value), the **maximum** (the highest value), the **range** (the difference between maximum and minimum), the **standard deviation** (a measure of variability), and **quartiles** (cut points located at the 25th, 50th, and 75th percentiles).

Inferential statistics enable us to make predictions about the population based on data drawn from the sample subjects. Inferential statistics have a greater potential for error compared to descriptive statistics because they are based on the probability that the observations of the sample subjects occurred randomly. Even if something is unlikely, it is still possible. The existence of that possibility means we can never be 100% certain that the observed outcome in a sample will predict an identical outcome in the population. Consider again the coin toss example where the outcome was heads for 75 coin tosses in a row. Although it is extremely unlikely this happened by chance, it is possible that it occurred naturally. If we claimed the coin toss was fixed in some way without having evidence, we would be guessing. We would have a chance of error.

Inferential statistics tell us if the difference in outcome between the treatment group and the control group was significant enough to *infer* that the treatment caused the outcome and it didn't happen simply because of random chance. Some examples of inferential statistics include *t*-test (a set of parametric tests for differences between two groups), **chi square** (a group of nonparametric statistics which test for differences between two or more groups), correlation (tests for relationships between variables), and **ANOVA** (tests for differences between multiple variables).

Understanding descriptive and inferential statistics can help you evaluate the statistical methods used in a study. Each statistical procedure has criteria that must be met in order for the test to be accurate. The criteria are based, in part, on several of the basic characteristics of the data. These characteristics include the data type, the sample size, the central tendency of the data, and the variance and shape of the data. An adequate sample size is needed in order for any statistical analysis to be valid. Sample size, central tendency, variance, and shape determine if parametric or nonparametric statistical tests should be employed.

Sample Size

Sample size is usually expressed as a count and often includes the total number of subjects in a study, the number of subjects in each group, and other counts (such as the number of males and females, the number within each age group, etc.). Other sample size numbers include the number of patients who begin a study and the number who complete it, or ratios such as the proportion of patients with a given level of disease severity. Ratios are valuable ways to describe a sample because they allow comparisons between groups in the study as well as comparisons between the sample and the population. For example, if 10% of the U.S. adult population has type 2 diabetes, then it would make sense that 10% of a random sample of U.S. adults would have type 2 diabetes. (When a value in a population is known, this value is referred to as a population **parameter.** Values calculated from a sample are referred to as *sample statistics*.) If a sample statistic differs greatly from a population parameter, the authors need to explain the reason for the difference.

Central Tendency: Mean, Median, and Mode

Central tendency is the phenomenon of typical values often occurring in the middle of a distribution. The greater the tendency toward the center, the more likely a distribution is normal in shape. Mean, median, and mode are all used to describe and evaluate the central tendency of a distribution. The *arithmetic mean* is the average of a variable and can only be reasonably calculated on interval, continuous, and ratio data. There are other types of means, such as the harmonic mean and the geometric mean. We will avoid discussing these two forms of mean for our purposes here. The majority of articles will report the arithmetic mean. Generally, it is safe to assume that when authors report a *mean* they are in fact giving the arithmetic mean.

An arithmetic mean only makes sense with normally shaped distributions. It is calculated by summing the values and dividing by the number of observations. The mean gives you a sense of the location of the center of a distribution. Sample means are often compared between groups. This comparison is frequently the outcome of interest in many studies. For instance diet/exercise studies frequently compare mean weight loss in one group to mean weight loss in another group. They test for statistically significant differences between the means of the two groups and determine if the diet/exercise regimen causes a greater amount of weight loss in the treatment group. Similarly, drugs for treating cholesterol will often compare the mean change in low-density lipoproteins (LDL), high-density lipoproteins (HDL), and triglycerides in the control group to these mean changes in the treatment group. If reductions in LDL and triglycerides are significantly greater in the treatment group, then the researchers report that the drug is effective. Because HDL is considered the *good* cholesterol, the researchers will look for a higher mean change in HDL level in the treatment group than in the control group. If this happens, the drug is reported to be effective.

What is the arithmetic mean for the set of fasting plasma glucose (**FPG**) observations shown in **Figure 5–12**? To answer this question, you add together all of the values and then divide by the number of values:

The sum of these values = 2,676
There are 22 values.
2,676/22 = 121.6

The arithmetic mean would be expressed as a whole number in this case, because the variables

FRG readings (mg/dL):							
70,	130,	90,	125,	140,	135,	90,	145,
140,	130,	120,	100,	76,	60,	90,	130,
145,	150,	140,	165,	160,	145		

Figure 5–12 Fasting Plasma Glucose Data

are reported as whole numbers. Hence, the mean is 122 mg/dL. In case you are interested, a score of less than 100 mg/dL is considered normal.[3] The impaired fasting glucose range, or pre-diabetic range, is 100–125 mg/dL. Measures of 126 mg/dL or higher are considered diabetic.

Another variable that gives information about the center of a distribution is the median. The *median* is the point at which a distribution is split in half, with 50% of observations above and 50% below. The median makes more sense than the mean with data that are skewed. For example, the average (mean) net worth of families in the United States in 2007 was $556,300, but the median net worth of families was $120,300.[4] The vast difference between the mean and the median is a result of the skew of this distribution.

Finding the median is a matter of arranging all observations from lowest to highest. If there is an odd number of observations, then the median is simply the one in the middle. If there is an even number of observations, then you average the two observations in the middle. **Table 5–2** shows our example data set again ordered from lowest to highest.

Notice that the mean (122 mg/dL) and the median (130 mg/dL) are different from one another. This could indicate a skewed distribution. We do not have quite enough information yet to make that decision, but this is reason to be suspicious. In a normally shaped distribution, the mean and median will be very close or even identical. When the mean and median differ, researchers must look closely at the shape of the distribution to ensure that they select appropriate statistical procedures. They need to run further tests on the data to determine the shape of the distribution. This is where visuals become helpful to researchers. A picture

Table 5-2   FPG Observation Counts from Lowest to Highest

60	1st	The lowest observation has been designated as the first and the highest observation has been designated as the 22nd item in the list. We did this in order to count the number of observations and to see where the middle is located.
70	2nd	
76	3rd	
90	4th	
90	5th	
90	6th	
100	7th	
120	8th	
125	9th	
130	10th	
130	**11th**	With 22 observations, the middle is at observations 11 and 12. There is an equal number of observations between the 1st and the 11th positions as there are between the 12th and 22nd positions. Each half has 11 observations.
130	**12th**	
135	13th	
140	14th	Because there is an even number of observations, the median is the average of the middle two. Item 11 is 130 and item 12 is also 130. The average of these two values is 130. Hence, the median for these data is 130 mg/dL.
140	15th	
140	16th	
145	17th	
145	18th	
145	19th	
150	20th	
160	21st	
165	22nd	

of the distribution will provide additional helpful information.

We will explore the use of visuals in a later section of this chapter using the same data set. The important point for you, as a user of healthcare research, is to look for statements in publications about the shape of the distribution. Authors should say something like, "The data set was found to satisfy the assumptions of normality" or "The data set was found to be skewed." If the data are found to be skewed, the authors need to also explain the reason for the skewed shape and discuss if the shape is to be expected.

The third measure of central tendency is the mode. The *mode* is the most frequently occurring value or values. In a normal distribution there will be only one mode, and it will occur at the same value or very close to both the mean and the median. The mode can be determined by counting the number of times each observation occurs. **Table 5-3** shows the counts for each observation for our FPG data.

Modes are sometimes determined by creating a chart, in this case a histogram. **Figure 5-13** shows what this would look like for our FPG data set. It is easy to see that the distribution is **multimodal.** The numbers 90, 130, 140, and 145 all occur three times. The FPG data shown in this histogram are clearly not normal in distribution, as evidenced by the multiple modes. Compare these data to the earlier histogram of IQ scores. The distribution of IQ scores that we discussed earlier (see **Figure 5-14**) was **unimodal** (having just one mode), and the mode appeared in the middle of the distribution. The most frequent values occurred between 60% and 64%.

Table 5–3 Frequencies of Observations in FPG Data

60	1	Notice that four observations occurred three times. This situation means that there are three modes in this distribution. The modes for this distribution are 90, 130, 140, and 145.
70	1	
76	1	
90	3	
100	1	
120	1	
135	1	
130	3	
135	1	
140	3	
145	3	
150	1	
160	1	
165	1	

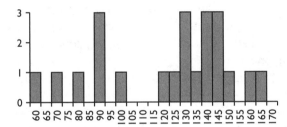
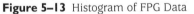

Figure 5–13 Histogram of FPG Data

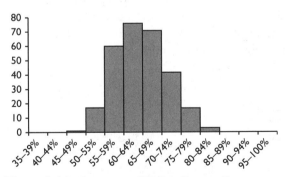

Figure 5–14 Histogram of IQ Test Percent Scores

The FPG data set does not have a clear center, but the IQ data set does have a discernible center. Sample size may be a related factor in the centrality of these two data sets. The FPG sample includes only 22 observations, whereas the IQ sample included 363 observations. The amount of variability in the data may cause a small sample to appear to be multimodal or skewed. As such, further examination of the sample data is needed. This brings us to the topic of variability as it relates to the shape of a distribution.

Variability and Shape

Variability tells us how far apart the observations in the data are from one another. This step is important in determining if a difference or a relationship between variables is significant. Standard deviation is a widely used measure of variability. Standard deviation represents how far the observations are from the center of the distribution. Standard deviation, mathematically, is the square root of the variance. **Variance** is the average distance of each observation from the mean (the sum of the squared divisions divided by n−1). It is important that the data have a normal distribution in order for this calculation to be accurate. As we have seen with our FPG data, the mean is not a good representation of the center of the distribution; hence, it might be inaccurate to calculate a standard deviation on the FPG data set.

A study on the efficacy of gastric restriction surgery to reduce metabolic diseases demonstrates the role of standard deviation.[5] The researchers used excess weight, measured in kilograms (kg), as a variable. We would expect there to be considerable variability in excess weight among adults in the study. The study included 165 adult patients (135 females and 30 males). The average amount of excess weight was 71 kg for females and 91 kg for males. The standard deviation was 19 kg for females and 35 kg for males. On average, each female's excess weight was just 19 kg different (higher or lower) than the mean for all females; while, on average, each male's excess weight was 35 kg different than the mean for all males. The variability was clearly very different between the sexes. The variability in excess weight was much greater among the male subjects.

Variability is important because it relates to precision. When the observations are close together, it is easy to see if one observation stands out. For instance, if the mean for the treatment group is more than two or three standard deviations different than the mean for the control group, many researchers consider the difference significant. Conversely, when the observations are highly variable it is difficult to see if one observation stands out. If the mean for the treatment group is one standard deviation different from the control group, it is difficult to state that the difference is significant.

For example, in the study we mentioned earlier (involving excess weight[5]) a much greater amount of excess weight change would be necessary for males than for females in order to see a significant difference. Again, the average amount of excess weight was 71 kg for females and 91 kg for males, and the standard deviation was 19 kg for females and 35 kg for males. If the females lost 38 kg in excess weight, this would be a difference of two standard deviations (SD):

$$38/19 = 2 \text{ SD}$$

However, if males lost 38 kg of excess weight the outcome would be just over 1 SD:

$$38/35 = 1.09 \text{ SD}$$

Weight loss of 38 kg for males would be much less meaningful than for females. A difference of 38 kg would not stand out as much among the males as it would among the females. Note that this applies strictly to the sample from this study. It is not a statement about weight loss in general.

Standard deviation can be affected by sample size. In the study we have been discussing, the number of females was 135, whereas there were only 30 males. The small sample size of males could explain the difference in standard deviation. With regard to this study, it is important to recognize that the sample size may be influencing the outcome among male patients and that the male and female patient data should not be combined because of the difference in standard deviation. Any conclusions about weight loss based on the combined data of males and females might be suspect because the two groups differed so much in standard deviation.

The shape of the distribution is another important characteristic. The shape of the distribution is influenced by the number of observations above and below the mean, the range between observations (in a bar chart or histogram this would be the height of the columns), how evenly the distribution curves out from the median to the tails, and the number of modes. As we mentioned earlier, a normal distribution has the characteristics of having approximately equal numbers of observations above and below the mean. A normal distribution also has the *bell curve* shape, which means that the columns are neither too short nor too tall and the columns taper down smoothly from the median to the low and high values. There is symmetry between the left and right sides of the distribution. The distance from the mean to the low value is about the same as the distance from the mean to the high value. The histogram in **Figure 5–15** shows a distribution of the heights of adult females involved in a study.

This histogram exhibits all of the characteristics of a normal distribution. It has a single mode (at 66 inches). The mode is at the same location as the mean and the median. The right and left tails are about the same distance from the median. The tails are symmetrical and have the classic bell shape. In this example, the variable of age is a continuous variable, so a histogram is the correct way to display the distribution.

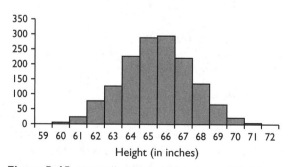

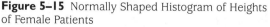

Figure 5–15 Normally Shaped Histogram of Heights of Female Patients

When reading studies, it is important to look for explanations from the authors about the variability of the data. For quantitative data sets in which the mean and median are close to one another, the distribution is unimodal, and the shape appears to be symmetric (in other words, it is a normally distributed data set), standard deviations should be reported for each variable. The authors also should report any differences in variability between groups that might influence or limit the outcome of the study.

Variability for qualitative data (categorical data, especially) cannot be measured using standard deviation. As with quantitative variables, the best way to view the shape of the distribution is to make a chart of the frequencies of observations (a bar chart for qualitative variables). Variability in qualitative data can be calculated in several ways. One of the most common calculations is the variation ratio.[6] A further discussion of variability calculations for categorical data is beyond the scope of our discussion here. It is sufficient for you, as a healthcare professional, to recognize that qualitative and quantitative variables have different tests for variability. If a study that uses a categorical variable reports a standard deviation, then you know right away to read very carefully because there may be a fundamental flaw in the data analysis. Additionally, you know to look for explanations from the researchers about the shape of the distribution.

Frequencies

Frequencies are perhaps the most common statistics reported. Frequencies are expressed as counts or as percentages (e.g., the number of patients with high blood pressure or the proportion of males and females) and are reported in narrative, tabular, or graphical forms. Tables, bar charts, and histograms are the most common ways to report frequency data. The frequencies related to demographic characteristics of a study sample should nearly always be reported in any research publication. This description should include the number of patients who completed the study, the number of males and females, the number of patients in each age group, the number of each race/ethnicity, and so on.

Frequencies should be reported for any variable that is informative and potentially influential. The frequency tables or charts are one of the fastest ways for you to determine if the study might apply to your patient. If the study included mostly females and your patient is male, you will see this quickly, and you might consider selecting a different article. Normally, the frequency distribution of the study sample is reported early in an article under a heading such as *Sample*.

Frequencies nearly always require grouping of observations in order to generate efficient displays of the data. For example, the heights of adult female patients in the chart we showed you earlier ranged from 59 inches to 72 inches. The frequency table for this chart is shown in **Table 5–4**.

However, not all frequencies can be reported using bins with an increment of one. The variable of measure may be too wide ranging for this to be possible. Look again at the FPG histogram we discussed in Figure 5–13, because it exemplifies this point.

Notice that the labels on the x-axis show bins in increments of five. If the bins were in increments of one, the chart would look very strange, with many empty bins. Furthermore, the values on the x-axis become illegible when there are many small increments. It is essential that the size of the bins makes sense for the data and that there is no overlap between them. Each observation must be counted only once, so it cannot fall into more than one bin. If a patient had an FPG of 129, then it would fit exclusively into the column above the label 125. It would be counted as falling between 125 and 129. Note that an observation of 130 would be displayed in the column above the label 130. Values of 125, 126, 127, 128, and 129 are included in the 125 bin. Values of 130, 131, 132, 133, and 134 would be in the 130 bin.

Proportions

Proportions are percentages and are used with nearly every type of data. Frequency tables, bar

Table 5–4 Frequency Table of Heights of Females

Height (in inches)	Count	
59	3	In the column on the left you see the categories for heights rounded off to whole numbers. It is highly unlikely that all of the women had heights that measured at exact 1-inch increments. So the heights had to have been rounded. There were three women who were 58.5 to 59.4 inches tall. They are all included in the first category, 59. Similarly, there are eight women in the 60 inches category. So, eight women were between 59.5 inches and 60.4 inches. Each of these height categories are referred to as *bins*. In this example, each bin is a 1-inch increment.
60	8	
61	26	
62	80	
63	129	
64	228	
65	290	
66	296	
67	222	
68	137	
69	68	
70	24	
71	6	
72	2	

graphs, and histograms are often reported with proportions. Proportions are also often referred to as *relative frequency*. Proportions can be easier to understand than frequencies when large samples are analyzed. However, one mistake often made with proportions is using them with small samples. They can distort the meaning of a finding. In a study, for example, if there were six cases of cancer in the exposed group and five cases in the nonexposed group, an author might state that there was a 20% increase in cancer among the exposed group, which sounds alarming. But to state that there was one additional case of cancer among those exposed may have an altogether different impact on you and your patients.

This example might be even more relevant to you if the study was reporting the effect of a treatment for heart disease and if the incidence of cancer was 5 out of 10,000 in the population at large. If the treatment could reduce the risk of death from stroke but increase the risk of cancer to 6 out of 10,000 would you consider it? The use of proportions and frequencies with regard to these kinds of statistics is vitally important to you and your patients.

Proportions are often used with categorical data to perform statistical tests. The chi-square test is often used to test for a difference between the observed proportion in the experimental group and the observed proportion in the control group. For example, the proportion of people who develop lung cancer among smokers would be compared to the proportion of people who develop lung cancer who are nonsmokers.

Five-Number Summary

A **five-number summary** is a shorthand way of reporting five commonly used descriptive statistics (minimum, lower quartile, median, upper quartile, and maximum). A five-number summary is a quick way to see the shape and range of a distribution. The values in a five-number summary can be calculated on ordinal, interval, continuous, or ratio data. The minimum and maximum are easy to recognize. The median can sometimes be easily visualized or can be identified with a simple calculation. The steps for finding the median are explained in the earlier section of this chapter under the heading *Central Tendency*.

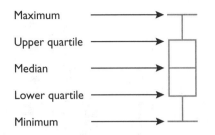

Figure 5–16 Five-Number Summary Displayed in a Box-and-Whisker Plot

The term *quartile* is used to indicate the division of the distribution into four equal parts. Twenty-five percent of the observations are located in each quartile. So, 25% of the observations are below the 25th percentile. Fifty percent of the observations are below the 50th percentile, and so on. The upper and lower quartiles in a five number summary are marked by the cut points of the 75th and 25th percentiles, respectively, on their upper limits. The box-and-whisker plot in **Figure 5–16** provides a visual for this concept.

The key concept for healthcare providers related to the five-number summary is to recognize what it tells us about the shape of a distribution. It shows us the range of the observations and if there is symmetry between the upper and lower halves. The box-and-whisker plot in Figure **5–16** is an example of a normally shaped distribution. This is evident by the location of the median visually in the center of the diagram. One could fold the diagram in half vertically at the median and the lines for the minimum and maximum would meet, as would the lines for the upper and lower quartiles.

VISUAL REPRESENTATIONS OF DATA

Visual representations are used with both descriptive and inferential statistics. Visual representations are descriptive in nature, however. Many readers look first at visuals such as charts and graphs before reading an article. Some readers look only at the visuals without reading the article itself. Because visuals can have a profound impact on the readers, it is important to know how visuals should be used and the ways in which they can misrepresent the data presented in a study.

We have mentioned several types of visual representations of data, including the bar graph, the histogram, and the box-and-whisker plot (also known as a box plot). You can evaluate, in part, the trustworthiness of a publication by the accuracy of the charts they use. There are countless ways to display data, more than we can mention in this text. However, several common types are widely used.

You can look for several characteristics in visual representations, regardless of the type of figure displayed, to help you determine if a publication is trustworthy. We will begin with the three types we have mentioned already: the bar graph, the histogram, and the box-and-whisker plot.

Bar Graphs

A *bar graph* is used to display frequencies or proportions of categorical data. As mentioned earlier, the distribution is divided into **bins**. The count or the percentage of values in each bin is represented by the columns in the chart. Two rules should be followed in bar charts. First, the bins should be of equal size, meaning that the range covered by each bin should be the same as every other. There are times when this rule has to be broken, such as when the number of cases in a bin is very small. Second, the bars in the chart should not touch one another. The gap between the bars means the data are categorical or ordinal, whereas in a histogram the columns in the chart touch one another to indicate the data are interval, continuous, or ratio.

Figure 5–17 is a bar graph showing ordinal data. It shows the counts for how many of each response was chosen on a survey. The columns in the bar chart do not touch one another, to indicate the nature of the data as ordinal. Another important aspect of this chart is the scale on the *y*-axis. The numbers range from 0 to 60, indicating the minimum and the maximum for the tallest bin. This gives the reader a realistic sense of the range and variability of the data.

A bar graph like this can be easily distorted by changing some aspect of the scale or by changing

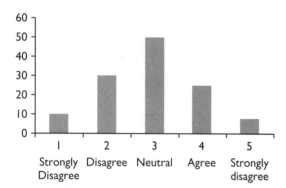

Figure 5–17 Bar Graph of Ordinal Data

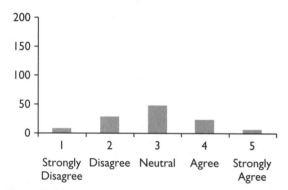

Figure 5–18 Bar Chart with Exaggerated Scale on Y-Axis

the widths of the columns or the gaps between them. Changing the scale on the y-axis can give a different impression of the data. In a version of the same chart (**Figure 5–18**), there appears to be little difference between the number of responses in each bin. There is little difference between the *agrees* and the *neutrals*, for example. However, by increasing the y-axis to 200, which is far above the maximum number of responses in a single bin, the chart has been crafted to convey a different message. It could say to you that few people responded to the survey, indicating that whatever question was asked was of little importance to the subjects.

Histograms

A histogram is similar to a bar graph; it plots the frequencies or proportions of observations in a data set. Where a bar graph reports ordinal or nominal data, a histogram reports interval, continuous, or ratio data. Histograms serve the additional function of showing the shape of the distribution.

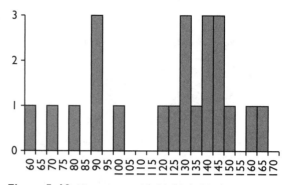

Figure 5–19 Histogram with Multiple Modes Ddisplaying Continuous Data

The distribution of this continuous data set is multimodal (**Figure 5–19**). It could also be described as skewed.

Histograms are important visuals for researchers and statisticians because they help them see if a data set has the characteristics of a normal distribution (unimodal, even distribution on either side of the median, a shape that resembles a bell with the tails on either side curving symmetrically to one another). Unfortunately, a journal article rarely has enough space to publish the histograms of the data tested in a study. As the reader, you will look for statements such as, "The main variables of the study were found to satisfy the assumptions of normality." If a histogram is provided, you can decide for yourself if the distribution looks normal and if the statistical tests chosen were appropriate.

Box-and-Whisker Plots

A **box-and-whisker plot** shows the shape of a distribution and the presence of outliers. These diagrams use little space to convey a great deal of information. They show the location of the median; the location of the upper and lower quartiles; and, in some data sets, the minimum and maximum. The *upper quartile* is the median of the upper half of the data set, whereas the *lower quartile* is the median for the lower half of the data set (**Figure 5–20**).

The T-bars that extend from the boxes are called *whiskers* (or *inner fences*). The T-bars extend to 1.5

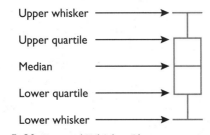

Figure 5–20 Box-and-Whisker Plot

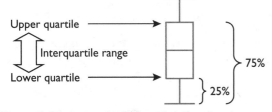

Figure 5–21 Box-and-Whisker Plot Showing the Interquartile Range

Figure 5–20 shows a normally shaped distribution. Another important value that is easily discernible from the box-and-whisker plot is the **interquartile range** (or **IQR**). Mathematically, the IQR is the upper quartile minus the lower quartile. Visually, the IQR is the distance between the two quartiles. (See **Figure 5–21**).

Box-and-whisker plots are often used to report on distributions that are non-normal in shape. They can be displayed vertically or horizontally (**Figure 5–22**). Also, it is common to display multiple box-and-whisker plots in the same diagram to show different groups at once. This strategy provides a great deal of information to the reader in a small amount of space.

Figure 5–22 is an example of a box-and-whisker plot from a hypothetical study showing the changes in levels of pain associated with three different treatments. Pain was assessed at baseline and again at 12 weeks. Group I was the control group. They received over-the-counter pain medication. Group II was an intervention group that received behavior modification therapy. Group III received both over-the-counter pain medication and behavior modification therapy.

times the height of the box or, if no observation has a value in that range, to the minimum or maximum values. If the data are distributed normally, approximately 95% of the data are expected to lie between the whiskers. The box-and-whisker plot in

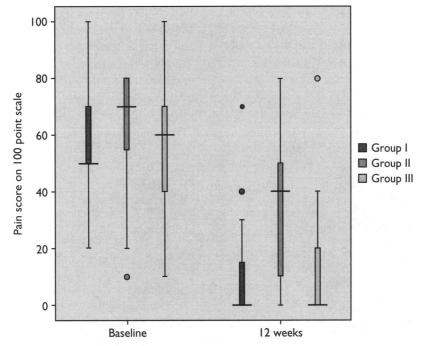

Figure 5–22 Diagram with Multiple Box-and-Whisker Plots

Note in the diagram, the small circles associated with several groups. These circles show unusual observations in the data set, that is to say, individuals with unusually high or low pain levels (outliers). **Outliers** are values that fall above or below the whiskers. You can see in this example that there were several outliers over the course of the study. There is one outlier in group II at baseline and there are three outliers after 12 weeks, two in group I and one in group III. This might indicate that the data were not normally distributed. Another potential clue about the shape of the distribution is the location of the median in each group. The median for group II at baseline is off center. For group I and group III, the median is off center at the 12-week point.

Although it is not clear if the data are normally distributed, it is clear that the pain levels improved in these patients over the 12-week trial. The question of normality in this example only becomes relevant if the authors perform inferential statistical tests, such as testing for significant differences in levels of pain reduction between groups at the end of the study.

The two types of inferential statistics are parametric and nonparametric. We discuss this further in the next major section of this chapter. Researchers need to use parametric tests if the data are normally distributed (and if the data satisfy the other assumptions of the statistical test being used). This box-and-whisker plot helps you see not only the results of the intervention, but it also gives you a sense of the shape of the distribution. You might see a statement like, "A test for distribution shape showed that the sample met the assumption of normality, allowing the use of ANOVA to test for significance in weekly FPG means." If no comment is made about testing for the shape of the distribution, then you would be left to wonder if they chose the appropriate inferential statistical test.

Pie Charts

A **pie chart** is a circular graph that includes 100% of the observations in a sample. The chart divides up a sample into proportions. Pie charts have limited use in biomedical statistics, because they are difficult to compare across groups or over time. They are most often used to display characteristics of the sample, such as the age distribution or the proportion of each race or ethnicity. A pie chart is most useful in demonstrating a disproportion between groups. **Figure 5–23** demonstrates the use of pie charts to show the disproportion of patients with healthy, borderline, high, or very high triglycerides between the control and treatment groups at the end of a study on exercise intervention. In this case, more patients were healthy and borderline in the treatment group than in the control group at the end of the study.

Some issues to consider with pie chart design is whether too many categories are used, if some

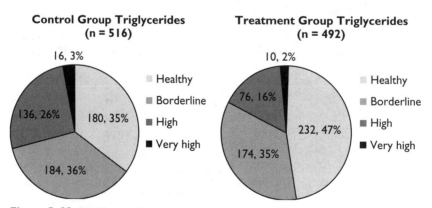

Figure 5–23 Pie Charts Showing Triglycerides in the Control Group Versus the Treatment Group at the Conclusion of a Study[*]
[*]Example not based on an individual study.

categories are not shown (because their proportions are too small to display), and whether or not the segments sum up to the whole. A pie chart should be used to represent 100% of the variable. If this cannot be done, then a different type of chart should be used. Additionally, subsets should not be summarized into categories in order to simplify a pie chart. Summarizing subsets into categories can hide useful or important information from the reader. Another problem that arises with pie charts, as well as other types of charts, is whether the categories are mutually exclusive. Each observation represented in a pie chart, as with a bar chart, must fall uniquely into only one category.

Some evidence suggests that pie charts are not as well understood as bar graphs. A 2006 study[7] found a 3.6-fold increase in correct point reading when readers were given a bar graph instead of a pie chart. Another study, however, found that both pie charts and bar graphs are poorly understood, with bar graphs having lower accuracy of interpretation scores than pie charts. The study examined decisions made by physicians with icon displays, tables, pie charts, and bar graphs and found that icon displays had the highest level of correct interpretation. (We describe icon displays in the next section.) Eighty-two percent of clinician researchers (n = 34) correctly interpreted icon displays, compared with 68% for tables, 56% for pie charts, and 43% for bar graphs.[8]

It is salient to note here that the studies performed on this topic are small and have not been reproduced. Hence, the evidence we provide in this discussion is not particularly strong. We were unable to locate a meta-analysis or a well-designed RCT of sufficient size on this topic. There is considerable agreement in the literature that visuals can be easily misinterpreted, but it is not clear which visuals are in fact the most correctly understood by readers.

Pie charts are often used in popular media despite their somewhat poor interpretability. This is important for clinicians, because these are the types of visuals that patients are likely to encounter. Several design issues with pie charts to watch for include the use of three-dimensional representation, breaking out sections of the chart, and using different sizes of circles for different groups.

The meaning of data can be dramatically influenced by design strategies. This problem is more common in popular literature than in academic literature, but it is something for you to watch for as a reader.

Icon Displays

Icon displays include Cates plots, visual analog scales, and generic icon displays. **Figure 5–24** is an example of a generic icon display. The circles in the diagram represent cases of lung cancer. The dark colored circles are those with lung cancer who currently smoke or who had a significant smoking history. The light colored circles are those with lung cancer who never smoked. In the lung cancer icon display, there are 100 icons, 90 of which are dark colored, indicating that 90% of people with lung cancer in this study were smokers or former smokers. The remaining 10 (10%) were those with lung cancer who were not smokers. The icon display typically has just two outcomes represented (e.g., positive/negative, survived/died, etc.). The dark colored dots are positive for smoking history, and the light colored dots are negative for smoking history.

The Cates plot is a special type of icon display (**Figure 5–25**) that includes more information. The distinguishing characteristics include the use of emoticons (facial expressions in the icons) and more than binary outcomes (positive/negative). In this example, three outcomes are possible: No side effects, severe side effects, and minimal side effects. A chart like this could be used to express outcomes

In the United States, cigarette smoking is associated with about 90% of lung cancers.

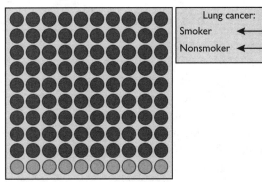

Figure 5–24 Generic Icon Display

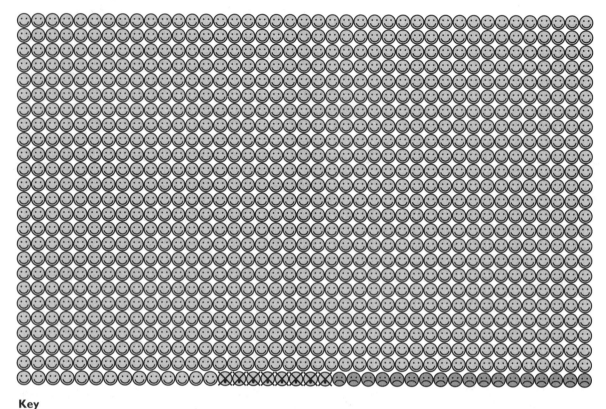

Key

☺ No Side Effects   ☹ Severe Side Effects   ⊗ Minimal Side Effects

Figure 5–25 Cates Plot

associated with a medication study. The chart has 625 total icons, with 599 no side effects (95.84%), 18 severe side effects (2.8%), and 8 with minimal side effects (1.2%). The smiley faces could indicate a good outcome from the medication. The frowny faces indicate severe side effects with the medication and, of course, the surprised faces with the x's through them indicate minimal side effects.

Scatter Plots and Dot Plots

Scatter plots and dot plots are sometimes confused with one another, but they are actually different types of graphs. A **scatter plot** usually shows relationships between variables (similar to a line graph), whereas a **dot plot** shows frequencies of observations (similar to a histogram). *Scatter plots* are used to look for relationships among continuous and ratio variables, usually in two or three dimensions (x/y or $x/y/z$). Scatter plots with more than

three dimensions can be overlaid when more than three variables need to be displayed. Such visuals, however, are rarely published, because they can be challenging for readers to interpret. The scatter plot in **Figure 5–26** shows the relationship between two variables such that the higher one variable, the higher the other (a positive association).

We can draw a line through the dots in this chart that would approximate the shape of the dots, starting in the lower left corner and going up toward the upper right corner. The closer the dots are in a scatter plot to forming a line, the stronger their association. This is the fundamental model behind the concept of correlation. We use correlation to determine if the value of x is associated with a specific value of y. When two variables have a strong correlation, they will resemble a line in a scatter plot. In this example, the two variables have a moderate correlation. We can see there is a tendency for a higher x value to produce a higher y

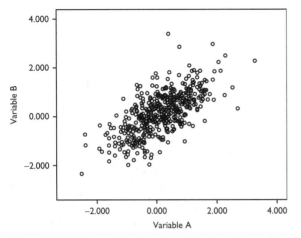

Figure 5–26 Scatter Plot Showing Relationship Between Variable A and Variable B

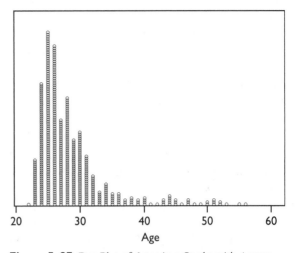

Figure 5–27 Dot Plot of Ages in a Study with 1-year Increments per Column

value, but it is not a perfect association. We could not with any accuracy predict the y value associated with a specific x value.

Dot plot are similar to histograms in that they are used to show frequencies, but they have the advantage of making it somewhat easier to see how many items are in each column. Also, dot plots can be drawn using a single increment in the x-axis rather than using bins (ranges of values); that is, a dot plot can show columns of dots rather than bins of frequencies. **Figure 5–27** demonstrates this usage.

As you can see, the age of the subjects in this study is right (positively) skewed, with the majority at approximately 25 years old. This hypothetical study was conducted in university student health centers, explaining the skew of the subjects' ages. Such a chart is useful to us as readers because it can help us determine if the data satisfy the assumption of normality. We can see immediately that this is not a normally shaped distribution, which would most likely require nonparametric statistical tests (if inferential statistics were being used). If parametric statistical tests were used, we know, because of this chart, to look for an explanation as to why parametric tests were appropriate. If there is no explanation, we are left to wonder if the statistics are valid.

Forest Plots

A **forest plot** is a special usage of box-and-whisker plots. It includes a series of box-and-whisker plots

with a trend line across the different plots. Forest plots are most often used in meta-analyses and systematic review articles to compare the results of different studies. The forest plot in **Figure 5–28** displays the results of five studies related to reduction of LDL cholesterol, the so-called "bad cholesterol." The five hypothetical studies compared a new drug (treatment) to a drug that is commonly used in the current standard of care (control). For example, Study 1 had whiskers that range from approximately 0.60 to 1.1. This means the relative risk for coronary events was between 0.60 and 1.1.

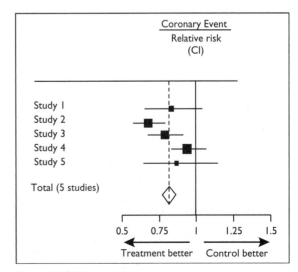

Figure 5–28 Forest Plot

The small black box in the center of the line for Study 1 indicates that the point-estimate for relative risk was approximately 0.80. This means that patients on the experimental medication in Study 1 had a 0.80 times (lesser) risk of a coronary event compared to the patients on the standard medication. Note that for all five studies, the black box associated with the relative risk point estimate is less than 1.0. In all five studies, the risk of a coronary event was lower for the experimental medication than the standard medication.

The dotted vertical line shows the mean relative risk across the five studies. The diamond at the bottom represents the **confidence interval** for the pooled relative risk number for the five studies.

Survival Curve

A **survival curve** is used to show the length of time until a bad event, such as death. Survival curves can include just one line or they can have multiple lines comparing different groups. The *x*-axis shows the length of time (it can be in hours,

weeks, months, or years, depending on the condition), and the *y*-axis shows the percentage of the group. **Figure 5–29** is an example of a survival curve published by the National Cancer Institute.[9] (This graph is public domain material and, as such, could be reproduced without permission.) In this example, there are five lines, although one of the lines is difficult to see because it matches another. Grade I and grade II forms of prostate cancer have nearly identical survival curves. The chart appears to show that close to 100% of patients diagnosed with grade I or grade II prostate cancer survive at least 120 months. Approximately 50% of patients diagnosed with grade IV prostate cancer are still alive at 120 months. We should note here that the publication goes on to show a significant difference in survival rate depending on the location of the cancer. The survival rate with grade IV cancer that is localized only to the prostate was 70% at 120 months, but with distant cancer (which means cancer found in a different area of the body) the survival rate at 120 months was approximately 5%.

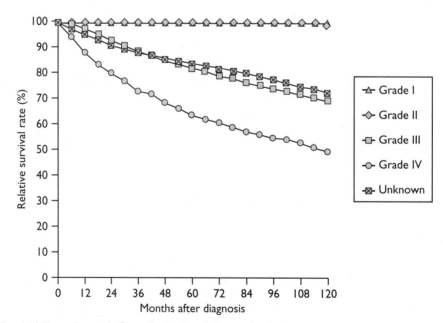

Figure 5–29 Survival Curve Example from the National Cancer Institute
Source: Adapted from Hamilton A, Gloeckler Ries LA. Cancer of the prostate. In: Ries LAG, Young JL, Keel GE, Eisner MP, Lin YD, Horner M-J (eds). *SEER survival monograph: Cancer survival among adults: U.S. SEER program, 1988-2001, patient and tumor characteristics.* National Cancer Institute, SEER Program, NIH Pub. No. 07-6215, Bethesda, MD, 2007. Available at: http://seer.cancer.gov /publications/survival/. Accessed March 20, 2012.

While by its name it is apparent that a survival curve indicates the percentage of patients surviving at progressing increments of time, the fundamental design of a survival curve is used for other purposes. This type of graph can be used to show duration of time cancer-free, and thus it could be referred to as a *cancer-free survival curve* or a *cancer recurrence curve*. Any event that is reported as a function of time can be displayed with this type of graph. For this reason, a survival curve is really just one type of **time-to-event curve.** Many types of time-to-event curves are possible, but the fundamental design concepts are essentially the same as the example given here of a survival curve.

CHAPTER SUMMARY

This chapter has reviewed the basic concepts of descriptive statistics. If you have good recollection of basic statistics, then you most likely did well on the Basic Statistics Background Knowledge Probe given at the beginning of the chapter. It has been our experience that many students have limited recall of basic statistics if they have only taken one course in the past. As with many domains of knowledge, statistics need to be used in order to really stick in your memory, and too few students have any occasion to use statistics outside of the one required class.

Even if you are not comfortable performing statistical calculations yourself, you still need to be able to read the statistics presented in healthcare research articles. Your ability to interpret the statistics presented in an article will greatly enhance your ability to determine which articles are of good quality and which ones are not. Many clinical decisions are informed by the publications you read as well as those read by your patients and your colleagues. In some cases, other people will have less education about statistics and research than you, and they will rely on you to avoid basing decisions on results from poorly designed or reported statistics. In addition to your knowledge of statistics, we recommend you have a statistician you can contact when you have questions.

Descriptive statistics summarize a data set but do not make predictions about a population. Making predictions, or more correctly, inferences, is the role of inferential statistics. Descriptive statistics will give you the basic values of a sample, such as how many subjects were in a study, their age groups, severity of illness, geographic locations, and so on.

In statistics, the two general types of data are qualitative and quantitative. The distinction between qualitative and quantitative data is based on the scale of the data. The term *scale* represents a set of attributes of each type of data, such as the distance between points, the presence of an absolute zero, and whether the points on the scale are ordered (fall into a sequential pattern where values next to one another are higher or lower). Qualitative data include categorical, nominal, and ordinal data scales. Interval, continuous, and ratio scales are considered quantitative data.

Data are categorical when each observation can be assigned to one unique category. When there are only two categories, the data are said to be binary, or dichotomous. Data become nominal when a numerical code is assigned to each category (e.g., 0 for male and 1 for female). An ordinal data scale is a series of nominal variables with each point on the scale being higher than the previous. A Likert scale is perhaps the most common example of an ordinal scale.

Interval scale data have four characteristics:

1. They are ordered, meaning each successive unit is higher or lower than the next.
2. The distance between each unit is equal, meaning that each unit represents the same magnitude of the variable.
3. The zero point of the scale is arbitrary. It does not represent the absence of the variable, but simply a point we have decided means zero.
4. Values in an interval scale can be added and subtracted, but it does not make sense to multiply or divide them.

Continuous and ratio data have all of the characteristics of interval data, but they also can take on any value within the intervals and there is an absolute zero. Continuous and ratio data do not have natural categories as do nominal and ordinal data. Ratio data, as the name implies, are ratios. Ratios can be calculated on continuous variables.

For most **parametric statistics** the observations need to satisfy the assumption of normal distribution. A normal distribution means there is a single center point which represents both the mean and the median (the tallest point is in the middle), the values are equally distributed over both sides of the mean, and, when drawn, the frequency distribution looks like a bell curve.

Qualitative data cannot satisfy the assumption of normality. As such, nonparametric statistical tests need to be used with qualitative data. Quantitative data types have the potential of satisfying the assumption of normality. If the quantitative data in a study are in fact normally distributed, then it is possible that parametric statistical tests can be employed. This depends on whether the data satisfy the other assumptions for the specific statistical test to be used.

The number of observations is an important consideration related to normality. The sample size needs to be sufficient to make a reliable decision about the shape of the distribution. A sample of more than 100 observations is considered sufficient, as a general rule of thumb, to determine if the population from which the sample was drawn is normally distributed. Sample size is usually expressed as a count and often includes the total number of subjects in a study, the number of subjects in each group, and other counts (such as the number of males and females, the number within each age group, etc.).

Descriptive statistics are calculated on qualitative as well as quantitative data. Normality and sample size are two examples of descriptive statistics. Other examples include the mean (the average), the mode (most frequent value or values), the minimum (lowest value), the maximum (highest value), the range (difference between the maximum and minimum), the *standard deviation* (a measure of

variability), and the quartiles (cut points located at the 25th, 50th, and 75th percentiles).

Another important descriptive characteristic of data is central tendency. Central tendency is the phenomenon of typical values often occurring in the middle of a distribution. The greater the tendency toward the center, the more likely a distribution is normal in shape. Mean, median, and mode are all used to describe and evaluate the central tendency of a distribution.

Variability is another important descriptive statistic. It tells us how far apart the observations in the data are from one another. Variability is important because it relates to precision. When the observations are close together, it is easy to see if one observation stands out. Standard deviation is a widely used measure of variability. Variance approximates the average distance of observations from the mean. Variance is the sum of squared deviations divided by n–1 (where n is the sample size). For a sample (as opposed to a population) variance is symbolized by a lower-case sigma with a superscript number 2 (σ^2), which stands for sigma-squared. Standard deviation and variance can be affected by sample size. Variability can only be measured on quantitative data.

Frequencies are descriptive statistics that give the count of observations in categories. Frequencies should be reported for any variable that is informative and potentially influential. Proportions are percentages and are used with nearly every type of data, but most often with frequencies. Frequency tables, bar graphs, and histograms are often reported with proportions. Proportions are also often referred to as relative frequency.

Five commonly used descriptive statistics are grouped in the five-number summary: minimum, lower quartile, median, upper quartile, and maximum. A five-number summary is a quick way to see the shape and range of a distribution. The values in a five-number summary can be calculated on ordinal, interval, continuous, or ratio data. The term quartile is used to indicate the division of the distribution into four equal parts.

Descriptive statistics are often reported through visual representations of data, such as frequency distributions, bar charts, histograms, box-and-whisker plots, pie charts, icon displays, scatter plots, dot plots, forest plots, and survival curves. You can evaluate, in part, the trustworthiness of a publication by the accuracy of the charts used. Visuals can be useful for a quick summary of the findings of a study. However, they can also misrepresent the results through design errors, whether intentional or accidental. It is essential for health professionals to read the article and not rely solely on the visuals to determine the quality of the research.

REFERENCES

1. Wiersma W, Jurs SG. *Research methods in education: An introduction*, 9th ed. Upper Saddle River, NJ: Pearson/Allyn and Bacon; 2009.
2. Motulsky H. *Intuitive biostatistics*. Oxford, UK; Oxford University Press; 1995.
3. National Library of Medicine, National Institutes of Health. Glucose test—blood. Available at: www.nlm.nih.gov/medlineplus/ency/article/003482.htm. Accessed March 12, 2012.
4. U.S. Census Bureau. Income, expenditures, poverty, and wealth. *Statistical Abstract of the United States*. 2011. Available at: www.census.gov/compendia/statab/cats/income_expenditures_poverty_wealth.html. Accessed March 15, 2012.
5. Wolf AM, Beisiegel U, Kortner B, Kuhlmann H-W. Does gastric restriction surgery reduce the risks of metabolic diseases? *Obes Surg*. 1998;8(1):9–13.
6. Weisberg HF. In Lewis-Beck M, Bryman A, Liao TF. (eds). *The Sage encyclopedia of social science research methods, volume 3*. Thousand Oaks, CA: Sage; 2004.
7. Muscatello DJ, Searles A, MacDonald R, Jorm L. Communicating population health statistics through graphs: A randomised controlled trial of graph design interventions. *BMC Med*. 2006;20(4):33.
8. Elting LS, Martin CG, Cantor SB, Rubenstein EB. Influence of data display formats on physician investigators' decisions to stop clinical trials: Prospective trial with repeated measures. *BMJ*. 1999;318(7197):1527.
9. Hamilton A, Gloeckler Ries LA. Cancer of the prostate. In: Ries LAG, Young JL, Keel GE, Eisner MP, Lin YD, Horner M-J (eds). *SEER survival monograph: Cancer survival among adults: U.S. SEER program, 1988–2001, patient and tumor characteristics*. National Cancer Institute, SEER Program, NIH Pub. No. 07-6215, Bethesda, MD, 2007. Available at: http://seer.cancer.gov/publications/survival/. Accessed March 20, 2012.

ANSWERS TO BASIC STATISTICS BACKGROUND KNOWLEDGE PROBE

1. d
2. a. ~68%; b. ~95%; c. ~99.7%
3. a
4. d
5. a
6. a. i; b. iii; c. ii
7. a
8. d
9. b
10. c
11. a. iv; b. ii; c. i; d. iii
12. a. vii; b. x; c. v; d. ix; e. i; f. vi; g. iii; h. ii; i. iv; j. viii
13. b
14. d
15. c
16. c
17. b
18. a. i; b. vi; c. x; d. ii; e. iv; f. v; g. iii; h. vii; i. ix; j. vii
19. a
20. b
21. a
22. d
23. c
24. c
25. b

Inferential Statistics

Bernadette Howlett, PhD

INTRODUCTION

Inferential statistics allow researchers to make inferences about a population based on results in a sample. Optimally, a sample of representative subjects is given an intervention and compared to a similar sample of subjects who receive the usual care, a placebo, or no intervention. Inferential statistics can be used to measure the accuracy of diagnostic procedures, the efficacy of treatment interventions, the impact of risk factors on a given outcome, or the efficacy of a preventive strategy to reduce the burden of disease. Inferential as well as descriptive statistics are used throughout healthcare research. The primary difference between inferential and descriptive statistics is generalizability. With inferential statistics, researchers attempt to generalize a phenomenon measured in a sample to the population represented by the sample. From the inferential perspective, if the sample is indeed representative, then the effects found in the sample subjects will be essentially the same for the population.

THE CLINICAL RESEARCH PROCESS

Before getting into the details of inferential statistics, we need to provide an overview of the clinical research process. This process is much the same regardless of the types of statistical tests performed, although not all studies are interventional. Each of the concepts addressed in this chapter represents part of the clinical research process (**Figure 6-1**). The three major phases of clinical research include: (1) identifying the need, (2) designing the study, and (3) performing the study. After the study has been completed, researchers monitor the phenomenon to determine if the outcomes of the study are the same in the long term.

Phase 1 begins with observing a phenomenon (e.g., in a study related to thyroid disease, patients exhibited symptoms of thyroid dysfunction despite having normal laboratory values)[1] and determining if research is needed based on a gap in knowledge. The gap is identified by performing a thorough review of the literature as well as reviewing information on research that is currently underway or that was completed but never published. In the thyroid dysfunction example, the researchers found a controversy in the literature regarding the treatment of patients with signs and symptoms of hypothyroidism whose TSH (thyroid-stimulating hormone) lab test was within the normal range.[1]

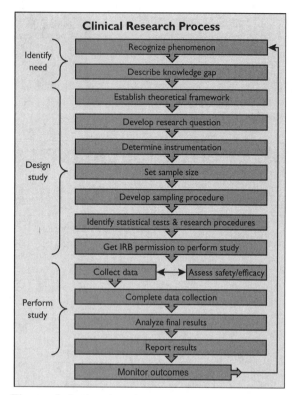

Figure 6–1 The Clinical Research Process

Once the gap has been identified and carefully described, researchers decide the research question and frame the question within a *theoretical framework*. The theoretical framework includes the major areas of investigation represented by the research problem. In the thyroid study, the framework included epidemiology of hypothyroidism, empirical treatment, and laboratory science.

Empirical treatment is when clinicians provide treatment based on the patient's history and physical exam, rather than on lab tests, imaging, or other studies. If a patient responds positively to the treatment, then the diagnosis is confirmed. In phase 2 of the clinical research process, after establishing the theoretical framework the researchers develop their research question. For the thyroid study, the question was: "What is the strength of the relationship between TSH and T4?" T4 is a thyroid hormone that circulates in the blood. The recommended procedure for diagnosis of hypothyroidism is to gather the patient's history, perform a physical exam, and measure the patient's TSH and

T4 levels.[2] The higher the TSH level, the lower the levels of thyroxine (T4) as well as tri-iodothyronine (T3). T3 is the biologically active form of thyroid hormone, and T4 is considered a prohormone.[3] One hundred percent of circulating T4 is produced by the thyroid gland, whereas only 20% of circulating T3 comes from the thyroid gland. The remaining 80% of T3 is produced by conversion of T4 into T3 in the peripheral tissues. Because the thyroid produces 100% of circulating T4, it is often tested alongside TSH.

TSH comes from the pituitary gland. It is the hormone that tells the thyroid gland to produce T4 and T3. TSH has an inverse relationship with T4 and T3. In hypothyroidism, the thyroid gland is not producing enough T4 and T3, so the body increases TSH levels to stimulate the thyroid gland to increase output. Hence, levels of TSH can indirectly indicate levels of T4 and T3. As such, the researchers recognized that TSH and T4 should be statistically correlated to one another.

The next step in phase 2 is determining the instruments to be used for data collection (*instrumentation*). For the thyroid study, the researchers determined that patient charts would be utilized in a practice where the routine procedure for thyroid testing included both a TSH test and a T4 test.

Once the instrumentation has been determined, a sampling frame is selected based on the research question, which leads to determining the necessary sample size. In the hypothyroid study, the sampling frame was a single internal medicine practice. This frame was based on access to patient charts and the resources available to the researchers to conduct the study. The study was considered a pilot project. In this example, a sample size was not calculated. However, if the study had been interventional or if it had been more than a pilot study, the researchers would need to have completed a sample size calculation.

The number of subjects needed in a study (sample size) is based on three major considerations: (1) the type of data to be collected, (2) the degree of effect required (effect size), and (3) the probability level to be used (alpha). The hypothyroidism study had both continuous (TSH, T3, T4) and categorical (sex, diagnoses, medications) variables. The effect size was based on the degree of association between TSH and T4 levels. The researchers deemed a correlation of .70 or higher as the minimum level of association. They selected 0.05 for the level of alpha.

Once the sample size is determined researchers proceed to selecting sampling procedures as well as the types of statistical tests to be used. Sampling procedures are driven by cost, time, and access to subjects. In the hypothyroid study, the researchers developed a process for randomly selecting up to 50 charts that met the inclusion criteria for the study. Certain charts were excluded based on age of the patient and medications being taken by the patient.

The types of statistical tests chosen for a study are based on several characteristics (i.e., assumptions), such as the sample size, the type of data, the variability of the data, and the shape of the data distribution. For the hypothyroidism study, the researchers chose to perform a correlation test as well as to calculate sensitivity and specificity. Once all of these decisions have been made, the researchers then need to gain approval from the appropriate Institutional Review Board (IRB) to perform research involving human subjects. After IRB approval is in place, the researcher moves on to phase 3—data collection, analysis, and reporting.

Clinical trials should be registered (such as with clinicaltrials.gov). Once a study is underway, the researchers may or may not continue to collect all of the data as planned. During the data collection phase, researchers monitor subjects to look for adverse events that might trigger an early stop of the study. Trials that end early are referred to as **truncated trials**. In designing a study, researchers establish specific adverse events that will cause them to stop the study before data collection is complete, such as an increase in mortality. Early stops can also happen due to positive treatment effects. If a treatment is having a significant positive effect early in a study, researchers might end the trial in order to allow the treatment to become available more quickly to the market and to make the treatment available to subjects in the control group. In the hypothyroid study, there was no need for an early stop because the research was retrospective and noninterventional.

Once data collection is complete, researchers have several important comparisons to make. First, they must determine if the treatment and control groups were similar to one another at the end of the study (to account for dropouts in each group). They should also compare the groups with the demographics of the population they are intended to represent. Sometimes the demographics at the end of data collection change sufficiently such that the study sample is no longer representative. Researchers should also examine the data for the shape of the distribution for each variable as well as the amount of variability to verify that the data satisfy the assumptions for the statistical tests to be performed. Researchers sometimes need to change the statistical tests at this point in the research due to reductions in sample size or unexpected outcomes in the data, such as increased variability or skewed shape of a distribution.

After this verification step, the researchers are able to run the statistical tests. When statistical tests are run, each test produces a test statistic with an associated p-value (probability that the test statistic represents normal variation) and confidence interval (the range in which the true population parameter can be found, with a given percentage likelihood). The concepts of sample size, sampling frame, sampling procedures, effect size, alpha, p-value, and confidence interval are discussed in the first half of this chapter. Explanations about different types of inferential statistics are presented in the second half of the chapter.

After publication, researchers should monitor the literature for any new information or contradictory results from other studies. Additional research should be performed if other studies have different outcomes or if new information emerges. This is not to say that the same researchers are expected to perform all future studies, but rather that researchers in the field of interest should continually monitor for new and different information. Some fields of interest have organizations that perform this function and publish research agendas to guide investigators and focus research funding.

One way for you to evaluate a research study is to look for evidence of the procedures that we have just outlined. In an optimal publication, every procedure would be sufficiently described such that you could replicate the study. Unfortunately, space limitations in journals usually result in exclusion of some of the needed information, and we have to do the best we can to evaluate the study based on the information provided. Sometimes there is not enough information, and we deem an article inadequate as a source to inform our healthcare decisions. Thankfully, a significant amount of information is available to us from many sources and we can seek more information when necessary.

PARAMETRIC AND NONPARAMETRIC STATISTICAL TESTS

Parametric and nonparametric statistical tests represent two forms of inferential statistics. Researchers must choose the statistical tests they use based on several important characteristics of the data, including the type of data, the shape of the distribution, and the variability of the observations in each sample. Parametric and nonparametric tests rely on different assumptions about these characteristics. If an inappropriate type of statistical test is used, the results can be incorrect or underpowered.

Parametric statistical tests are those that assume that the data meet all of the following criteria:

- Ratio or interval scale.
- Normal in shape (or nearly normal).
- Sufficient sample size.
- If there is more than one group, each group has the same (or nearly the same) amount of variability, the same shape, and the same (or nearly the same) sample size.

Nonparametric statistical tests assume that the data meet all of the following criteria:

- Nominal or ordinal scale.
- Non-normal shape (skewed).
- Small sample size.
- If there is more than one group, the groups have differing variability, shapes, or sample sizes.

Assumptions

This brings us to the concept of assumptions. Each statistical test has a set of parameters that govern its application called *assumptions*. There are many places in life where assumptions matter. For example, if you pick up a hammer, the assumption of this tool is that a nail is to be driven or removed. The tool is not designed to be used for other functions, such as tightening or loosening a screw. In inferential statistics, every test has specific uses. The independent-samples *t*-test, for instance, is used for testing the difference in means between two independent measures. It is used with ratio or interval, normally distributed, independent variables, whose groups have similar variation. Note that there are six assumptions for the independent samples *t*-test:

1. Each variable has a sufficient sample size to enable accurate measurement of a mean.
2. The data are ratio or interval scale (which is necessary to calculate a mean).
3. There are only two measurements to be compared.
4. The two measures are independent of one another.
5. The variation within the data set for each variable is similar between the two measures.
6. Each data set has a normal-shaped distribution.

If all of the above assumptions are not met, then the *t*-test might not be accurate.

Another commonly used type of *t*-test is the paired-samples *t*-test. It has the same assumptions as the independent-samples *t*-test, with one exception: The paired-samples *t*-test assumes that the two measurements are related. For example, if a study compared patients' systolic blood pressure prior to treatment and after treatment, then a paired-samples *t*-test could be used (if the data satisfied the other five assumptions). The two measures of systolic blood pressure in this case would be related. They would be two measures of the same person at two different times. This approach is also often referred to as a *pre/post-test* or as a *within-subject test*. The pre/post-test and within-subject designs are very common types of statistical tests in healthcare research.

Many types of statistical tests are available. A discussion of the assumptions of all tests is well beyond the scope of this chapter. What is important for you at this time is to recognize that authors should verify that the data they use meet the assumptions of the statistical tests they use. They should include a statement in their articles explaining that the data were checked for satisfaction of the tests' assumptions. Here is a good example from an article where the authors explain which statistical tests were used:

> Categorical data was analyzed using chi-square test. When data met the assumption of normality, independent-samples t-tests were used to examine group differences on neuropsychological measures. When basic assumption for parametric tests, i.e. normal distribution, was violated, Mann-Whitney U nonparametric tests were used.[4]

Look for statements like these in the articles you read to determine if the authors have been thorough and careful. An explanation of the statistical procedures used in a study generally belongs in the methods section of an article. This type of explanation allows you to critique the research and even replicate the study if you wanted to do so.

There is a great deal to know about biostatistics. We encourage you to maintain a working relationship with a statistician. When you are not sure of the assumptions of a given statistical test, look it up in a reliable resource first, but if you find the explanation difficult to interpret, give your statistics expert a call.

SAMPLING

Possibly the most important characteristic of a healthcare study is the selection and inclusion of subjects, or *sampling*. The subjects sampled for a study must experience the phenomenon of interest (e.g., have high blood pressure) and must include appropriate variability (representing the population). The study sample must be drawn from a frame of subjects that can reasonably represent the true population. It would be perfect if we could simply study the entire population, in which case sampling would be unnecessary. A sample is used

because researchers cannot access the entire population. Consider type 2 diabetes. Approximately 25.8 million people in the United States have this diagnosis.[5] The number of people with type 2 diabetes and their geographic distribution across the country makes a population study simply impossible. In most instances researchers are limited by time, money, and space. They must study a sample of the population as a result.

The sample needs to include subjects from each subgroup based on gender, race/ethnicity, geographic location, age, income, education, severity of illness, and insurance status, because these variables can influence the outcome of the study. Men and women sometimes respond differently to a given treatment and sometimes have different health problems. In well-designed studies, researchers will check that the proportions of each subgroup in the sample are similar to the proportions in the population. Additionally, the researchers will check that each group in the study is similar to one another in terms of demographics and baseline characteristics. The control group and the treatment group, for example, should have the same proportion of males and females, the same distribution of age groups, and have the same severity of disease.

The researchers also need to analyze changes to the groups as a result of subjects dropping out of a study. If a disproportionate number of males, for example, dropped out of a study in the treatment group compared to the control group, it might indicate that males in the treatment group were experiencing a side effect. Researchers should make comparisons of the group characteristics before the study begins and at the end of the study. In longer duration studies, these group comparisons should also be made at certain intermediate points during the study, such as at the end of each treatment phase.

Researchers need to know demographic details about the population of interest to determine the necessary characteristics of the sample subjects. The proportion of men and women in a sample should be close to the known proportion in the population. The distribution of age in the sample should be similar to the age distribution in the population for the question of interest. Consider a study on the *incidence* (new diagnoses) of lung cancer. The sample should include proportions of males and females, age levels, economic status, education level, and insurance status similar to the proportions of those in the population.

For example, the rate of smoking is much lower in the western United States (15.9%) than in the Midwest (21.7%).[6] According to the CDC, young adults, those aged 18 to 24 years, are far more likely to smoke than people 65 and older (10.2%). There is a difference between males (21.5%) and females (17.4%) as well. Level of education is strongly associated with smoking: the more years of education, the lower the percentage of smokers. For example, 28.4% of people with less than a high school diploma smoke, but only 9.1% of people with a bachelor's degree or higher smoke. Among those in the middle (with a high school education or some college), more than 20% smoke.

We could have a lengthy discussion here about the apparent association between completing college and nonsmoking, but that would lead us astray from the main point. The point is that a study on smoking behavior would have to include a sample with similar proportions as those reported by the Centers for Disease Control and Prevention (CDC). Imagine researchers intended to study the effect of a public awareness smoking cessation campaign on adults. If the population of the study was mainly working professionals with college degrees, then the sample would most likely not represent the population.

Researchers generally must rely on sources such as the CDC, the WHO (World Health Organization), and the U.S. Census Bureau to determine the basic characteristics of a population. In their publications, researchers should explain the characteristics of the population and the source upon which their reported characteristics were based. This information belongs in a section of the article called "Sample." Not every journal will use this heading, so you might have to read closely to locate the description of the study sample. A well-written article will compare the study sample to the population and will provide a table outlining the demographics of the study subjects. In a well-written article, the researchers will describe the frame from which the sample was drawn and the method of assigning subjects to groups.

Sample Size

The number of subjects in a sample is referred to as the *sample size*. The overall size of a study sample is of critical importance. The sample must be large enough to include all of the variability in the population and to be sufficiently powered to detect the effects of different variables. Furthermore, the sample should also not be too large. It is possible for a sample to be so large that the study increases its risk of error. As the sample size gets larger, there can be an increased chance that the researchers will see a statistically significant result that is of no clinical importance.

The authors should report the results of a *sample size calculation* that was used in advance of data collection to determine the necessary minimum number of observations required for their study. A sample size calculation will typically be reported in the *Sample* section of the article. If there is not a heading called "Sample," then you can scan for the term *sample size*. If you have an electronic version of the article, then you can simply use the search feature to locate this term. Any study that uses a sampling strategy and that calculates inferential statistics should include a sample size calculation.

The sample size needs to be sufficient not only for the overall study, but for the subgroups within it. There needs to be a large enough number of males and females, of each race/ethnicity, and with each level of education, income, and insurance status so that each category can be analyzed and compared. Well, in the perfect world each study would have a sample of this kind. This is the ideal. Very large randomized control trials can sometimes achieve this objective. All too often, however, studies are not able to achieve a large enough sample size for every subset. This is especially true when the subsets are combined, such as comparing women to men at each income level, education level, and insurance status.

Imagine a study on smoking broken down according to gender, income, education, and health insurance status. Let's say that the sample size calculation for a study indicated that 100 subjects were needed and the researchers planned to make a subgroup comparison. They wanted to know if there was an interaction between gender and income. Is there a difference between men and women in smoking behavior based on income and/or education? For the sake of discussion, we will say that the lowest income group is individuals who earn less than $10,000 per year.

This means that each subgroup (gender + income + education) should have 100 people. The researchers would also need to control for health insurance status, because it is commonly known to affect outcomes. So, there would need to be at least 100 women with less than a high school education who *do not* have health insurance. There would need to be at least 100 men with less than a high school education who *do not* have health insurance. There would need to be at least 100 men and 100 women with less than a high school education who *do* have health insurance. There would need to be at least 100 women and 100 men with a high school diploma who do *not* have health insurance. And so on, and so on.

The following diagram series (**Figures 6–2, 6–3, and 6–4**) demonstrates how a study starting with a sample of 1,600 subjects might ultimately be divided into subgroups where one or more of the subgroups

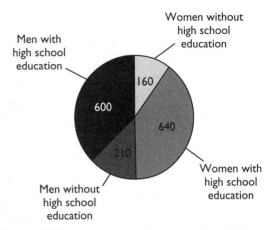

Figure 6–3 Sample Divided by Sex and by High School Education

drops below the desired sample size. Again, we set the desired sample size at 100.

In Figure 6–2, the 1,600 subjects have been divided into male and female members. In this invented example, there are 800 men and 800 women.

In Figure 6–3, each group of 800 women and 800 men has been subdivided into those with and without a high school education. The sample size remains above 100 for each group.

In Figure 6–4, the sample has been further divided by insurance status. At this level of subgroup analysis, the sample size has dropped below the 100 minimum established at the beginning of the study. There are only 80 men without a high school education who are without health insurance, and there are only 48 women without a high school education who are without health insurance.

The overall study sample size needs to be large enough to enable subset analysis down to the lowest level of comparison or the authors need to report that such analyses could not be performed. This is often the case, as you can imagine, because the sample size requirement can balloon quickly with each subset. The solution to the problem for many studies is to perform different subset analyses in each study. Later, when enough studies have been conducted, a meta-analysis can be undertaken to examine the small subset results.

n = 1,600

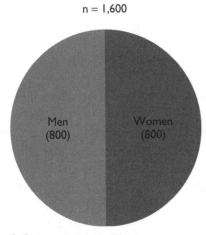

Figure 6–2 Sample Divided by Sex

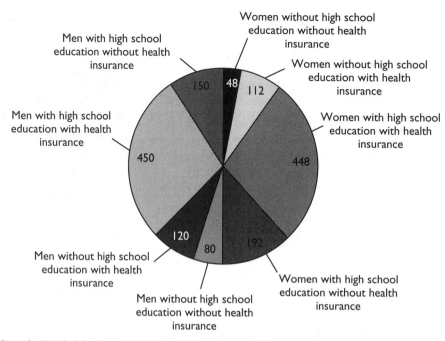

Figure 6–4 Sample Divided by Sex, High School Education, and Insurance Status

Effect Size

Another important and related consideration to the sample size in a study is the effect size of the intervention. The term **effect size** has several meanings in statistics. In this case, we are referring to the expected amount of clinically important effect, which is used in a statistical power calculation. **Power calculations** are used for determining sample sizes (among other things). A power calculation should be conducted before data are collected in order to guide the sample size determination. A power calculation utilizes effect size, alpha, and a third value referred to as *power*. A minimum of 0.80 (80%) power is usually recommended. According to GraphPad, "Power is the fraction of experiments that you expect to yield a 'statistically significant' *p*-value. If your experimental design has high power, then there is a high chance that your experiment will find a 'statistically significant' result if the treatment really works."[7]

In power analysis, the concept of effect size is similar to the concept of clinical significance. It is possible to have an intervention with a small clinical effect to nonetheless have a statistically significant result. Just because a statistically significant difference or relationship occurs in the data, it does not mean that the outcome has clinical significance. For instance, returning to the example of the TSH/T4 correlation study[1] (n = 50), the regression analysis showed a statistically significant association between TSH and T4, resulting in a *p*-value of 0.013. This *p*-value by itself would be interpreted to mean that there is a statistically significant relationship between TSH and T4 levels, meaning that if TSH is normal than we can expect T4 to be normal. Statistically this should be true. However, the clinical picture with the patients did not reflect this statistical result. The patients exhibited the signs and symptoms of hypothyroidism even though their lab test results were in the normal range.

Another example of effect size comes from the REFOCUS clinical trial, which examined community-based mental health teams as a pro-recovery intervention. In the study, researchers set an effect size of 0.40, or 40%, as measured by the Questionnaire about the Process of Recovery (QPR).[8] By *personal recovery*, the authors are referring to a process of regaining active control over one's life even with limitations caused by illness. The effect size of 40% means that the intervention needed to achieve a change in QPR score of 40% or greater in order for the treatment to be deemed sufficiently effective. The authors determined, based on the effect size (0.40) and level of alpha (0.05), that the sample size needed to be at least 336 subjects. This information is helpful to us, as readers of the study, because we can easily see if the sample size was large enough or if the sample size was significantly greater than necessary, which has its own problems. The researchers designed the sample, therefore, to include 435 subjects: 225 receiving the intervention and 210 in the control group.

Determining a clinically meaningful effect size in advance of a study can be a matter of an educated guess or a matter of extensive research. With certain diagnostic instruments, research has been performed to determine the effect sizes that researchers should use for specific conditions. For example, an instrument used in cancer research in Europe is the European Organisation for the Research and Treatment of Cancer Quality of Life Questionnaire Core 30 (EORTC QLQ-C30).[9] This instrument is one of the most widely used instruments for assessing quality of life for patients with cancer. Cocks et al.[9] reported that results from this survey instrument had been analyzed inconsistently across studies, making results difficult to apply to patient care. The authors explained:

> [A]lthough studies using the QLQ-C30 were reported to a high standard, clinical interpretation of QOL differences was lacking (62% not addressing clinical significance). There was an over-reliance on statistical significance to determine impact on QOL. Where clinical significance was addressed, it was most common to assume that 10 points was clinically significant (however, fewer than 25% of the RCTs used this method). Reporting of sample size calculations was also lacking. Twelve RCTs specified QOL as a primary end point; however, only seven detailed the sample size calculation. There was no consistent basis for these calculations.[9]

Because of the lack of consistency and difficulty in interpreting data resulting from research using the QLQ-C30, the researchers performed a systematic review and meta-analysis that combined the results of 152 studies.[9] They determined, among other things, that an effect of a 9-point change on the cognitive functioning scale and a 19-point change on the role functioning scale was needed in order to achieve a clinically significant finding. As such, researchers can now apply these effect size values to more accurately calculate the necessary sample size. The researchers published guidelines for the sample size calculations for clinical trials utilizing the QLQ-C30 instrument.

Two clinically useful conclusions can be drawn from this study. First, when assessing quality of life for cancer patients, an improvement of 10 points on the overall QLQ-C30 scale is associated with clinically meaningful change. Also, an 11-point improvement on the social subscale, or a 13-point improvement on the pain and fatigue subscales, indicates a clinically meaningful change. Second, when reading publications of clinical trials, look for results of a sample size calculation and the associated effect size utilized. The effect size will offer additional guidance on the meaningful treatment effect you should look for in patients.

Well-designed and well-written studies will include a statement about sample size and effect size. For example, in a study comparing two medications for treatment of eczema, the researchers stated, "Calculations showed that 56 participants were needed for a study with 80% power and 5% significance level . . . We aimed to recruit 66 patients to allow for a 15% dropout rate."[10]

Unfortunately, the researchers were able to recruit only 38 study participants. However, the reporting of the sample size calculation is a strength of this publication because it enables us to quickly determine if the sample size of 38 patients was sufficient for the question under consideration. Another strength of this publication was the baseline comparison reported on the study groups:

> Patients randomized to prednisolone (n = 21) and ciclosporin (n = 17) did not differ significantly in any of these characteristics at baseline. Mean age was about 30 years, slightly more than half of all patients were male (55%), and the majority of patients (74%) had comorbid allergic rhinitis and/or asthma indicating extrinsic eczema. Mean SCORAD at baseline was

57Æ6 and 54Æ7 units in the prednisolone and ci-closporin group, respectively. Mean baseline DLQI [Dermatology Life Quality Index] was 19 units in both groups reflecting highly impaired health-related quality of life due to eczema.[10]

Sampling Frame

The *sampling frame* is "a list or other record of all the elements in the population from which the sampling units are drawn. It defines your accessible population, which might be different from your target population, depending on how good your sampling frame is."[11] For example, it is common to use a telephone directory to draw names for a sample. Researchers might decide to select every 100th name in the white pages to consider for study inclusion. In this case, the telephone book is the sampling frame. The sample section of an article should describe the sampling frame utilized. The sampling frame should enable researchers to draw a representative sample of the population under study.

Sampling Fraction

The **sampling fraction** is simply "the size of the sample as a percentage of the population from which it was drawn."[11] The sampling fraction should be sufficient to draw subjects representing all of the relevant variation with regard to influencing and confounding factors.

Simple Random Sample

Many methods for selecting subjects are available once the sampling frame has been established. The method considered the most valid is the **simple random sample**. It is a form of probability sampling (which means that each individual has a known probability of being selected) that allows every member of the population to have an equal chance of being selected for the study.[11] It is designed to avoid duplicate sampling, which means that the same subject cannot be selected more than once, and to ensure that the sample includes all of the variability in the population.

Simple random sampling is often difficult to carry out because it is not possible to gain access to a complete list of all members of a population. Imagine researchers wanted to study drug interactions between aspirin and sertraline (which is a serotonin reuptake inhibitor used to treat depression and several other mental health conditions). In order to draw a simple random sample, the researchers would need a list of all people taking both medications. Such a list surely does not exist. For this reason, researchers would begin with a sampling frame that includes subjects who they deem representative of the population.

The typical procedure for drawing a simple random sample is to use a random number generator and to assign a random number to each individual in the sampling frame and then select every *n*th individual. The *n*th individual means a predetermined number, such as every 25th, every 50th, or every 1,000th individual, and so on. The number used depends on the size of the sampling frame and the distribution of population characteristics, such as the prevalence of a given health condition. Many statistics textbooks have random number tables that can be used. Several statistical software packages also have the ability to generate random numbers. When reading the sample section of a research article, look for an explanation of the sampling frame used and the method for selecting individuals from within it.

For example, consider drawing a random sample from a package of candies that contains 100 pieces divided into six colors (red, green, blue, yellow, orange, and brown). Now imagine that the researchers know from many other studies and from the candy manufacturer that the distribution of colors is as shown in **Table 6–1**.

Based on this information, there would be a 10/100 chance of drawing a red candy; that is, a 1 in 10 chance. The same is true for drawing a blue candy. There is a 5/100, or a 1 in 20, chance of

Table 6–1	Distribution of Candy Colors				
Red	10%	Green	5%	Blue	10%
Yellow	20%	Orange	25%	Brown	30%

drawing a green candy. However, for a brown candy the chance is 30/100, or 3 in 10. The choice of which *n*th number to use in the random sampling process differs between the colors. Researchers might be comfortable drawing every 10th candy, expecting they would draw some brown candies after three or four selections. However, if they used the option of every 10th candy for the color green, they would have to draw many more times from the sample. For a study involving the green candies, researchers might choose every 5th candy rather than every 10th. Of course, with only 100 candies in the sampling frame, they might choose to study the entire group.

Stratified Random Sample

In a **stratified random sample** the sampling frame is divided into *strata* (groupings) and a random sample is drawn from each stratum.[11] For example, with the colored candies, the researchers may want to ensure that every color is represented in the study, in which case they would utilize the stratified random sample. They would first divide the sampling frame (the bag of candy) into strata according to color and then draw a simple random sample from each stratum. When using this technique, it quickly becomes evident that the sampling frame might be too small. Just one bag of 100 candies has only 5 greens, 10 reds, and 10 blues. A random sample from each group might not produce a sufficient sample size. This situation would likely lead the researchers to increase the sampling frame to include enough packages to allow for large enough numbers in each group.

Consider a study on epidemiology of cervical cancer. Researchers would be interested in ensuring that the sampling frame included women of all ages as well as ethnicities and geographic regions. A study of this kind would require a stratified random sample.

Multistage Sampling

A **multistage sampling** procedure occurs in one or more steps (stages). This procedure often is used when dealing with very large sampling frames

and when researchers want to ensure that every subgroup is included. For instance, in the previous example about cervical cancer a multistage approach might be needed.

In the first stage, the researchers might start by creating clusters that divide the United States into regions and then randomly sample states from the regions. Then, in the second stage, they might create clusters in which the cities and towns are divided according to population density and degree of rurality. This second stage would ensure that urban, suburban, and rural communities of various sizes are included in the final sampling frame. Next, the researchers would draw a simple random sample of cities and towns to include in the next stage of the process. In the third stage, the researchers might divide the communities into voting districts, which tend to be drawn along ethnic population parameters. For this final stage, a simple random sample of voting districts would be randomly selected. At the end of the process, the researchers would have a set of voting districts across the United States that represents various regions, population densities, and ethnicities. The next step would likely be to randomly draw subjects from the sampling frame.

The following outline lists the steps in the multistage process described above:

1. Divide the United States into geographic clusters and randomly select states from each cluster.
2. Stratify cities and towns in the selected states into population density and rurality groups, then randomly select cities and towns from each group.
3. Stratify selected cities and towns into ethnic groups by voting districts and randomly select districts from each ethnic group.

Nonprobability Sampling

A recent study comparing the brand version of the drug enoxaparin (Clexane) to a biosimilar version (Cutenox) exemplifies the use of a nonrandom sample, or **nonprobability sample**.[10] Enoxaparin, is a low-molecular-weight heparin class of drug.

It is used for prevention of blood clots in the legs of patients who are on bedrest.[12] This drug is often administered to patients who undergo hip replacement, knee replacement, or stomach surgery. Enoxaparin is administered by subcutaneous injection. In the study, the drugs were administered once daily to healthy volunteers.

The researchers looked for differences in immune response between the two groups in a sample of 40 patients. The study was intended to determine if further research was needed. Because of the type of treatment, the quantitative response variable, and the nature of the research question, a random sample was not necessary. It is unlikely that the patients could have altered the outcome of the study based on this design. Furthermore, the authors did not make a generalization about the use of the drug in patient care. Instead, they looked for a difference between the two drugs that would warrant further research. This type of study is performed because of the relatively low cost involved in order to provide evidence to support the greater expense of a large, double-blind, randomized control study. In this study, the authors did find sufficient evidence to recommend further research.

Several types of nonprobability sampling procedures are available, including convenience sampling, purposive sampling, and snowball sampling.

Convenience Sampling

Convenience sampling means that the researchers base the sampling frame on individuals to whom they have easy access. Convenience sampling is used in quantitative types of research, such as observational studies and survey studies. For example, researchers might choose three hospitals for a study on pharmaceutical errors because the hospitals are part of the same system, they are geographically close to one another, and the researchers have previously performed studies involving the three hospitals. In such a study, the researchers would be interested in describing the errors made in these hospitals, but not drawing inferences about pharmaceutical errors in general.

Purposive Sampling

Purposive sampling is a strategy in which "the researcher's knowledge of the population and its elements is used to hand-pick the cases to be included in the sample."[13] Purposive sampling is typically used in qualitative research studies, such as grounded theory, phenomenology, ethnography, and biography. A purposive sampling procedure is often necessary when there are few cases of a specific problem, such as with a rare diagnosis, or when researchers are interested in the experiences of specific subjects. For example, a study on perceptions of persons with schizophrenia relating to body weight was performed at an outpatient clinic.[14] The purpose of the study was to understand the experiences of persons with schizophrenia with regard to weight and lifestyle. The qualitative nature of the research question indicated a need to perform interviews. As such, a purposive sampling strategy was employed.

In purposive sampling, the goal is to ensure that multiple perspectives are represented. Also, the identification of subjects emerges as the study progresses. After completing the first interview, researchers gain insight into the phenomenon of interest and make adjustments to the selection criteria. They will purposely seek the next participant to have either a similar or a different perspective. For example, they might first select a female participant and then for the second interview select a male because there is likely to be a difference in perspectives between the two sexes. Based on emerging data from the first and second interview, they might purposely select another male and another female for the third and fourth interviews. Atypical antipsychotic medications have a side effect of weight gain.[15] As such, they might purposely select subjects who have gained weight because they have experience with the phenomenon of weight gain as well as the phenomenon of taking atypical antipsychotics.

In Digel's study[14] on experiences among those with schizophrenia who were taking atypical antipsychotics, the purposive selection procedure included male and female patients as well as "participants who identified themselves as under-weight, normal weight and overweight . . . as well as persons at varying points of care. Participants' recovery stage ranged from newly discharged, to active day hospital members, to infrequently fol-lowed outpatients."[14]

Snowball Sampling

Snowball sampling is a type of purposive sampling used in quantitative research when the researchers are interested in studying a population that is dif-ficult to identify, such as gang members, IV drug users, or illegal aliens, to name a few. Those identi-fied initially are asked to identify others who might be able to provide data. The researchers then con-tact them and determine if they experience the phe-nomenon of interest and meet the study's inclusion criteria. If they are a good fit, they are added to the sample, and then those added are asked to identify other acquaintances, and so on, until a sufficient sample size is achieved to attain statistical power. The difference between the purposive sample and the snowball sample is the characteristic of statisti-cal power.

ALPHA (PROBABILITY)

Alpha (α) is the probability of a *Type I error*. It is often referred to simply as *probability*. It is the chance that a researcher will incorrectly reject the null hypothesis. Consider a study comparing two medications, we will call them SuperStatin and BogusStatin. Research convention dictates that the null hypothesis should allow for the pos-sibility that either drug is superior to the other, meaning that the null hypothesis must state that the drugs are equal, as represented by the follow-ing shorthand:

$$H_0: SuperStatin^{LDL-C} = BogusStatin^{LDL-C}$$

H_0 (referred to as "H-naught") is the null hypo-thesis. For this example, the comparison made between the drugs is their ability to reduce LDL cholesterol, hence the superscript LDL-C.

If the statistical test shows that one drug reduces LDL cholesterol significantly more than the other, then the researchers can reject the null hypothesis. The two drugs are not equal. However, there is a chance that the test statistic was purely the result of random chance and not the result of the drug. The percentage of this risk is alpha, the probability of a Type I error.

When designing a study, researchers establish the amount of risk they are willing to take with regard to making a Type I error. The most com-mon levels of alpha are 0.05, 0.01, and 0.001. That is to say, the most common percentages of risk researchers are willing to tolerate are 5%, 1%, and 0.1%. Researchers should identify the level of alpha selected in a study and explain if other simi-lar studies also utilized the same alpha level.

$\alpha < 0.05$ means that there is a less than a 5% chance that the test statistic represents normal variability.

$\alpha < 0.01$ means that there is a less than a 1% chance that the test statistic represents normal variability.

$\alpha < 0.001$ means that there is a less than 0.1% chance that the test statistic represents normal variability.

The level chosen for alpha is based on conven-tions for the discipline, the level of alpha used in similar studies, and the severity of the outcome. If the outcome is death or some other severe con-sequence, the level of alpha will likely be very low. Researchers are not as willing to risk a Type I error when the outcome is very hazardous. However, using a very low alpha has its own problems. It is possible to have a significant result that is missed. This is called a *Type II error* (incorrectly failing to reject the null hypothesis).

Researchers should explain if the hypothesis was one of equality, such as the example given above, or one of inequality. For example, the null hypoth-esis could have been that one drug was superior to the other, which would be indicated by the fol-lowing shorthand:

$$H_0: SuperStatin^{LDL-C} > BogusStatin^{LDL-C}$$

It is rare for researchers to perform statistical tests based on an inequality, because it generally violates research conventions. However, it is possible and should be clearly explained. The issue of testing equalities versus inequalities has an effect on how alpha is applied.

Alpha Halves

Alpha halves is the risk of a Type I error when a test of equality is performed. If equality is tested, then the researchers assume that either group could turn out to be superior, in which case alpha should be divided in half. When a test of equality is performed, it is referred to as a *two-tailed test*, meaning that there are two sides. The test could show that the experimental treatment is better, or it could show that it is worse. If you think of this in terms of a number line, it means that the mean for the experimental group could be to the left of the mean for the control group or that it could be to the right of the mean of the control group (**Figure 6–5**).

The mean of the control group (Cr) is placed at the center. The symbol $\bar{x}$ (which is pronounced as "x-bar") represents the mean of a sample, whereas the mean for a population would be signified by the Greek letter μ (*mu*, which is pronounced "myoo"). Think of Cr $\bar{x}$ as zero on the number line. The experimental group is signified by *Tx*, which means "treatment." Thus, the mean for the treatment group is denoted as Tx $\bar{x}$. Figure 6–5 shows

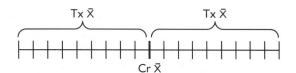

$$\text{Tx } \bar{x} \qquad \text{Tx } \bar{x}$$

$$\text{Cr } \bar{x}$$

Figure 6–5 Number Line with Two Tails

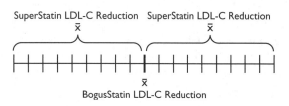

SuperStatin LDL-C Reduction   SuperStatin LDL-C Reduction
$\bar{x}$ $\bar{x}$

$\bar{x}$
BogusStatin LDL-C Reduction

Figure 6–6 Number Line Showing Two Possible Outcomes for SuperStatin vs. BogusStatin

that the mean for the treatment group would be either higher (to the right on the number line) or lower (to the left on the number line) than the mean for the control group. Either outcome is possible. Each segment of the number line on either side of the control group mean is a "tail." This shows why a test of equality is referred to as a *two-tailed test*.

So, returning to the example of comparing Bogus-Statin and SuperStatin, if BogusStatin was the standard-of-care treatment, then it would be the treatment received by the control group, and the researchers would compare the ability of each medication to lower LDL cholesterol **(Figure 6–6)**. Once again, the null hypothesis would be a statement of equality:

$$H_0: \text{SuperStatin}^{\text{LDL-C}} = \text{BogusStatin}^{\text{LDL-C}}$$

Imagine that both groups started at an average of 130 mg/dL of LDL cholesterol (which would put them in the high-cholesterol range) and that the average cholesterol lowering for the control (BogusStatin) group was 10 mg/dL. Because the experiment is testing equality, the researchers accept the possibility that the treatment (SuperStatin) group could have a greater effect on cholesterol lowering compared to the control or a lesser effect on cholesterol lowering compared to the control.

If alpha is set at 5%, then the probability of a Type I error should be shared by both possible outcomes. This means that the *p*-value associated with the test statistic needs to be half of alpha in order to be deemed significant.

Alpha halves is $\frac{\alpha}{2}$. If alpha is set at 0.05, then alpha halves is $\frac{0.05}{2}$, or 0.025. If alpha is set at 0.05, then the *p*-value for the test statistic must be less than 0.025 in order to be statistically significant. If the *p*-value for the test statistic is not less than 0.025, then the result is not considered statistically significant when alpha is set at 0.05. If alpha is set at 0.01, then alpha halves = $\frac{0.01}{2}$, or 0.005. In this case, the *p*-value for the test statistic must be less than 0.005 in order to achieve statistical significance.

The Normal Curve

The number line represents the base of the normal curve. If we think of this concept of alpha halves in terms of the normal distribution, then we can think of alpha as the percent of naturally occurring results that fall in a specific area of the curve. The normal curve (**Figure 6–7**) includes all of the "normal" results that occur in the population, even those that might represent only a very small proportion of the population. The farther a test statistic falls to the left or to the right, the less probable the outcome. There is a lower and lower percentage of results as the test statistic moves away from the center of the number line. These percentages are represented by the curve. Keep in mind that although the percentages of outcomes are very small in the tails of the number line, these rare results are still possible and can occur naturally.

Half of all naturally occurring results will fall below the mean/median (as shown in **Figure 6–8**). Let's consider height. The average height of adult males in the United States is 69.5 inches.[16] This means that 50% of adult males are less than or equal to 69.5 inches. Of course, it also means that 50% are greater than or equal to 69.5 inches. It is possible for a man to be significantly taller or shorter than 69.5 inches. In other words, normal variation can include a man who is 85 inches tall or a man who is 48 inches tall, but the majority of men will be closer to the average of 69.5 inches. The farther we get away from the mean, the fewer observations there will be until we reach a point where there are no observations. For example, there will be no observations at 120 inches (10 feet tall) or 12 inches.

The standard deviation for height among men is 3 inches. *Standard deviation* is the square of the average amount the observations deviate from the mean. By definition, in a normal distribution about 68% of the results are within one standard deviation from the mean. This means that the majority of men are between 66.5 and 72.5 inches tall, as shown in **Figure 6–9**.

Because height is a normal distribution, a small percentage of men are much taller or much shorter than the mean. About 16% of men are above 72.5 inches tall and about 16% of men are less than 66.5 inches tall, as shown in **Figure 6–10**.

Approximately 2.5% of observations in a normal distribution are more than two standard deviations below the mean and approximately 2.5% of observations are more than two standard deviations above the mean, as shown in **Figure 6–11**.

Continuing out to three standard deviations, 0.15% of observations will be more than three

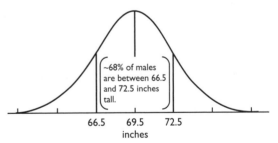

Figure 6–9 Sixty-eight Percent of Males Are Within One Standard Deviation

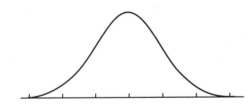

Figure 6–7 Normal Curve

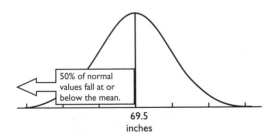

Figure 6–8 Fifty Percent of Values Fall Below the Mean/Median in a Normal Distribution

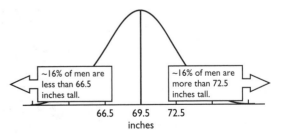

Figure 6–10 Proportion of Men Above One Standard Deviation and Below One Standard Deviation

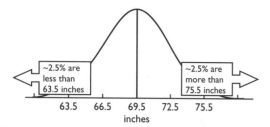

Figure 6–11 Proportion of Men Above and Below Two Standard Deviations

standard deviations below the mean and another 0.15% will be more than three standard deviations above the mean.

The 68-95-99.7 Rule

The pattern just discussed is often referred to as the *68-95-99.7 rule*. As you can see in **Figure 6–12**, 34.1% of observations fall between the mean (signified by x̄) and one standard deviation below the mean (signified by –1σ). Sigma (σ) is the Greek letter used to symbolize the standard deviation of a population. Also, 34.1% of observations fall between the mean and one standard deviation above the mean (+1σ). When you add together all of the observations that fall between –1σ and +1σ, you get approximately 68%.

Following this logic, if you add all of the values that fall in between –2σ and +2σ you get 13.6% + 34.1% + 34.1% +13.6%, which adds up to approximately 95%. If you add all of the proportions between –3σ and +3σ, then you find that the total is approximately 99.7% of the observations.

The farther we get from the mean, the smaller the percentage of observations that are part of the normal distribution. As you can see from Figure 6–12, only 0.15% of observations are more than three standard deviations above the mean, and only 0.15% are three standard deviations below the mean. If the test statistic were to be more than three standard deviations above the mean, there would only be a 0.15% chance that this result was part of the normal population.

This is one reason that setting alpha at 0.05 is widely accepted. When alpha is set at 0.05, the researchers are allowing for the possibility that the test statistic could represent a naturally occurring value that lies in the territory on the curve beyond two standard deviations. Approximately 95% of the values are between –2σ and +2σ, meaning that the remaining 5% are those values that are either two standard deviations above or two standard deviations below the mean. This is also another reason for performing a two-tailed test (testing equality). When researchers choose 0.05 for alpha, they presume that if the test statistic lies to the right 2σ that the result is due to the intervention and the test statistic is not one of the normal values that also lie in that area of the curve. If they are incorrect, then they will have made a Type I error.

In the example of men's heights, the CDC found the average height of men in the United States to be 67.5 inches; that is, x̄ = 67.5 inches. Height can be a helpful diagnostic indicator, such as in Marfan syndrome, which is a connective tissue disorder that affects the skeletal and cardiovascular

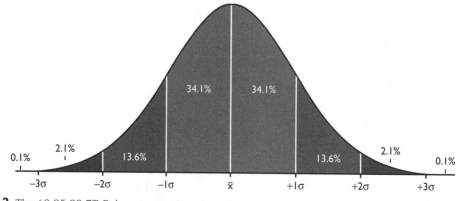

Figure 6–12 The 68-95-99.7% Rule

systems, the eyes, and the skin.[17] According to the National Library of Medicine:

> *Marfan syndrome is caused by defects in a gene called fibrillin-1. Fibrillin-1 plays an important role as the building block for elastic tissue in the body. The gene defect also causes too much growth of the long bones of the body. This causes the tall height and long arms and legs seen in people with this syndrome.*[17]

If researchers were interested in whether the heights of patients with Marfan syndrome differed from the general male population, they could use the data from the CDC as a basis of comparison. The CDC's number becomes the expected mean. If Marfan syndrome patients were 76 inches tall on average (and if alpha was set at 0.05), then the researchers could conclude that the Marfan patients were significantly taller than average, because 76 is more than two standard deviations above the mean.

TEST STATISTICS

Throughout the discussion on alpha we mentioned the term *test statistic* several times. The **test statistic** is the numerical outcome of a significance test. Each significance test produces a test statistic, such as a *t*-score, an F ratio, or a chi-square score. When a *t*-test is performed, then the test statistic will be a *t*-score. When an ANOVA test (or one of its variants) is performed, then the test statistic will be an F ratio. And when a chi-square test is performed, the resulting test statistic will be a chi-square score. Hence, when the mean of one group is compared to the mean of another group, as in a *t*-test, the result of the test is a *t*-score. Test statistics also have associated *p*-values (and in most cases a confidence interval, too). The test statistic is derived from sample data.

The *p*-value associated with the test statistic tells you the probability that the test statistic came from the normal population. If the test statistic is less than alpha (for a one-tailed test) or less than alpha halves (for a two-tailed test), then researchers deem the test statistic to be significantly different from the mean. Optimally, authors should report the test statistic, the *p*-value, and the confidence interval. For instance, imagine with the example

of BogusStatin versus SuperStatin that SuperStatin lowered LDL cholesterol by 20 mg/dL. Earlier we described BogusStatin as lowering LDL cholesterol by 10 mg/dL. The authors should report whether the difference between the BogusStatin group and the SuperStatin group was statistically significant in the following manner:

> *SuperStatin reduced LDL-C 20 mg/dL (n = 50), while BogusStatin reduced LDL-C by 10 mg/dL (n = 50). The distribution of each group met the assumption of normality, and the data fit with the assumptions for a t-test. The difference between the two treatments was significant (t = 1.987; df = 99; p = 0.015; 95% CI: 20 mg/dL ± 3 mg/dL).*

In this example, ***df*** means **degrees of freedom**, which is the number of observations minus one (i.e., n − 1). This indicates that there were 100 observations (100 participants in the study). The test statistic in this example is the *t*-score (t = 1.987). This example includes the confidence interval as well. It is rare to find explanations of statistical findings that are as complete as the example we provided. In many instances, only the test statistic being compared, the *p*-value, and the confidence interval are reported. The above example would more likely be reported as follows:

> *SuperStatin reduced LDL-C (20 mg/dL) significantly more (p = 0.015; 95% CI: 20 mg/dL ± 3 mg/dL) than BogusStatin (10 mg/dL).*

THE *P*-VALUE

We have mentioned the term *p*-value multiple times. The **p-value** (often expressed simply as a lowercase letter *p*) is similar to alpha in that it also reflects the percentage of chance that the outcome occurred naturally, representing normal random variation. Alpha is set ahead of time as the amount of risk the researchers are willing to take that their test statistic is indeed the result of normal variation and not the result of the intervention. The *p*-value is the percentage of risk that the test statistic itself represents normal variation. For a test statistic to be deemed statistically significant, the *p*-value must be less than alpha. In other words, there must be a lower risk that the test statistic represents normal variation than the researchers set in advance as the amount of risk they would tolerate. For example, let's say that researchers set alpha at 0.05. This means that they are willing to take a 5% risk that the test statistic will result from normal variation. In order for the test statistic to be deemed statistically significant, the *p*-value associated with the test statistic must be less than 5%. If a two-tailed test was performed, then the *p*-value would have to be less than 0.025 in order to be significant. **Figure 6–13** displays the **area under the curve (AUC)** represented by 0.025 (2.5%) in each tail, which is located at approximately 1.98 standard deviations above and below the mean.

CONFIDENCE INTERVALS

This brings us to the concept of confidence intervals. A *confidence interval* gives you information about the variability of the outcome. Confidence intervals are highly useful in that they help us contend with the reality that no two experiments will come out identically no matter how carefully the researchers designed the studies. For example, if you tossed a coin 100 times, it might land on heads 53 times. Then, if you repeated the experiment with the same coin, it might land on heads 45 times. There is a range of results you would expect that would not surprise you. In fact, it would surprise you, most likely, if you did the 100 coin tosses 10 times and all 10 times you got heads on exactly 50 tosses. We expect the outcome to vary a little from one experiment to the next, no matter how similar the experiments.

A confidence interval helps us predict how widely the results will vary when the experiment is performed repeatedly. If you performed many 100-coin-toss experiments, you would find that the number of heads (with a fair coin) will range from 45 to 55. A confidence interval tells us the probability that the test statistic will fall within a specific range. A 95% confidence interval tells us that 95% of the time the test statistic will fall within the given range, or some might say that we are 95% confident that the true value of the population falls within the given range (although this phrasing is disputed, it is often used).

Looking at the SuperStatin versus BogusStatin example again, SuperStatin reduced LDL-C (20 mg/dL), which was significantly more (*p* = 0.015; 95% CI: 20 mg/dL ± 3 mg/dL) than BogusStatin (10 mg/dL). The outcome was 20 mg/dL with a 95% confidence interval of plus or minus 3 mg/dL. This means that if the experiment were run many times, we would expect the outcome to range between 17 mg/dL and 23 mg/dL 95% of the time. Or we might say that we are 95% confident that the true LDL-C lowering value of SuperStatin is between 17 mg/dL and 23 mg/dL.

The range of the confidence interval is useful because it helps us determine if the outcome is sufficiently narrow. If the 95% confidence interval had been ±10 mg/dL, then the difference between SuperStatin and BogusStatin would be unclear. If this

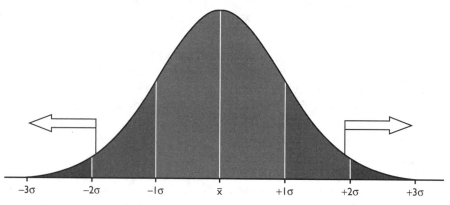

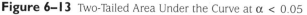

Figure 6–13 Two-Tailed Area Under the Curve at α < 0.05

was the case, then the range for SuperStatin would be 10 mg/dL to 30 mg/dL. Notice that at the low end the value is the same as BogusStatin at 10 mg/dL. With a 95% confidence interval of 10 mg/dL, it is possible that the two drugs are actually not different at all. It is also possible that SuperStatin lowers LDL-C by as much as 30 mg/dL. The range of the confidence interval is very wide in this case, and it should give us pause. With a wide confidence interval, we would want to learn more information about these drugs before making any treatment decision.

The rules to follow with confidence intervals are that the range for the interval should not include zero and the range should not include the outcome of the control group. In the above example, the confidence interval of 20 mg/dL $\pm$ 10 mg/dL contained the outcome of the control group (10 mg/dL), because 20 mg/dL minus 10 mg/dL equals 10 mg/dL.

INFERENTIAL STATISTICS

As we said earlier, *inferential statistics* are used to make predictions based on probability. Inferential statistics focus on the probability that the observed outcome happened by random chance. The lower the probability of random chance explaining the outcome, the more likely the outcome was caused by the intervention. The three main categories of inferential statistical tests are differences, relationships, and models.

Tests for Differences

A **test for differences** compares a statistic, such as a mean or a proportion, between two or more groups. For example, many studies on cholesterol treatments compare the mean LDL cholesterol level in the experimental group to the mean LDL cholesterol level in the control group. (Usually these studies also compare the mean HDL levels between the two groups.) An epidemiological study might compare the proportion of people with tooth loss in a region with fluoridated water to the proportion of people with tooth loss in a region without fluoridated water. The central question in tests for differences is whether there is a statistically significant

difference between the compared variables. Tests for differences can be used in three different ways:

1. To compare independent groups
2. To compare different points of time for the same subjects (referred to as *pre/post, self-controlled,* or *correlated group* design)
3. To compare different areas of the body on the same subjects (referred to as *within subject, self-controlled*, or *correlated group design*)

Pre/post, within-subject, self-controlled, and correlated group designs are all types of **repeated measures tests**. When a test for differences is used to compare variables that are from different groups that do not influence one another, the measures are said to be *independent,* whereas repeated measures tests are used when the variables being compared are not independent. Several examples of parametric statistical tests used to test for differences include the independent-samples *t*-test, the one-sample *t*-test, the paired-samples *t*-test, and ANOVA (analysis of variance). Other tests for differences are available, but these four are widely used, so we will explain them here in a little more detail.

Independent-Samples t-Test

The *independent-samples t-test* is an example of a test used to compare the means of two independent groups. The following study demonstrates usage of the independent-samples *t*-test. A nursing team[18] used the independent-samples *t*-test to compare the levels of anxiety, depression, and suicidal ideation between patients with different severities of obsessive compulsive disorder (OCD). The response variables were anxiety, depression, and suicide. The instruments used to measure the response variables included the Beck Anxiety Inventory (BAI), the Beck Depression Inventory II (BDI-II), and the Beck Scale for Suicide Ideation (BSS). The predictor variable (severity of OCD) was measured using the Yale-Brown Obsessive Compulsive Scale (Y-BOCS).

This means that three independent-samples *t*-tests were performed: (1) comparing mean anxiety between the two OCD groups, (2) comparing mean depression between the two OCD groups, and (3) comparing suicidal ideation between the two OCD groups. The central question of the study was whether the mean levels of anxiety, depression, or suicide ideation were different between subjects with high- versus low-severity OCD. High-severity OCD was defined as a Y-BOCS score above 15, whereas low-severity OCD was defined as a Y-BOCS score of 15 or less. The study included a convenience sample of 128 outpatients with OCD. The researchers found that patients with high-severity OCD had significantly higher levels of anxiety, depression, and suicidal ideation.[18]

The independent-samples t-test was used because the groups being measured were independent of one another. The levels of anxiety, depression, or suicidal ideation in one group have no effect on these levels in the other group. When reading this article, it would be important to look for discussion regarding the other assumptions about the t-test. Not only do the groups need to be independent of one another, but the shape of the distributions for all of the measures need to be normal, they need to have similar variability, and they need to have similar sample sizes. One assumption we can be sure was satisfied based on reading just the abstract was that there were only two groups. If the article is well written, and the study well designed, then the researchers will state that tests for normality showed that the response variables met the assumption of normality.

One-Sample t-Test

A **one-sample t-test** is a quantitative test that compares the mean score of a sample to the known mean (normative or expected) value from a trustworthy source. This test is used when a normative value derived from a previously known, and trustworthy, source is the basis of comparison for a variable measured among the experimental group. The normative value takes the place of a control or placebo group. Typically the normative value is based on a measure that is regularly

reported by an authoritative organization, such as the CDC or the WHO. The central question in a one-sample t-test is whether there is a difference between the experimental group(s) and the known normative value.

For example, a study published in 2012 compared a sample of 111 adult stroke survivors to national averages on level of disability and quality of life.[19] The subjects completed two surveys: the World Health Organization Disability Assessment Schedule (WHODAS II) and the Short-Form Health Survey (SF-36). These same surveys are administered annually to a random sample of healthy people in the United States. The mean results of the national surveys were used as the normative values in the study. The central question of the study, therefore, was whether stroke patients differed from the population in terms of level of disability (WHODAS II) and quality of life (SF-36). The results of the study showed that both the WHODAS II scores and the SF-36 scores were significantly lower for the stroke patients compared to the national norms. They also found the lower the WHODAS II score, the lower the SF-36 score, meaning the worse the disability from the stroke, the lower the quality of life. The researchers also found that employed persons had a higher quality of life and lower disability levels.

A one-sample t-test would be needed for a study like this one because the researchers do not have access to the original data file with the raw scores of the national surveys. They had access only to the mean scores from the national survey. If they had access to the original data file, they would have been able to use an independent-samples t-test.

Paired-Samples t-Test

A *paired-samples t-test* is a type of repeated measures test where measures are taken over time and the results are compared from one point in time to another. If there are only two measures, then this is referred to as a *pre/post paired-samples t-test*. The paired samples t-test is sometimes also referred to as a *dependent-, related-, or correlated-samples* t-*test* because the two measures are in some way dependent on or related to one another. The distinguishing characteristic of this test is that it looks for a difference within the same group at different points in time.

A study published in 2011[20] used the paired-samples t-test to determine the efficacy of a medication for the treatment of nocturia (awakening from sleep during the night because of the need to urinate before getting a full night's sleep; that is, 6 to 8 hours[21]). The study was a double-blind, placebo-controlled design. A total of 60 patients were included in the study. Thirty patients were in the experimental medication group, and 30 were in the placebo group. The patients included in the study were men older than age 60 who complained of two voids per night. The study lasted for 8 weeks.

The incidents of nocturia were assessed at 4 weeks and again at 8 weeks. The 4- and 8-week intervals represent the repeated measures in this study. The initial number of incidents represents the preliminary measure. The main objective of the study was to determine whether the incidence of nocturia changed over time. A paired-samples t-test was needed because the variable being measured (incidents of nocturia) was within the same sample of people. The variables were not independent, but rather they were related.

The initial mean incidence of nocturia for the experimental group was 2.6, whereas the mean incidence of nocturia for the control group was 2.5. At the end of 8 weeks, the mean incidence of nocturia for the control group was 2.3 but for the treatment group the incidence was 1.6. A paired-samples t-test showed that the change from 2.6 to 1.6 incidents was statistically significant.[20] The study indicates that the medication might be helpful in reducing the number of times per night a man older than age 60 gets out of bed during the night to urinate. This could be important to patients if the nocturia is resulting in less sleep, lower quality sleep, waking another person in the bed, or otherwise impacting quality of life.

We feel that it is important to note with this example that the incidence of nocturia might not fit the definition of evidence that matters. Based on the abstract, it appears the researchers did not measure any variables that meet the definition. As a reader of this article, it would be important for you to determine if putting a patient on this medication was worth the cost and side effects (if any). When interviewing a patient with this complaint, you should ask about the impact nocturia is having on his sleep and quality of life. After the patient has been on the medication for a sufficient length of time, you should ask again about sleep and quality of life. You should also ask about side effects and whether the patient feels the medication is making a meaningful difference.

ANOVA

ANOVA stands for *analysis of variance*. The ANOVA test is similar to the independent-samples t-test. It is used as a test to compare means between independent variables with similar variance and normality of distribution. Whereas the t-test compares just two means, an ANOVA test can be used to compare multiple groups. For example, a study could have more than a control and one treatment group. It is not uncommon for studies to have more than two groups.

A study published in 2011 demonstrates the use of the ANOVA test.[22] The researchers performed a randomized clinical trial evaluating the efficacy of three treatment options for painful temporomandibular joint clicking. The temporomandibular joints (abbreviated TMJ) are the joints where the upper temporal bone, which is part of the cranium, meets the lower jaw bone (the mandible). The term TMJ is often used incorrectly to refer to temporomandibular joint disorder, which is correctly abbreviated TMD.[22]

This study examined painful clicking of the TMJ. In this study, 60 patients were randomly assigned to one of three treatment options: (A) anterior positioning splint therapy, (B) physical therapy, or (C) physical therapy in addition to splint therapy. The study showed a significant difference in the level of pain between the three groups. The patients in group A (anterior positioning splint therapy) showed the greatest reduction in pain compared to group B and group C. ANOVA was used because more than two groups were compared.

There are two additional facts you need to know about ANOVA. First, an ANOVA test needs to be accompanied by a post hoc test as well as a test called a Bonferonni test. An ANOVA test shows whether there is a significant difference between groups, but it will not tell you which specific groups were different. In other words, the ANOVA test gives only a yes or no result. Was there a significant difference, yes or no? A problem with performing multiple comparisons is that the risk of error for each comparison increases the overall risk for error. The Bonferroni test accounts for the multiple comparisons performed, bringing the risk of error back into the acceptable range.

In order to determine which group or groups differ, a post hoc test must be performed. Several versions of the post hoc test can be used to identify which group differed from which. One example is Tukey's Honestly Significant Difference test; another is Scheffé's method. We will not go into all of the alternatives. What is important is to look for the use of a post hoc test whenever ANOVA is used with more than two comparisons. Tukey's test is the most common.

In the TMJ clicking study[22] the authors used Tukey's test. They found that group A was significantly different from group B, and group A was also significantly different from group C. Furthermore, it showed that group B and group C were not different from one another. Only the treatment given to group A showed a significant reduction in pain. The researchers compared the amount of change in level of pain from baseline to posttreatment. The ANOVA test was used to determine if the degree of change

in pain scores differed between the three groups. They used the mean score on a Visual Analogue Scale (VAS). The scale included a low-end self-rating of 0 for "pain free" and a high-end self-rating of 100 for "maximum pain."

The researchers calculated a mean VAS score for each group as well as a standard deviation. **Table 6–2** presents the pre/post VAS mean score and standard deviation for each group as reported in the results section of the article.[22] The three treatments compared in the study were: (I) anterior splint positioning therapy, (II) physical therapy, and (III) combination of the two (physical therapy + anterior positioning splint therapy).

The information in Table 6–2 tells us that all three groups experienced improvement in the amount of pain reported by patients. However, this is not enough information to determine if the reduction in pain was statistically significant or which group experienced the most significant pain reduction. In order to determine if the amount of pain reduction was significantly different between groups the researchers used an ANOVA test (specifically the one-way ANOVA).

The ANOVA test showed that there was a statistically significant difference between the groups. However, the ANOVA test by itself does not identify which specific groups were different from the others. Thus, the researchers used Tukey's test to find the answer. They then reported, "We found a significant difference between groups I and II ($p < 0.05$). Although a difference between groups II and III was observed, it did not reach a significant level."[22]

In other words, group I had a significantly greater improvement than group II, but, compared to group III, group I was not significantly different. Furthermore, although group III had greater pain reduction than group II, the difference was not

Table 6-2 VAS Mean Scores and Standard Deviations from the TMJ Clicking Study

Group I: Anterior Positioning Splint Therapy		Group II: Physical Therapy		Group III: Physical Therapy + Anterior Positioning Splint Therapy	
Pre	Post	Pre	Post	Pre	Post
59 ± 20.75	11 ± 16.61	61 ± 21.74	36.50 ± 27.20	53.57 ± 27.63	12.86 ± 23.01

statistically significant. As such, the authors concluded, "The results of the present study indicate that anterior positioning splints can provide better improvement of TMD than other modalities."[22]

When multiple comparisons are made, it is important for authors to account for the probability of the Type I error in each comparison. If one comparison is made in a study in which alpha was less than 0.05, then there is a 5% chance of a Type I error (of incorrectly rejecting the null hypothesis). This chance exists with each comparison, meaning the more comparisons made, the greater the total risk of a Type I error. If five comparisons are made, the total risk of a Type I error is 25%. The *Bonferroni correction* is a procedure that accounts for multiple comparisons.

The Bonferroni correction divides the error risk (alpha) across all of the comparisons. For example, if alpha is set at 0.05 and six comparisons are made, then the required level of significance becomes $\frac{0.05}{6}$, meaning that the *p*-value associated with the test statistic would have to be less than 0.0083 in order to achieve statistical significance. The important lesson for you, as the reader of research articles, is to look for a statement about the use of the Bonferroni correction whenever more than two comparisons are made. If the Bonferroni correction is not used, the authors need to explain why.

In the TMJ example, the correction was not used. It is possible they did not use it because the Bonferroni correction increases the risk of Type II error.[23] However, the authors did not provide an explanation about their failure to use the Bonferroni correction. It is not clear from the information provided if the Bonferroni correction was warranted. As mentioned earlier, the authors said, "We found a significant difference between groups I and II ($p < 0.05$). Although a difference between groups II and III was observed, it did not reach a significant level."[22] Their explanation did not include the actual *p*-values associated with the Tukey's tests. This is unfortunate, because we could determine for ourselves if the result was significant enough to satisfy the Bonferroni rule if we knew the *p*-value.

The *p*-value would need to be less than $\frac{0.05}{3}$, or 0.0167. If the *p*-value was less than 0.0167, then we would know that it was significant enough to satisfy the rule even though the Bonferroni correction was not used. Thus, we are left to wonder if the anterior position splinting therapy was truly superior to the other treatments in terms of pain relief.

Chi Square

Chi square is a group of tests generally used with qualitative or non-normal data. There are chi-square tests that can be used to compare independent measures as well as tests to look for differences or for relationships. The chi-square test statistic is usually signified by the symbol χ^2. The most common use of the chi-square test is to test for differences between two groups of count data;[23] for example, the number of subjects in the treatment group who survived compared to the number of subjects in the control group who survived. This usage is similar to the independent-samples *t*-test. Another common form of chi square is to compare the count of a variable in the sample to an expected value that is theoretically expected, such as a known parameter from the population.[23] This usage is similar to the one sample *t*-test. Chi-square tests such as the Pearson chi-square test and the Mantel-Haenszel chi-square test can be used to test for relationships.

Chi-square tests are often referred to as **goodness-of-fit tests** because they can test if the sample distribution fits with a theoretical distribution. With a goodness-of-fit test, the bigger the chi-square statistic, the poorer the fit between the sample group and the theoretical distribution. As with all inferential statistics, each type of chi-square test has a set of assumptions that must be met in order for the test to produce valid results. Chi-square tests are often employed in making comparisons between groups with regard to demographic factors such as the age distribution of the sample compared to the population and compared to the control group. The goal, typically, is for the experimental group, the control group, and the population not to differ from one another in terms of demographics or severity of disease at baseline, meaning the chi-square test shows that they fit with one another.

For example, in a randomized control trial published in 2012 researchers evaluated the efficacy of quadriceps muscle neuromuscular electrical stimulation (NMES) as an adjunct to standard rehabilitation in patients receiving total knee arthroplasty (TKA).[24] Arthroplasty is a type of surgery to relieve pain and restore range of motion by realigning or reconstructing a joint.[25] TKA involves total replacement of the knee joint. The most common indication for TKA is severe osteoarthritis of the knee associated with significant loss of joint space, pain, and limited range of motion.[26] The procedure is used after conservative treatment strategies have failed. According to the authors, more than 687,000 TKAs are performed every year in the United States. The authors further state that, "one month after TKA, quadriceps muscle strength drops 50% to 60% of preoperative levels, despite the initiation of rehabilitation within 48 hours after surgery."[24]

The 66 subjects (age 50 to 85 years) included in the study were randomly assigned to control (standard rehabilitation alone) or experimental (standard rehabilitation plus NMES initiated 48 hours after TKA) groups. The study lasted for 52 weeks and included measures taken at baseline and at 3.5, 6.5, 13, 26, and 52 weeks. The researchers measured quadriceps and hamstring muscle strength, functional performance, and knee extension active range of motion. The chi-square test was used to compare the treatment and control groups to one another in terms of baseline characteristics.

Two chi-square comparisons were made: the proportion of men and women in each group and steps per day (measured with a pedometer). The treatment group was 42.9% male, and the control group was 48.4% male. The treatment group completed an average of 5,133 steps, whereas the control group completed 4,842 steps during baseline testing. **Table 6–3,** which is derived from the publication, shows the statistical results of the comparisons made between the control and treatment groups at baseline.

The *p*-value reported for each comparison indicated that there was no significant difference between the control and treatment groups in terms of the proportion of men and women or the number of steps the subjects could take. The number of steps is a measure of functioning and is intended to represent the severity of symptoms. By including this information, the researchers are letting us know that the study began with two groups who were similar to one another.

Tests for Relationships

Tests for relationships are used to determine if variables change in relationship to other variables, (e.g., arthritis incidence increases with age or heart disease increases with incidence of diabetes). A positive relationship exists when an increase in one variable is associated with an increase in another. A negative relationship exists when an increase in one variable is associated with a decrease in another. The stronger the association between variables, the more likely the relationship is significant, meaning that it cannot be explained by random chance. Tests of association usually involve a *correlation analysis* of some kind. The most straightforward test for relationships is the *correlation coefficient*.

Correlation tests are used to determine if the association between two variables indicates a potential causal relationship. You most likely

Table 6-3 Chi-square Results from Baseline Comparisons Between Groups

Variable	NMES Group		Control Group		*p*-value
	n	**%**	**n**	**%**	
Women	20	57.1	16	51.6	0.65
Men	15	42.9	15	48.4	
	n	**x̄ (SD)**	**n**	**x̄ (SD)**	
Pedometer	25	5,133 (3,109)	18	4,842 (3,757)	0.79

learned in previous studies the concept "correlation is not causation." It is important to remember this concept, but it is also important to recognize that with sufficient, well-designed research a consistent correlation might be pointing to a causal relationship. It is that causal relationship that guides clinicians to take action.

A powerful example of correlation is the relationship between cigarette smoking and lung cancer. For many years the argument that correlation does not mean causation was used successfully to resist acceptance of the dangers of smoking tobacco. In a history of research on smoking and lung cancer, White cites a 1954 statement from a group of cigarette manufacturers in the United States acknowledging "the increased incidence of cancer of the lung in recent years," but denying that there was any proof that smoking was responsible.[27] For several decades in the early 1900s, researchers disagreed about whether there was a legitimate increase in the incidence of lung cancer.

By the early 1950s, the dramatic increase in lung cancer was accepted, but it would require another decade of rigorous research and vigorous debate before the relationship would be accepted as causal. White explains in 1957 that the United States Surgeon General stated that excess smoking was "one of the causative factors in lung cancer." In 1959, the Surgeon General finally published a statement accepting the strength of the association between lung cancer and cigarette smoking: "The weight of evidence at present implicates smoking as the principal etiological factor in the increased incidence of lung cancer."[27] Note the shift in language from referring to cigarette smoking as "one of the causative factors" to "the principal etiological factor." It was not until 1966 that the American Medical Association published an article in the *New England Journal of Medicine* agreeing with the Surgeon General that cigarette smoking was a hazard. The moral of this story is that correlation might very well be indicative of causation and resistance to accepting the possibility of a causal relationship can result in significant harm to individuals. We must continue to recognize that correlation does not automatically indicate causation, but causal relationships might be possible.

Regression Analysis

The last major category of statistical tests includes those that check if multiple variables in a study are associated. These tests often focus on relationships among several variables that best explain a specific response. A **regression analysis** determines the line that best fits within a set of coordinates. It is the line that comes the closest to all of the dots on a scatter diagram.

Regression analysis can include multiple variables and often includes the identification of a model that accounts for multiple variables at one time. For example, we know that age, sex, weight, and family history are all associated with the likelihood of developing type 2 diabetes mellitus. However, considering only one of these predictor variables is not sufficient. It is the combination of them that produces the greatest predictive value. As each variable is added to the model, the regression line fits better. Another example is the Framingham Calculator, which is a tool clinicians can use to determine a patient's 10-year risk of having a heart attack. This calculator takes into account age, sex, total cholesterol, HDL cholesterol, smoking, systolic blood pressure, and whether the patient is currently being treated for high blood pressure. These seven variables when combined have a far greater predictive value than any one of them alone or any combination of them with less than seven variables.

The goal of regression analysis is to identify the combination of predictor variables that best explains the variability in the response variable. In simple linear regression, the researchers test only for the degree of association between one predictor variable and one response variable. In regression analysis, the model of multiple predictor variables that have the highest correlation with the response variable is determined. Different combinations of the predictor variables are placed into a model and compared to the response variable. This procedure is performed until all reasonable combinations have been tested and the model with the greatest degree of correlation is identified. This process can lead to a fishing expedition where any variable is placed into the model. It is important that researchers determine ahead of time which variables are expected to have some degree of contribution to the model and justify their explanatory power. One could put the color of leaves into a model that explains the development of rheumatoid arthritis, for example, and an anomalous association might be found in the data. When reading a study that includes regression analysis, look for an explanation from the authors about the selection of predictor variables that were tested in the model. These variables should make sense.

Pearson Product-Moment Correlation Coefficient

The **Pearson product-moment correlation coefficient**, also referred to as *Pearson's correlation coefficient* and symbolized by a lowercase *r*, is a test for relationship between two variables that are interval or ratio data types. It is a particular type of regression analysis that is used very often. This test is used so often that sometimes the term correlation is used to refer to it even though there are many types of correlation tests (such as Spearman's rho or Kendall's tau).[11] If authors identify a test simply as a "correlation," then it is up to us as readers to determine if the two variables included in the test were indeed of the appropriate scale (i.e., interval or ratio). When Pearson's correlation coefficient is used, it is important for authors to display a scatter diagram to help readers visualize the degree of association between the two variables, as shown in **Figure 6–14**. In this example from a study coauthored by one of the authors of this book, the diagram is showing a weak negative association between TSH and T4.[1] The line between the coordinates is a linear regression line (line of best fit) showing the best fit for the coordinates.

It is not uncommon for statistically significant correlations to be found in data that are in fact not strongly associated. The dots on the scatter diagram

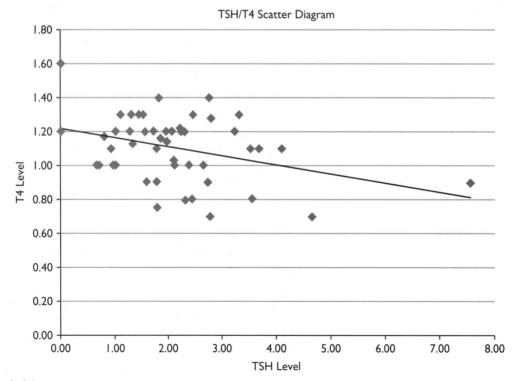

Figure 6–14 A Scatter Diagram Including the Line of Best Fit (Linear Regression)

should approximate a line if the association is to be meaningful.

A correlation coefficient will range from −1.0 to +1.0, meaning that the two variables can have a perfect negative association (−1.0) or a perfect positive association (+1.0). A perfect negative association means for every one point the X variable increases the Y variable decreases by one point. A perfect positive association means for every one point the X variable increases the Y variable increases by one point. When this happens, the dots formed by these X/Y coordinates will form a perfect line. A correlation coefficient of zero means there is no association between the predictor and response variables.

A rule of thumb employed with correlation tests is that an r of at least 0.755 is considered a strong positive association (whereas −0.755 would be a strong negative association). A so-called *weak* relationship would be at an r of 0.160 or less.[11] When reading a study that utilizes a correlation test such as Pearson's correlation coefficient, be careful to look at the r value and not just the p-value. The p-value might indicate a statistically significant result even when the r value is not indicative of a strong association.

Along with an r value, authors should report the **coefficient of determination**, which is r^2 (the correlation coefficient squared). The coefficient of determination tells us the proportion of the variability in the response variable that is explained by the variability in the predictor variable. The higher the percentage, the stronger the association. Thus, a correlation coefficient of +1.0 or −1.0 would have an r^2 of 100% because $1.0^2 = 1.0^2$ and $−1.0^2 = 1.0$. However, a correlation coefficient of 0.755 would produce an r^2 of 0.570, which means that a correlation coefficient of 0.755 represents a coefficient of determination of 0.570 (57% of the variation in the response variable is explained by variation in the predictor variable).

RELIABILITY AND VALIDITY

The instruments used in research must be consistent (**reliable**) and accurate (**valid**). To be reliable, the instrument must provide the same result from one use to the next. Consider the scale used in the clinic to weigh patients. If a patient is weighed then steps off the scale and is weighed again, the two results should be consistent. The greater the degree of consistency, the more reliable the scale. Validity has to do with whether the instrument measures what it is intended to measure and if it does so both within itself as well as in comparison to other methods of measurement. These are issues of accuracy. If the same scale weighs people consistently, it may still be wrong. It could be calibrated to 5 pounds instead of zero, thereby adding 5 pounds to every person's weight. For this reason, other methods of measurement must be compared to one another in order to ascertain if the instrument is accurate. These issues of validity and reliability apply to both descriptive and inferential statistics.

Factor Analysis

Factor analysis is a procedure for combining items in a survey instrument to represent a single concept (called a *construct* or *domain*). A survey is broken down into domains (also called subscales) that include multiple questions. A certain number of items need to be included in each domain in order for the domain to be considered valid. Each of the items in a domain must be conceptually as well as statistically related.[11] The statistical test for relationships among the factors in a survey is referred to as *factor analysis;* "Factor analysis is done by finding patterns among the variations in the values of several variables; a cluster of highly intercorrelated variables results in a factor."[11] Thousands of questionnaires are used in healthcare research, as well as in clinical practice. It is important that authors include explanations in their articles about the validity of the instruments they use as well as the results of factor analysis studies that demonstrate the instruments measure what they purport to measure.

Many phenomena are not directly observable. For this reason survey instruments are used. Consider the difference between a broken bone and anxiety. The bone fracture can be observed on x-ray, or even visual inspection, but anxiety is an internal experience that clinicians cannot observe directly. Instead, we ask patients to complete a survey, which is used to assess anxiety. Such surveys are composed of multiple factors, also known as *subscales* or *constructs*. Each subscale has multiple questions, because no single question is sufficient for diagnostic purposes. Imagine asking a patient, "Do you have anxiety?" Each patient has different feelings. What one patient experiences as harmful anxiety, another might experience as mild or even helpful anxiety.

For example, the Maslach Burnout Inventory Human Services Survey (MBI-HSS) is used to measure level of burnout as an occupational issue among human services workers (such as health professionals, educators, and social workers).[28] The survey contains 22 questions. The questions are divided into three constructs: emotional exhaustion, depersonalization, and personal accomplishment.[29] Emotional exhaustion represents feelings that workers are no longer able to give of themselves at a psychological level. Depersonalization represents negative, cynical attitudes and feelings toward patients. Personal accomplishment is associated with feelings of accomplishment and personal achievement. When experiencing burnout, human services providers tend to perceive themselves negatively in terms of personal accomplishment. The Emotional Exhaustion subscale has nine items. The Depersonalization subscale has five items, and the Personal Accomplishment subscale has eight items.

Previous and New Instruments

In the methods section of an article, the authors should identify the instruments used to collect data. When a study uses survey and self-report data, then the instruments need to be validated. Researchers sometimes use previously developed instruments, whereas at other times they develop the instruments for their research. There are slightly different considerations for readers when researchers use previously developed instruments compared to when they develop new ones. In either case, the instruments need to be validated. Validity

testing should include factor analysis to determine if the items included in each subscale group together statistically. In other words, if five items are grouped together to measure depersonalization, as in the MBH-HSS, then there should be a trend that shows consistency among the responses to those items.

A test called Cronbach's alpha is used to measure the degree of association among items in a survey. This test can be used when all survey items fall into a single domain or it can be used to test the correlation among items of the subscales within an instrument. Usually, results of Cronbach's alpha are reported along with the result of factor analysis testing. Cronbach's alpha can be used with items that have more than two responses. The Kuder-Richardson (KR-20) test is a similar test used in the same manner, but applied to items that have dichotomous responses (such as correct/incorrect).

If an instrument has been used in prior research, then the authors can refer to the validation and factor analysis that was performed on the instrument in the past—if indeed these steps were completed. With previously validated and factor-analyzed instruments, there are two strategies researchers should use. First, they should reference earlier publications. Second, they should perform confirmatory validity and factor analysis with their own data. When researchers report the use of a previously validated instrument, it is essential that they describe the prior validation studies and reference them so that readers can locate them. The researchers should describe the similarities and differences between their study and the prior instrument validation research.

For example, in studies utilizing the Maslach Burnout Inventory Human Services Survey (MBI-HSS) researchers should report the validity of the instrument overall as well as the validity of the constructs within the instrument. Because the MBI-HSS has been evaluated in multiple studies, the validity of the instrument is easier for researchers to establish. The MBI-HSS was tested on postsecondary educators, social service workers, medical professionals, and mental health workers.[29] Researchers employing the MBI-HSS with any of these groups have a defensible reason for doing so because the instrument has been validated with these groups of people. However, if researchers were to use the instrument with an untested group, such as fast food workers for example, then the prior validation research might not be applicable. The validation assessment would need to be performed again with the present sample of subjects.

It is advisable, even when using a validated instrument with a group for whom it was validated, that researchers perform a confirmatory analysis to verify that the instrument is valid with the present sample. Validating an instrument with the current subjects helps researchers avoid any mistakes that might have occurred in earlier validation research, and it helps researchers identify any unusual patterns in the present study. If the factor analysis performed on the present group of subjects results in different factors, then the researchers might have new or different information to add to the body of knowledge about the group under study in comparison to other previously studied groups.

A study completed by Bell, Davison, and Sefcik[28] utilized the MBI-HSS to measure burnout among emergency medicine physician assistants. In utilizing earlier research with the MBI-HSS, the authors referenced three studies of emergency medicine physicians that also used the MBI-HSS. In addition to these references, the researchers provided four references to studies using the MBI-HSS with other healthcare worker populations. In this example, the researchers referenced earlier research demonstrating the applicability of the instrument with the group they studied. However, they did not mention if they performed any confirmatory analysis on the instrument's reliability and factors. The similarity between emergency medicine physicians and physician assistants might be sufficient for us as readers to accept that the instrument was appropriate for this study, but if they had performed validity and factor analysis testing we would not have to rely on that assumption.

When researchers develop and utilize their own instrument, it is critical that they report the results of instrument validity and factor analysis. Furthermore, the researchers should clearly identify the instrument as being newly developed. Before usage with the subjects of interest, researchers should perform several phases of instrument testing, including face validity testing, internal consistency testing, and external validity testing. They should explain the reason for creating a new instrument, namely that there was not an instrument already available or the cost of available instruments prohibited the completion of the study.

Additionally, separate studies should be conducted in order to develop the instrument so that it measures what it is intended to measure without redundancy. This means that there should not be more items on a survey than needed. Factor analysis allows researchers to determine which items provide the maximum information without overestimating subjects' responses. With the MBI-HSS, for example, the researchers were able to reduce the number of questions through multiple factor analysis studies and synthesize the instrument to the smallest number of questions.[29] The fewer the number of questions, the more likely subjects are to complete the survey and to remain focused while answering questions. However, it is possible to have an insufficient number of items and not collect enough information. A rule of thumb for construct validity is that instruments include at least three to four items per domain.

CHAPTER SUMMARY

Inferential statistics allow researchers to make inferences about a population based on results from a sample. These inferences lead to conclusions, such as whether a new drug is safe in comparison to a placebo, if a new treatment is as effective as the usual care, or if one diagnostic procedure is as accurate as another, and so on. A number of considerations must be taken into account when designing a research study with regard to inferential statistics, including sampling procedures (sample size, effect size, and the nature of the sampling frame), the type of sampling (simple random sample, multistage sampling, nonprobability sampling, convenience sampling, purposive sampling, and snowball sampling), the type of data (parametric or nonparametric), the level of alpha set in the design of the study, the *p*-values and confidence intervals associated with the resulting test statistics, and the types of tests performed (differences, relationships, regression analysis, reliability, validity, factor analysis, and so on.).

The type of data, the sample size, the shape of the distribution, and the type of research question determine the type of statistical test performed. Each statistical test has a set of characteristics referred to as assumptions that determine its usage. Researchers should determine the statistical tests to be used during the planning phase of the study and verify that the data meet the assumptions of the tests. This verification step should occur at the start of the study and at important end points, depending on the duration of the study.

The statistical test produces a test statistic, a *p*-value, and usually a confidence interval. The *p*-value for the test statistic is compared to alpha to make the determination of significance. If the *p*-value associated with the test statistic is less than alpha (or alpha halves), then the result is deemed statistically significant. Alpha halves should be used for studies in which a test of equality is performed, in which case the *p*-value of the test statistic must be less than half of alpha in order to be deemed statistically significant. The confidence interval tells us the range in which the true population

parameter exists with a given percentage likelihood. For example, a 95% confidence interval tells us that the test statistic will fall within the given range 95% of the time. The more narrow a confidence interval, the more trustworthy the test statistic.

Inferential statistics encompass a variety of statistical test categories, including tests for differences, tests for relationships, regression analysis, reliability and validity, factor analysis, and more. Each category includes numerous types of statistical tests that each apply to specific situations and types of data. Every statistical test has a set of assumptions that must be met in order for the test to produce valid results. Researchers should test the data from a study for satisfaction of these assumptions and report the results of assumption checks. It is important for clinicians to have professional relationships with research design experts and statisticians who can assist with interpretation of the statistics presented in publications and presentations. Furthermore, the better your understanding of statistics and research design, the more you will glean from the publications you read and the presentations you attend—and the better you will be able to engage in an evidence-based practice.

EXERCISES

Matching

Match the vocabulary term to its definition.

Vocabulary Terms	Definitions
1. Factor analysis	A. A type of repeated measures test where measures are taken over time and results are compared from one time point to another.
2. Sample size	B. A procedure for combining items in a survey instrument to represent a single concept (called a construct or domain).
3. Confidence interval	C. The probability of a Type I error.
4. Effect size	D. Data that are assumed to be (any one or more of the following): nominal or ordinal scale; non-normal shape (skewed); small sample size; or if there is more than one group, the groups have differing variability, shapes, or sample sizes.
5. *p*-value	E. A sampling procedure that occurs in one or more steps.
6. Inferential statistics	F. A group of tests used with nonparametric data.
7. Stratified random sample	G. The numerical outcome (such as a *t*-score, an F ratio, or a chi-square score) of a significance test.
	H. The rule of a normal distribution that states the proportion of observations between -1σ and $+1\sigma$ is 68%, -2σ and $+2\sigma$ is 95%, and -3σ and $+3\sigma$ is 99.7%.

8. Independent-samples *t*-test
   I. A form of probability sampling that allows every member of the population to have an equal chance of being selected for the study.

9. Sampling frame
   J. A quantitative test that compares the mean score of a sample to the known mean (normative or expected) from a trustworthy source.

10. Paired-samples *t*-test
   K. Statistical tests that assume the data to have all of the following characteristics: continuous or interval scale; normal in shape (or nearly normal); sufficient sample size; and if there is more than one group, each group has the same (or nearly the same) amount of variability, the same shape, and the same (or nearly the same) sample size.

11. Alpha
   L. The number of subjects included in a study.

12. Nonparametric data
   M. A test for relationship between two variables that are continuous, interval, or ratio data types.

13. Multistage sample
   N. The risk of a Type I error when a test of equality is performed.

14. Chi square
   O. A test that compares a statistic, such as a mean or a proportion, between two or more groups.

15. Test statistic
   P. The set of parameters that govern the application of each statistical test.

16. 68-95-99.7 rule
   Q. A type of purposive sampling used in quantitative research when the researchers are interested in studying a population that is difficult to identify. Those identified initially are asked to identify others who are then added to the sample, and then those added are asked to identify other acquaintances, and so on, until a sufficient sample size is achieved to achieve statistical power.

17. Simple random sample
   R. A test to compare means between independent variables with similar variance and normality of distribution with more than two groups.

18. One-sample *t*-test
   S. The probability that the test statistic will fall within a specific range.

19. Parametric statistics
   T. An element in a power calculation that includes the expected amount of effect.

20. Pearson product-moment
   U. The percentage of chance that the test statistic occurred naturally, representing normal random variation.

21. Alpha halves
   V. A type of statistics that allows researchers to make inferences about a population based on results in a sample.

22. Test of differences
   W. A procedure through which the sampling frame is divided into groupings based on a characteristic and a random sample is drawn from each.

23. Assumptions
24. Snowball sample
   X. An inferential statistical test used to compare the means of two independent groups.

   Y. A list or other record of all the elements in the population from which the sampling units are drawn.

25. ANOVA

Multiple Choice

1. The authors of a study set alpha at 0.05. If the null hypothesis was a test of equality, what is alpha halves?
   a. 0.05
   b. 0.01
   c. 0.10
   d. 0.025
   e. It cannot be determined based on the information provided.

2. What percentage of observations in a normal distribution fall between –2 SD and +2 SD?
   a. 50%
   b. 68%
   c. 95%

    d. 99.7%

    e. None of the above

3. A p-value of 0.060 resulted from a test for inequality (a one-tailed significance test). The p-value was statistically significant. What level of alpha must have been used?

    a. 0.05

    b. 0.01

    c. 0.0010

    d. 0.10

    e. None of the above

4. Identify the test statistic in the following statement: "Prevalence of hypercholesterolemia was not different between men and women. Chi-square value was 2.93 (p = 0.23)."

    a. 2.93

    b. Prevalence

    c. 0.23

    d. Hypercholesterolemia

    e. There is no test statistic included in this statement.

5. A p-value of 0.040 resulted from a test for equality (a two-tailed significance test). The p-value was statistically significant. What level of alpha must have been used?

    a. 0.05

    b. 0.01

    c. 0.10

    d. 0.001

    e. None of the above

6. "Prevalence of hypercholesterolemia was not different between men and women. Chi-square value was 2.93 (p = 0.23)." Based on this statement, if alpha was set at 0.05 and the test was one of equality, which of the following is true of the result?

    a. It is not statistically significant.

    b. It is statistically significant.

    c. The result is not given.

    d. The result is equal between men and women.

    e. It is an example of a paired-samples t-test.

7. If the Pearson correlation coefficient is r = 0.86, what is the coefficient of determination?

    a. 0.05

    b. 68%

    c. 0.025

    d. 0.86

    e. 0.74

8. Identify the p-value in the following statement: "Prevalence of hypercholesterolemia was not different between men and women. Chi-square value was 2.93 (p = 0.23)."

    a. Men and women

    b. 2.93

    c. 0.23

    d. Chi square

    e. There is no p-value in this statement.

9. Based on the confidence interval and the other details provided below, which of the following statements is true?

    • HDL-C levels (mg/dL) for SuperStatin increased by 20%

    • HDL-C levels (mg/dL) for BogusStatin increased by 15%

    • p = .02; MD = 5% (95% CI: $+/-$ 3%)

    • α < 0.05

    a. Although the difference is statistically significant, the confidence interval indicates that the two treatments might not be different if the study was performed again.

    b. The confidence interval supports the statement that SuperStatin increases HDL-C significantly more than BogusStatin.

    c. The confidence interval supports the statement that BogusStatin increases HDL-C significantly more than SuperStatin.

    d. The confidence interval provides no additional information than the p-value about the difference between these treatments.

    e. The confidence interval indicates that a one-tailed test must have been performed.

10. In a study looking at sleep-disordered breathing among patients with normal versus high triglycerides, the researchers found that those with high triglycerides had 3.92 greater odds (p < 0.001) of experiencing sleep-disordered breathing compared to those with normal triglycerides (95% CI: 2.98–5.16). Which of the following statements is true?

    a. Although the difference is statistically significant, the confidence interval indicates that the two groups might not be different if the study was performed again.

b. The confidence interval supports the statement that those with high triglycerides are significantly more likely to experience sleep-disordered breathing, even if the study was repeated many times.

c. The confidence interval supports the statement that those with high triglycerides are not more likely to experience sleep-disordered breathing if the study was repeated.

d. The confidence interval provides no additional information than the p-value about the difference between the two groups.

e. The confidence interval indicates that alpha was set at 0.05.

REFERENCES

1. Evans K, Howlett B. Thyroid hormone level correlations in a sample of patients at an internal medicine practice. March 2012. National Conference on Undergraduate Research 2012. Ogden, UT.

2. Chakera AJ, Pearce SHS, Vaidya B. Treatment for primary hypothyroidism: Current approaches and future possibilities. *Drug Des Devel Ther*. 2012;6:1–11.

3. BMJ Evidence Center. *Thyroid function testing*. Updated October 21, 2011. Available at: http://bestpractice.bmj .com. Accessed May 15, 2012.

4. Wehling E, Lundervold AJ, Standnes B, Gjerstad L, Reinvang I. APOE status and its association to learning and memory performance in middle aged and older Norwegians seeking assessment for memory deficits. *Behav Brain Funct*. 2007;3:57.

5. American Diabetes Association. Diabetes statistics. January 26, 2011. Available at: www.diabetes.org /diabetes-basics/diabetes-statistics/. Accessed January 29, 2012.

6. Centers for Disease Control and Prevention. Summary health statistics for U.S. adults: National Health Interview Survey, 2010. *Vital Health Stat*. 2012;10(252). Available at: www.cdc.gov/nchs/data /series/sr_10/sr10_252.pdf. Accessed May 12, 2012.

7. GraphPad. Quick answers database: Relationship between statistical power and beta. FAQ 1711. Available at: www.graphpad.com. Accessed May 23, 2012.

8. Slade M, Bird V, Le Boutillier C, Williams J, McCrone P, Leamy M. REFOCUS Trial: protocol for a cluster randomised controlled trial of a pro-recovery intervention within community based mental health teams. *BMC Psychiatry*. 2011;11:185.

9. Cocks K, King MT, Velikova G, Martyn St. James M, Fayers PM, Brown JM. Evidence-based guidelines for determination of sample size and interpretation of the European Organisation for the Research and Treatment of Cancer Quality of Life Questionnaire Core 30. *J Clin Oncol*. 2011;29(1): 89–96.

10. Gomes M, Ramacciotti E, Hoppensteadt D, et al. An open label, non-randomized, prospective clinical trial evaluating the immunogenicity of branded enoxaparin versus biosimilars in healthy volunteers. *Clin Appl Thromb Hemost*. 2011;17(1):66–69.

11. Vogt WP, Johnson RB. *Dictionary of statistics and methodology: A nontechnical guide for the social sciences*. 4th ed. Los Angeles: Sage; 2011.

12. National Institutes of Health. MedlinePlus: *Enoxaparin injection*. Last reviewed September 1, 2010. Available at: www.nlm.nih.gov/medlineplus /druginfo/meds/a601210.html. Accessed January 23, 2011.

13. LoBiondo-Wood G, Haber J. *Nursing research: Methods and critical appraisal for evidence-based practice*. 6th ed. St. Louis: Mosby; 2006.

14. Digel A. *Perceptions of persons with schizophrenia relating to their weight*. A thesis submitted to the School of Nursing at Queen's University in Kingston, Ontario, Canada.

15. Kaplan A. Consensus panel urges monitoring for metabolic effects of atypical antipsychotics. *Psychiatric Times*. 2004;21(4):1–6.

16. Ogden CL, Fryar CD, Carroll MD, Flegal KM. CDC. Mean body weight, height, and body mass index, United States 1960–2002. *Adv Data Vital Health Stat*. 2004;347:1–18.

17. National Library of Medicine. *Marfan syndrome*. Last reviewed May 20, 2010. Available at: www .ncbi.nlm.nih.gov/. Accessed May 28, 2012.

18. Hung TC, Tang HS, Chiu CH, Chen YY, Chou KR, Chiou HC, Chang HJ. Anxiety, depressive symptom, and suicidal ideation of outpatients with obsessive compulsive disorders in Taiwan. *J Clin Nurs*. 2010;19(21–22):3092–3101.

19. Cerniauskaite M, Quintas R, Koutsogeorgou E, et al. Quality of life and disability in patients with stroke. *Am J Phys Med Rehab*. 2012;91(13 Suppl 1):S39–47.

20. Rezakhaniha B, Arianpour N, Siroosbakhat S. Efficacy of desmopressin in treatment of nocturia in elderly men. *J Res Med Sci*. 2011;16(4): 516–523.

21. The Cleveland Clinic. Diseases and conditions: *Nocturia*. Available at: http://my.clevelandclinic .org/disorders/nocturia/hic_nocturia.aspx. Accessed February 12, 2012.

22. Madani AS, Mirmortazavi A. Comparison of three treatment options for painful temporomandibular joint clicking. *J Oral Sci.* 2011;53(3):349–354.

23. Porta M. (Ed). *A dictionary of epidemiology.* 5th ed. Oxford, England: Oxford University Press; 2008.

24. Stevens-Labsley JE, Balter JE, Wolfe P, Eckhoff DG, Kohrt WM. Early neuromuscular electrical stimulation of improve quadriceps muscle strength after total knee arthroplasty: A randomized controlled trial. *Phys Ther.* 2012;92(2):210–226.

25. Farlex. The free dictionary. Arthroplasty. Available at: http://medical-dictionary.thefreedictionary.com/arthroplasty. Accessed May 24, 2012.

26. Palmer SH, Cross MJ. *Total knee arthroplasty.* Updated February 24, 2012. Available at: http://emedicine.medscape.com. Accessed May 24, 2012.

27. White C. Research on smoking and lung cancer: A landmark in the history of chronic disease epidemiology. *Yale J Biol Med.* 1990;63:29–46.

28. Bell RB, Davison M, Sefcik, D. A first survey measuring burnout in emergency medicine physician assistants. *JAAPA.* 2002;15(3):40–55.

29. Maslach C, Jackon SE, Leiter MP, Schaufeli WB, Schwab RL. *Maslach burnout inventory.* Menlo Park, CA: Mind Garden; 1986.

ANSWERS TO EXERCISES

Matching

1. B
2. L
3. S
4. T
5. U
6. V
7. W
8. X
9. Y
10. A
11. C
12. D
13. E
14. F
15. G
16. H
17. I
18. J
19. K
20. M
21. N
22. O
23. P
24. Q
25. R

Multiple Choice

1. d
2. c
3. d
4. a
5. c
6. a
7. e
8. c
9. a
10. b

APPLICATIONS OF EVIDENCE-BASED PRACTICE

INTRODUCTION

The second section of this text shifts the focus from providing foundational concepts to exploring concrete applications of evidence-based practice (EBP). First, we present a chapter on epidemiology (Chapter 7), followed by chapters on assessment and diagnosis (Chapter 8), treatment, harm, and prevention (Chapter 9), and pharmaceutical information (Chapter 10). Finally, the text closes with a culminating chapter that synthesizes the textbook overall (Chapter 11). Several overarching concepts in Part II apply to multiple chapters in this section of the text. As such, we will address them here.

ETHICAL PRINCIPLES IN BIOMEDICAL RESEARCH

Before we get into the application chapters of this book, note that one concept applies to all of these chapters: research ethics. When research designs are unethical we are presented with two questions. The first is whether to use the results of the research to inform clinical decisions. The second is whether the results of such studies are valid. For example, from 1932 to 1972 the Public Health Service in Alabama conducted a study on the progression of syphilis, which is often fatal if left untreated.[1] The researchers enrolled 399 African American adult males who had contracted the disease as well as 201 men who were free of the disease. They did not tell the subjects if they had the disease, and they did not provide treatment. In the first 8 to 10 years of the study, no definitive treatment was available for the disease.

By the mid-1940s, however, a standard treatment for syphilis was readily available (penicillin).[1] The intention of the **Tuskegee syphilis study**, as the study came to be called, was to understand the incidence and progression of the disease. The study was closed in 1972 after *The New York Times* ran stories about the study based on accounts provided by a whistleblower (Peter Buxtun), who had been working to get the study closed since 1966. It is estimated that between 28 and more than 100 of the subjects died from the disease and that many others were infected with it, including the men's wives and some of their children who contracted the disease in utero. Accurate records were kept; therefore, the numbers of deaths and infections resulting from the study are not known.

Findings from the study were published numerous times over its 40-year course.[1] The questions for us today include the following: Should the results of the Tuskegee syphilis study be used to improve our strategies for diagnosing and treating the disease? What rights do the survivors and their descendants have in deciding if the results should be used? Should the publications from the study be retracted? Many healthcare workers, policy makers, and researchers have read the publications of the Tuskegee syphilis study. If you were a reader of a publication in which it appeared that unethical practices had been utilized, what would you do? What choices would you have?

Unfortunately, many published examples of unethical research practices are available, such as the research performed by Dr. Josef Mengele in the Auschwitz Nazi concentration camp. Another salient example offered by Grodin and Glantz[2] related to diagnostic research was a study conducted by Arthur Howard Wentworth in 1896. Wentworth performed lumbar punctures on 45 children to determine if the procedure had an "unfavorable response." The first child on whom he attempted this procedure had a "questionable case of tubercular meningitis." She was free of the disease. He deemed the procedure harmless despite the pain it caused. However, he also demonstrated the diagnostic value of the procedure. It must be emphasized that these procedures were performed on children for whom there was no indication for the test. The children's parents had not been informed and had not given their permission.

Many of the regulations associated with biomedical research, as well as organizations such as the Food and Drug Administration (FDA), have come into existence as the result of harmful or questionable studies. In 1974, the National Research Act was signed into federal law. In 1979, the National Commission for the Protection of Human Subjects of Biomedical and Behavioral Research published a report entitled the Belmont Report.[3] The commission was created in response to news articles revealing the 40-year study in Tuskegee,[4] Alabama, that had followed men with syphilis without providing treatment or informing the patients, or their spouses, of the men's diagnosis.

Even after penicillin became available to treat syphilis in 1947, the men in the study were not offered the medication. In 1968, concerns were raised with the CDC about the Tuskegee syphilis study.[4] However, in 1969 the CDC affirmed the need for the research, with the official support of local medical societies (the American Medical Association and National Medical Association), and the study was allowed to continue.

A federal panel had been instituted in 1972 in response to the Associated Press articles and had recommended that the study be stopped because the harm to the subjects and their family members far outweighed the benefits of the research. In November of 1972, the study was discontinued by the Assistant Secretary for Health and Scientific Affairs. Five years later the Belmont Report was released and has been publicly available ever since.

When you read health-related research publications, you should evaluate the research in terms of the ethical principles and standards outlined in the Belmont Report. The Belmont Report[3] detailed three ethical principles for biomedical research as well as three applications of the standards. The three basic ethical principles include:

1. Respect for persons
2. Beneficence
3. Justice

The report also detailed three essential applications of these ethical principles:

1. Informed consent
2. Assessment of risks and benefits
3. Selection of subjects

According to the report, the three ethical principles are explained as follows:[3]

> *Respect for Persons. Respect for persons incorporates at least two ethical convictions: first, that individuals should be treated as autonomous agents, and second, that persons with diminished autonomy are entitled to protection. The principle of respect for persons thus divides into two separate moral requirements: the requirement to acknowledge autonomy and the requirement to protect those with diminished autonomy.*
>
> *Beneficence. Persons are treated in an ethical manner not only by respecting their decisions and protecting them from harm, but also by making efforts to secure their well-being. Such treatment falls under the principle of beneficence. The term "beneficence" is often understood to cover acts of kindness or charity that go beyond strict obligation. In this document, beneficence is understood in a stronger sense, as an obligation. Two general rules have been formulated as complementary expressions of beneficent actions in this sense: (1) do not harm and (2) maximize possible benefits and minimize possible harms.*
>
> *Justice. Who ought to receive the benefits of research and bear its burdens? This is a question of justice, in the sense of "fairness in distribution" or "what is deserved." An injustice occurs when some benefit to which a person is entitled is denied without good reason or when some burden is imposed unduly. Another way of conceiving the principle of justice is that equals ought to be treated equally. However, this statement requires explication. Who is equal and who is unequal? What considerations justify departure from equal distribution? Almost all commentators allow that distinctions based on experience, age, deprivation, competence, merit and position do sometimes constitute criteria justifying differential treatment for certain purposes. It is necessary, then, to explain in what respects people should be treated equally. There are several widely accepted formulations of just ways to distribute burdens and benefits. Each formulation mentions some relevant property on the basis of which burdens and benefits should be distributed. These formulations are (1) to each person an equal share, (2) to each person according to individual need, (3) to each person according to individual effort, (4) to each person according to societal contribution, and (5) to each person according to merit.*

In practice, these principles require that subjects be properly informed and that their consent be secured prior to participating in the study. The Belmont Report explains, "Respect for persons requires that subjects, to the degree that they are capable, be given the opportunity to choose what shall or shall not happen to them. This opportunity is provided when adequate standards for informed consent are satisfied."[3] The information provided through the informed consent process must fully disclose the procedures, risks, and benefits of the study (except under certain circumstances), be comprehensible to the subject, and ensure that the subject is aware of his or her right to withdraw from the study without negative repercussions.

One exception exists regarding informed consent, which allows researchers to deceive the subjects about the true purpose of a study. In some instances it is necessary to withhold the study's purpose or research question from subjects in order to avoid bias. For example, if self-reported data are utilized (such as pain scales) subjects might respond differently when they know the purpose of the study. There are guidelines that researchers must follow when utilizing deception. The deception cannot itself increase the risk of harm, and subjects must be informed upon completion of the trial about the true study purpose.

The investigator must be sure the subject understands the purpose of the research, other than when an approved deception is used, as well as the nature and scope of both risks and benefits for participating. In preparing for the study, the investigator must perform a systematic assessment of risks and benefits and disclose them to a review board, which has authority to approve or disapprove the study before any subjects are recruited.

Lastly, the selection of subjects for a study must be fair. Potentially beneficial research should be equally available to all individuals, and potential harm must be risked equally by all individuals. Disparities might not exist based on social, racial, sexual, or cultural biases. Furthermore, certain groups, such as institutionalized individuals, children, and pregnant women, are considered *vulnerable* and must be given special consideration. Their inclusion in research must be carefully considered and justified. The Belmont Report explains:[3]

> *Social justice requires that distinction be drawn between classes of subjects that ought, and ought not, to participate in any particular kind of research, based on the ability of members of that class to bear burdens and on the appropriateness of placing further burdens on already burdened persons. Thus, it can be considered a matter of social justice that there is an order of preference in the selection of classes of subjects (e.g., adults before children) and that some classes of potential subjects (e.g., the institutionalized mentally infirm or prisoners) may be involved as research subjects, if at all, only on certain conditions.*

You can read the full Belmont Report online. As of the writing of this chapter, the Belmont Report is located at www.hhs.gov/ohrp/humansubjects/guidance/belmont.html#xrespect.

The offer to participate in a study must be free of coercion and undue influence. Coercion can involve excessive enticements to participate in research, such as free health care, free products, or even money. Incentives are allowed, so long as they do not create undue influence. Institutional Review Boards (IRBs) review the incentives offered to subjects and make the determination as to whether they represent undue influence.

Another potential source of undue influence can come from the clinician–patient relationship. Patients might agree to participate in a study simply because their provider suggested it to them. There is greater power differential in the clinician–patient relationship than in the relationship between a patient and an unknown researcher. As such, the IRB reviews materials and procedures utilized for recruitment of subjects in order to avoid undue influence and ensure that patient autonomy and self-determination are maintained. An IRB helps researchers ensure compliance with the three basic ethical principles and the three essential applications of the principles from the Belmont Report, as well as other human protection codes or standards.

The Tuskegee syphilis study was sadly not the first instance of harmful biomedical research, nor the last. The Nuremberg Code was established in 1947 in response to horrific experiments performed by Nazi doctors. The Nuremberg Code[5] includes

10 principles for medical research, such as informed consent, lack of coercion, and the need for benefits to outweigh harm. In response to the harm caused by thalidomide, in 1962 the U.S. Congress passed the Kefauver-Harris amendments[6] to the 1938 Food, Drug and Cosmetic Act, which strengthened the government's ability to oversee drug testing and created a legal requirement for informed consent. Unfortunately, the Tuskegee syphilis study proceeded for 10 more years after the Kefauver-Harris amendments because of its noninterventional research design, in spite of laws and international codes in place at the time.

In 1981, FDA regulations were revised to enable the agency to provide oversight of IRBs. The 1974 National Research Act required implementation of IRBs, and the 1981 regulations provided a standardized and centralized means for governing them. IRBs are groups empowered with approval or disapproval of proposed human subject research.[6] Any research institution receiving federal funding must have IRB policies and procedures in place. Researchers must receive IRB approval before implementing research involving human subjects. Other types of research also require IRB approval, such as animal research. Among other considerations, IRBs evaluate proposed research in terms of the criteria outlined in the Belmont Report. Every publication of research involving human subjects should identify the IRB that approved the study and provide the approval number.

ROLE OF THE FOOD AND DRUG ADMINISTRATION

Drug manufacturers as well manufacturers of medical devices must register with the **FDA (Food the Drug Administration)** and gain approval prior to marketing their products. FDA approval is required for most medications, for many medical devices, and for many other products (such as vaccines, blood and biologics, and radiation-emitting products). Those items falling under FDA regulation must be researched via preclinical as well as clinical trials for safety and efficacy before they are approved for human use. The FDA categorizes clinical trials into five types: Treatment Trials, Prevention Trials, Diagnostic Trials, Screening Trials, and Quality of Life Trials. The FDA website[7] explains its regulatory role as follows:

> *Some products—such as new drugs and complex medical devices—must be proven safe and effective before companies can put them on the market. The agency also must approve new food additives before they can be used in foods. Other products—such as x-ray machines and microwave ovens—must measure up to performance standards. And some products—such as cosmetics and dietary supplements—can generally be marketed with no prior approval.*

At the heart of all FDA's medical product evaluation decisions is a judgment about whether a new product's benefits to users will outweigh its risks. No regulated product is totally risk-free, so these judgments are important. The FDA will allow a product to present more of a risk when its potential benefit is great—especially for products used to treat serious, life-threatening conditions.

The FDA reviews the results of laboratory, animal, and human clinical testing done by companies to determine if the product they want to put on the market is safe and effective. The FDA does not develop or test products itself. The agency does this premarket review for new human drugs and biologics (such as vaccines, blood products, biotechnology products, and gene therapy), complex medical devices, food and color additives, infant formulas, and animal drugs.

The FDA has streamlined its review process for medical products in recent years to help speed up the availability of important new treatments to patients. For example, the average review time for an innovative new drug is now only 6 months, and some have been approved even faster.

Manufacturers must complete clinical trials as deemed necessary by the FDA. These clinical trials are registered and posted online at ClinicalTrials.gov. You might find the information on the ClinicalTrials.gov website helpful in determining how a given FDA regulated treatment was studied prior to marketing the product. ClinicalTrials.gov is a useful resource when you are learning about a new treatment, diagnostic, prevention, or screening tool. The process of gaining FDA approval typically involves a minimum of four phases of study, and sometimes also requires a fifth phase. The phases are defined by the National Institutes of Health as follows:[8]

- In **Preclinical trials**, testing is performed with experimental drugs in the test tube or in animals. Preclinical trials include testing that occurs before trials in humans may be carried out.
- In *Phase I trials*, researchers test an experimental drug or treatment in a small group of people (20–80) for the first time to evaluate its safety, determine a safe dosage range, and identify side effects. Phase I trials are initial studies to determine the metabolism and pharmacologic actions of drugs in humans, the side effects associated with increasing doses, and to gain early evidence of effectiveness; they may include healthy participants and/or patients.
- In *Phase II trials*, the experimental study drug or treatment is given to a larger group of people (100–300) to see if it is effective and to further evaluate its safety. Phase II trials are controlled clinical studies conducted to evaluate the effectiveness of the drug for a particular indication or indications in patients with the disease or condition under study and to determine the common short-term side effects and risks.
- In *Phase III trials*, the experimental study drug or treatment is given to large groups of people (1,000–3,000) to confirm its effectiveness, monitor side effects, compare it to commonly used treatments, and collect information that will allow the experimental drug or treatment to be used safely. Phase III trials are expanded controlled and uncontrolled trials after preliminary evidence suggesting effectiveness of the drug has been obtained, and are intended to gather additional information to evaluate the overall benefit-risk relationship of the drug and provide an adequate basis for physician labeling.
- In *Phase IV trials*, postmarketing studies delineate additional information, including the drug's risks, benefits, and optimal use. *Postmarketing* means after the treatment has been marketed to the public. Postmarketing studies are important because they add information about how the general population responds to a treatment, as opposed to the highly selected set of subjects included in earlier-phase clinical trials. Postmarketing studies tend to be quasi-experimental, with fewer controls. As such, patients with more complex

health problems can be included in postmarketing research. A treatment can be recalled after FDA approval as a result of postmarketing research.

REFERENCES

1. Heintzelman CA. The Tuskegee syphilis study and its implications for the 21st century. *The New Social Worker*. 2003;10(4). Available at: www.socialworker.com/tuskegee.htm. Accessed May 15, 2012.
2. Grodin MA, Glantz LH (eds). *Children as research subjects: Science, ethics, and law*. Oxford: Oxford University Press; 1994.
3. U.S. Department of Health and Human Services. The Belmont Report. April 18, 1979. Available at: www.hhs.gov/ohrp/humansubjects/guidance/belmont.html. Accessed September 11, 2012.
4. Centers for Disease Control and Prevention. U.S. public health service syphilis study at Tuskegee. Updated June 15, 2011. Available at: www.cdc.gov/tuskegee/timeline.htm/. Accessed September 11, 2012.
5. U.S. Department of Health and Human Services. The Nuremburg Code. [ND]. Available at: http://history.nih.gov/research/downloads/nuremberg.pdf. Accessed September 11, 2012.
6. Sparks J. Timeline of laws related to the protection of human subjects. June 2002. Available at: http://history.nih.gov/about/timelines_laws_human.html. Accessed September 11, 2012.
7. U.S. Food and Drug Administration. About FDA product approval. Updated February 26, 2009. Available at: www.fda.gov/NewsEvents/ProductsApprovals/ucm106288.htm. Accessed September 11, 2012.
8. National Institutes of Health. Understanding clinical trials. Updated September 20, 2007. Available at: http://clinicaltrials.gov/ct2/info/understand/#Q18. Accessed September 11, 2012.

Epidemiology in Evidence-Based Practice

Gloria A. Jones Taylor, DSN, RN; Barbara J. Blake, PhD, RN, ACRN;
and D. Dennis Flores, BSN, ACRN

INTRODUCTION

Epidemiology is "the study of diseases in populations and the evaluation of interventions at a population level, as a method of solving the problems of diseases in individuals."[1] This chapter provides a brief history of epidemiology and describes the types of studies used to perform epidemiological research, the limitations of the study types, the functions of epidemiological research (such as establishing risk factors and determining a prognosis), statistics commonly reported in epidemiological studies, the role of risk factors (such as demographic, sociocultural, and geographic variables), and how to locate epidemiological studies. Understanding the statistics reported in epidemiological research is key to engaging in evidence-based practice (EBP). As such, a significant portion of the chapter focuses on statistics that are commonly reported in epidemiological studies. This chapter also provides examples of their use in published research. The statistics discussed include sensitivity, specificity, positive predictive value (PPV), negative predictive value (NPV), relative risk (RR), the odds ratio (OR), attributable risk (AR), attribut-

able risk percent (AR%), population attributable risk (PAR), population attributable risk percent (PAR%), incidence, prevalence, and confidence intervals.

HISTORY OF EPIDEMIOLOGY

Around 400 B.C., Hippocrates postulated on the relationship between disease and the physical environment—a significant break from the supernatural explanations of disease causation at that time.[2] In its modern form, epidemiology is primarily concerned with identifying important factors or variables that influence health outcomes.[3] In essence, epidemiologists are medical detectives tasked with figuring out the who, what, where, when, and how of disease causation.[4] Epidemiology practitioners borrow concepts and methods from other disciplines, including biology, sociology, and statistics, to identify factors related to a health issue within a defined population.[5,6] The ultimate goals of epidemiological studies include disease control, elimination, or eradication.

The Industrial Revolution in the mid-nineteenth century marked unprecedented economic growth in England. With business booming and labor in high demand, people in the countryside moved to the increasingly crowded streets of London to earn a living. The conditions in those areas became deplorable, because waste disposal, sanitation, and water quality were not being addressed effectively. The dominant belief then was that whenever somebody fell ill, a sickening vapor called *miasma* was the culprit. Assumed to emanate from decaying by-products of urban living, people regarded this noxious air as the cause of any and all physical maladies.[7]

The word *epidemiology* was first introduced around 1850 during the early years of the London Epidemiological Society.[7] *Epidemiology* comes from the Greek words, *epi*, which means "upon"; *demos*, pertaining to "people"; and *logos*, which is "the study of." In many ways, the early days of epidemiology represented the first concrete application of EBP. For example, out of the slums of working-class neighborhoods in London arose a cholera outbreak. This compelled **John Snow**, a physician, to track the residences of persons who became sick and died. From his meticulous accounting, a pattern emerged that eventually led to closure of the Broad Street water pump, which was identified as the source of contaminated water. In Victorian London, this pioneering man established the first examples of epidemiology's utility. Two years after Snow's cholera outbreak studies (1848–1849 and 1853–1854), legislation mandated that all water companies in London use sand filters and chlorine to disinfect the water. However, it would take another 26 years before Robert Koch would identify the organism causing these outbreaks, *Vibrio cholerae*.[8]

Sir Austin Bradford Hill, a British medical statistician, developed criteria on the association between disease and the environment, which became the seminal guideline for causation, *The Environment and Disease: Association or Causation?* Hill was instrumental in the introduction of randomized clinical trials as the "gold standard" when conducting research to test the efficacy of a proposed health intervention. In the 1950s, he was active in exploring the link between cigarette smoking and lung cancer.[9]

Epidemiological studies are relied upon when addressing disease and transmission patterns. Methodological investigation of the history and characteristics of persons living with HIV/AIDS provided evidence that the transfer of infected blood through transfusions, needle sharing, and sexual contact were the primary methods by which HIV was transmitted.[10] Over time, knowledge of disease distribution has become a necessity for effective planning and delivery of health care. Diminishing resources and tension between a population's healthcare demands and limited supply has underscored epidemiology's indispensability.

The Healthy People Program

One of the most ambitious applications of epidemiological research is exemplified by the Healthy People program. The goal of this federal program is as follows:

> *Healthy People provides science-based, 10-year national objectives for improving the health of all Americans. For three decades, Healthy People has established benchmarks and monitored progress over time in order to:*

- *Encourage collaborations across communities and sectors.*
- *Empower individuals to make informed health decisions.*
- *Measure the impact of prevention activities.*[11]

The program is in its third decade and has included four decade-long initiatives: Healthy People 1990, Healthy People 2000, Healthy People 2010, and Healthy People 2020.

Epidemiological research provides the foundation for measuring the effectiveness of Healthy People initiatives, and it informs the selection of Healthy People objectives. Healthy People 2020 includes nearly 600 objectives with over 1,300 measures.[11] Federal, state, and private funding of health research and public health intervention programs are determined in large part by the Healthy People objectives. This program both informs and drives not only funding, but also policy. The U.S. Department of Health and Human Services' prevention efforts are derived from this national health initiative, including efforts such as the Tobacco Control Strategic Action Plan, the Initiative on Multiple Chronic Conditions, and the Public Health System, Finance, and Quality Program (to name a few). To learn more about Healthy People 2020, visit www.healthypeople.gov.

Healthy People 2020 features 42 health topics. The following are several examples of Healthy People 2020 objectives:[11]

- *Adolescent Health Objective AH-1:* Increase the proportion of adolescents who have had a wellness checkup in the past 12 months.
- *Cancer Objective C-1:* Reduce the overall cancer death rate.
- *Diabetes Objective D-1:* Reduce the annual number of new cases of diagnosed diabetes in the population.
- *Healthcare-Associated Infections Objective HAI-1:* Reduce central line–associated bloodstream infections (CLABSI).
- *Nutrition and Weight Status Objective NWS-1:* Increase the number of states with nutrition standards for foods and beverages provided to preschool-aged children in child care.
- *Oral Health Objective OH-1.1:* Reduce the proportion of young children aged 3 to 5 years with dental caries experience in their primary teeth.
- *Sleep Health Objective SH-1:* Increase the proportion of persons with symptoms of obstructive sleep apnea who seek medical evaluation.

Each objective is supported by epidemiological research. For example, regarding Sleep Health Objective SH-1, the Healthy People website reports that, "25.5 percent of persons with symptoms of obstructive sleep apnea sought medical evaluation in 2005–08 (age adjusted to the year 2000 standard population)." This information was derived from research by the National Health and Nutrition Survey (NHANES), the Centers for Disease Control and Prevention (CDC), and the National Center for Health Statistics (NCHS).

IMPORTANT EPIDEMIOLOGICAL CONCEPTS

There are several important concepts to epidemiology, including case definition, web of causation, and the epidemiological triad of disease. These concepts are foundational to the field of epidemiology. Each term is defined and explained below.

Case Definition

A **case definition** is a set of standard criteria for classifying whether a person has a particular disease, syndrome, or health condition.[12] It is a working definition that researchers have agreed upon as the basic unit of study. A case definition provides parameters for comparing cases across time and place. During outbreaks of disease, the case definition is tentative, because modifications might be carried out as more accurate data are compiled.[13]

Case definitions are essential for tracking the number of people afflicted with a particular illness, often called **disease surveillance**. In 1982, for example, the CDC simply defined AIDS as: "A disease, at least moderately indicative of a defect in cell-mediated immunity, occurring in a person with no known cause for diminished resistance to that disease."[14] Subsequent revisions to this definition were made in 1987, 1993, and 2000 as the HIV virus was identified, antibody tests were developed, and clinical evidence reflective of a suppressed immune system (opportunistic infections and depressed CD4 T-lymphocyte counts) were included.[15]

Another example of a case definition comes from research into the association between cigarette smoking and lung cancer. When researchers wanted to know the relationship between smoking and lung cancer, it quickly became apparent that an accepted definition of *smoking* was needed. If subjects in a study smoked one cigarette per week for a year, their lung cancer outcomes were quite different from those who smoked a pack of cigarettes every day for 25 years. Additionally, people smoked different types of substances and by different means of administration. If one study included subjects who used chewing tobacco and another included subjects who used cigars, the lung cancer incidence would be very different, and different conclusions would be drawn. In order for the results of research to make sense, the researchers must use consistent and well-thought-out definitions. These definitions are also referred to as *operational definitions*.

Web of Causation

The **web of causation** posits that there is no singular reason for the occurrence of a disease. Rather, a compendium of factors predisposes an individual to meet criteria for a particular case definition. For example, sedentary lifestyle might not on its own lead to obesity. Nutrition is an important factor that contributes to obesity, as do genetics. When considering causation you need to take into account all of the factors (the web of causation) in order to arrive at an appropriate diagnosis and course of care.

Under the web of causation paradigm, each possible cause might increase the likelihood of exhibiting symptoms of the disease but might be neither necessary nor sufficient for its occurrence.[16] Instead of equating one cause to one disease, you, as a health professional, will have to identify multiple factors that have caused your patient to become ill. Epidemiology will arm you with data that will identify the health risks that those under your care will have.

The Epidemiological Triad

The **epidemiological triad** is another way to view the origins of some diseases by identifying the agent, host, and environment (**Figure 7–1**).[17] For example, pulmonary tuberculosis is often caused by the agent *Mycobacterium tuberculosis*; however, exposure alone does not always cause a person to become ill. Factors such as the host's susceptibility come into play; these include nutritional status and the quality of a person's immune system. Furthermore, significant environmental factors, such as poverty and crowded living conditions, add layers that determine health outcomes. As a future healthcare professional, you will have to ameliorate

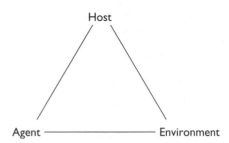

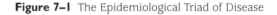

Figure 7–1 The Epidemiological Triad of Disease

these layers of factors to prevent disease occurrence; the possession of sound epidemiological evidence will be imperative to your practice.[2]

DISEASE OCCURRENCE

An epidemiological study identifies the relationship between individual characteristics and disease, with the occurrence of a foodborne outbreak being the classic example.[6] Often the reason for a foodborne outbreak can be identified by comparing the **attack rates (AR)** of persons who became ill after consumption of a given food item with persons who did not consume that food. An attack rate is similar to an incidence rate. It represents an increased occurrence of disease among people over a short period of time.

When one talks about a disease being **endemic** to a specific locale, it is marked by a persistently stable level of disease occurrence within a geographic area or population. Malaria is said to be endemic in low-income tropical countries. Cases reach **epidemic** proportions when there is a level of disease that exceeds what is normally expected. Special emphasis is placed on the time period, geographic region, and specific characteristics of the affected population.[18] The term **pandemic** is used when an epidemic is widespread over several countries or continents. Examples include the influenza pandemic of 1918–1919 and today's HIV/AIDS global epidemic.[19] The term **syndemic** is used to describe "two or more afflictions, interacting synergistically, contributing to excess burden of disease in a population" (e.g., insomnia and anxiety).[20]

Types of Outbreaks

It is important to know how infectious agents spread through a population. Two major categories of infectious disease outbreaks are common-source outbreaks and propagated epidemics. A **common-source outbreak** is when an agent or toxin from a single source simultaneously affects exposed individuals.[12] It is further classified as a **point-source outbreak** when that one source of infection results in a very rapid increase in the number of cases, such as in the cholera epidemic during John Snow's time in London. Usually, as in the case of the cholera epidemic, once you remove the common source the epidemic quickly subsides.[8]

Conversely, a **propagated epidemic** arises when an infectious agent infects one person who then transmits the disease to another person.[8] This can occur through direct or indirect contact. An example of direct contact is the transmission of HIV through sexual contact. Transmission of an infectious disease through indirect contact requires that the agent be able to survive on surfaces, such as doorknobs, handrails, and telephone buttons, or in food for an extended period of time. An example of indirect contact is the transmission of the *norovirus* (which causes severe vomiting and diarrhea) through contaminated food. Propagated outbreaks usually last longer than common-source outbreaks and have rises and falls in the number of new infections. Examples of propagated outbreaks are influenza epidemics, which can be caused by different strains of a virus.[8]

APPLICATIONS OF EPIDEMIOLOGY

The application of epidemiology to clinical care can be broadly classified into seven areas. Valanis[4] delineated each area's utility to everyday clinical practice:

1. Investigation of disease etiology
2. Risk identification
3. Identification of syndromes and disease classification
4. Differential diagnoses and planning clinical treatment
5. Effective surveillance of health status of populations
6. Community diagnosis and the planning of health service
7. Evaluation of health services and public health interventions

As a healthcare professional in training, you may already be familiar with a few of these functions.

Epidemiology has always been involved with the *investigation of disease etiology*. Through the identification of a causative agent and by determining the natural history of disease, you will be able to develop interventions for control or eradication. Obtaining a patient's medical history is an example and crucial step in this process.

Risk identification refers to ascertaining the factors that predispose someone to a specific disease. A more thorough discussion of risk is found later in this chapter. Whether one considers the web of causation or the epidemiological triad, a knowledgeable healthcare professional can prevent disease progression by addressing the "red flags" that have been identified prior to any epidemiological studies.

The *identification of syndromes and disease classification* are within the realm of clinical practice. The treatment of emerging diseases and of new syndromes can be achieved more quickly once broad clinical categories are narrowed based on observed symptoms. Whereas all vascular diseases were once classified together, epidemiology has enabled healthcare professionals to distinguish between cerebrovascular and cardiovascular diseases based on distinct conditions.

The study of disease distribution in a population is also useful for *differential diagnoses and planning clinical treatment*. Data from incidence reports aid health practitioners in specifying which among similar diseases afflict individuals with given risk factors and exposures. Consequently, the correct diagnosis allows for choosing the appropriate treatment plan.

Applying epidemiological data also allows for the *effective surveillance of the health status of populations*. **Surveillance** is the ongoing systematic collection, analysis, and interpretation of health data.

These data allow researchers to determine trends and norms in a population. With established historical trends and health records, deviations from the norm can be identified. When this occurs, alerts are sent out to warn those most at risk and to address the needs of persons already affected. An example of this type of publication is the *Morbidity and Mortality Weekly Report* published by the CDC. It provides information on recent instances of disease and death.

Community diagnosis and the planning of health services are feasible after analyzing epidemiological data. The blueprint for allocation of services and distribution of resources is then based on the overall health of the community.

Finally, the *evaluation of health services and public health interventions* is based on epidemiological findings. The success of health measures implemented at the population level can be validated by reports from the field. For example, one way of evaluating the effectiveness of vaccination campaigns against polio in India would be close monitoring of annual mortality and morbidity reports attributed to poliomyelitis through use of confirmed laboratory tests. Reports from community health centers are routinely used to measure program efficacy and determine subsequent funding, replication, or elimination.

SOCIOCULTURAL CONSIDERATIONS

Social and cultural considerations are important within the context of epidemiology. Although epidemiology examines disease and disease occurrence within populations, these parameters cannot be isolated from behavioral considerations. The social context for disease occurrence can be related to societal factors (rules and institutions) such as occupation, access to health care, poverty, public policy, political concerns, and religion. Any one of these can contribute to disease occurrence. These factors are considered *social determinates of health*. For example, exposure to pathogens can be influenced by occupation and the use of personal protective equipment, which might be influenced by rules and regulations.[21,22]

Culture is central to behavior and is strongly associated with health outcomes, because culture represents beliefs and values that shape behavior and is composed of systems of meaning and patterns of behavior. Systems within a culture are locally determined and can be temporally specific, unequally distributed, sometimes contradictory, and in many instances influenced by power. The study of culture and epidemiology is considered an integrated framework. Your ability to understand and interpret the role culture plays in health is important. It helps researchers understand the how and why of the association of the variables related to health. For example, pain is perceived and classified differently by people of different cultures, and consumption of certain foods can be deemed acceptable or unacceptable.[23,24]

There is a great deal to know about the social and cultural determinants of health and their impact on public health. A full discussion of this topic is beyond the scope of this chapter. However, this is a vital topic that, hopefully, will be fully explored in your curriculum. Throughout your career you will benefit from paying attention to research regarding social and cultural determinants of health. The Healthy People 2020 program includes an objective related to social determinants of health, "to create social and physical environments to promote good health for all."[11]

GEOGRAPHY AND DEMOGRAPHY

Epidemiology is dependent on geography and demography. Geography studies the land, atmosphere, and the inhabitants in a specific area; that is, it addresses the physical environment and the people. **Medical geography** shares a common goal with epidemiology in that they both have a goal of understanding the disease process to improve health. Medical geography focuses on the interplay of human behavior and the environment related to health outcomes, problems of disease, and disease control, which is similar to epidemiology. The basic difference is that medical geography addresses the spatial context of health-related issues; specifically, the location of disease occurrence and contributing environmental factors.[25] As previously discussed, geography played a role in stopping the London cholera epidemic in the mid-1800s. Dr. John Snow collected data (death records and interviews) and documented that most of the deaths associated with the outbreak were near the Broad Street water pump. These data were presented to officials, the pump handle was removed (thereby preventing usage of water from that pump), and the number of deaths due to cholera declined.[26]

Demography informs epidemiology because it focuses on the people per se. It focuses on their distribution, person-characteristics (age, gender), and those factors that influence the population, such as birth and death rates and migration patterns.[27] Combined, demography and epidemiology, "both explore the dynamics and characteristics of geographically-defined populations and, as such, take a global view of human activities and events, including health."[28] Both address the role that human behavior plays in health, historical human events (birth, death, and fertility as indicators of health and disease), and prediction of health and future events within a social context. Of importance, according to Wallace, both epidemiology and demography have a "heritage of applied problem solving," such as determining the transmission of communicable disease.[28] However, a distinct difference is that epidemiology engages in randomized and quasi-population experiments to validate phenomena and to test health interventions. Geography and demography are both important to epidemiology. Together they form a complete picture for the investigation of the health of populations.

INCIDENCE AND PREVALENCE

To understand the patterns of disease, health problems, or event occurrences within a population or community, researchers use the epidemiological measures of prevalence and incidence. **Prevalence** represents the proportion of cases observed in a population within a specific time period.[19] As an example, let's say that there were 1,000 women living with breast cancer in Small Town, USA, in 2010.

These women represented all of the known cases. However, this count included women who were newly diagnosed and those who were diagnosed with breast cancer prior to 2010 and still alive. Therefore, the incidence within 2010 would be *only those individuals diagnosed within that year*. One way of thinking about prevalence and incidence is that prevalence represents all cases and incidence reflects only the new cases. Keep in mind that both occur within a specific time period. Therefore, when reading these numbers look for the researcher's explanation about the context of time, which can be **point prevalent** (specific date) or **period prevalent** (month or year). For example, during a 2-year period, the period prevalence equals the point prevalence at the beginning of the interval plus the incidence (new cases) during the interval. **Figure 7–2** depicts the relationship between prevalence and incidence.

Prevalence includes all people during a defined period of time with a given diagnosis. **Incidence** is the new diagnoses during the defined period of time. The diagram demonstrates that incidence adds to the number of cases (thereby increasing prevalence) and recovery or death reduces prevalence. Prevalence and incidence are calculated as rates. The numerator represents the number of persons with the phenomenon under investigation, and the denominator is the number of persons within the population who are susceptible (can acquire the phenomenon under investigation). The formulas are shown in **Figures 7–3** and **7–4**.

Returning to the example of breast cancer we mentioned earlier, in 2010 there were 1,000 women living in Small Town, USA, who had breast cancer. To

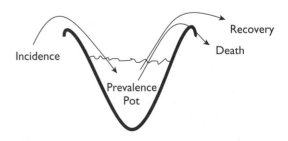

Figure 7–2 Relationship Between Incidence and Prevalence

Prevalence:

Number of the defined group of people with a given diagnosis or exposure
Number of people in the defined group during a specified period of time

Figure 7–3 Prevalence Formula

Incidence:

Number of the defined group of people with newly acquired diagnosis or exposure
Number of people in the defined group during a specified period of time

Figure 7–4 Incidence Formula

calculate prevalence, the researchers need to determine how many women lived in the town in 2010. (Note that this is an example of period prevalence.) For the sake of discussion, let's say that there were 40,000 women in the town. This means that the prevalence is 1,000/40,000, or 0.025, which is 2.5%.

The result of the calculation is converted into a percentage. Often researchers create a rate by multiplying the result by 1,000, 10,000, or 100,000. This facilitates comparison of rates across populations.

To calculate the incidence rate, the researchers would need to determine how many of the cases of breast cancer were *newly diagnosed* in 2010. Let's say 64 new cases of breast cancer were diagnosed in Small Town, USA, in 2010. Thus, to calculate the incidence rate they would divide 64 by 40,000. The incidence rate of breast cancer would be 0.16%.

When reviewing prevalence and incidence rates, you must consider their accuracy. Almost nothing is 100% accurate; however, you can ask yourself the following: Were the data collected as precisely as possible? Is the diagnosis accurate? Are the cases new or old? Do the data represent the population from which the individuals were drawn? Should cases be excluded related to specific age, gender, or ethnicity? Reflecting on these questions will help you determine if accurate data were used for the analysis.

RISK FACTORS AND SCREENING

Risk factors and *screening* are important aspects of epidemiology. Within EBP, investigators examine the relationship between risk factors and onset of disease. Risk factors associated with a disease can be genetic or environmental, or both. Within the context of environment, social and behavioral considerations can be included. For example, prolonged grief disorder recently has been associated with the violent and traumatic loss of a significant other. Individuals with prolonged grieving cannot accommodate the loss and fail to return to their preloss level of function. They develop protracted depression and anxiety, which interfere with daily functioning and can cause reduced quality of life. Persons affected are known to develop suicidal ideation, cancer, immunological dysfunction, hypertension, and other conditions. Therefore, prolonged grief is a risk factor for other health conditions.[29,30]

Engaging in a personal behavior, such as cigarette smoking, can increase the risk for developing lung cancer and heart disease. Current estimates indicate that 90% of lung cancer is associated with cigarette smoking and secondhand smoke.[31] Smoking is also associated with heart disease, the number one cause of death in the United States. In addition, smokers are four times more likely to die of heart disease.[32] On a positive note, modifying a risk factor, such as smoking, can play an important role in disease prevention and reduce healthcare costs. Your awareness of the association between risk factors and disease will prove an important tool in diagnosis, treatment, and prevention activities in your clinical practice.

Risk factors for many chronic and infectious diseases have been identified. Typically with an infectious disease, once the risk factors have been identified preventive measures can be implemented. For example, malaria is prevalent in tropical and subtropical areas of the world. The risk of infection, and thus the prevalence and incidence of the disease, can be significantly decreased by sleeping with an insecticide-treated mosquito net placed around the bed. However, for chronic disease there might be multiple causes, or what is known as the *web of causation* (interaction of multiple factors in producing disease), which was discussed earlier in this chapter.

Coronary heart disease is an example of a disease that has a web of causation. It has multiple risk factors, including high cholesterol, lack of physical activity and exercise, smoking, obesity, diabetes, and hypertension. In addition, a person's age, gender, and heredity are also risk factors; however, these cannot be changed. Therefore, it is difficult to isolate one risk factor as being the primary reason that a particular individual develops heart disease.[19,33] Further, addressing only one risk factor may not have sufficient impact on prevention or treatment.

When risk has been determined, **screening** is used to identify early signs and symptoms of a disease or health problem associated with a population at risk for a specific disease or event. This is done so that early treatment or intervention can be initiated, which has the potential to decrease morbidity and mortality and contribute to positive health outcomes.[34] It is well known that early detection of disease saves lives; a common example is cancer. When malignant tumors are detected at an early stage, the mortality is low for many cancers. Breast cancer is a classic example of screening to reduce mortality. According to the American Cancer Society:

> In the U.S., death rates from breast cancer in women have been declining since 1990, due in part to early detection by mammography screening and improvements in treatment. Currently, 60% of breast cancers are diagnosed at a localized stage, for which the 5-year survival rate is 98%. Further reductions in breast cancer death rates are possible by improving regular use of mammography screening and providing timely access to high-quality follow up and treatment.[35]

Screening activities can also include other conditions, such as disability. A well-known example is the Denver II (formerly Denver Developmental Screening Test, DDST). This test is used in pediatric settings to screen for developmental delays in children from birth to 6 years of age. The tool has been available since the early 1960s and has demonstrated its ability to detect and monitor developmental problems.[34,36]

Although there are numerous screening tests, you need to remember that a screening test's value is determined by its ability to delineate between a problem and nonproblem. When you are using a screening test, be mindful of its sensitivity, specificity, and predictive value.

EPIDEMIOLOGY BIOSTATISTICS

Sensitivity and Specificity

The general definition of **sensitivity** as it is used in medical biostatistics is the ability of the test to be positive given that the person tested has the disease/problem; similarly, **specificity** is the ability of the test to be negative given that the person does not have the disease/problem.[37] It is important to recognize that these terms have other meanings. In laboratory research, sensitivity refers to the ability of an analytical technique to measure only the substance of interest. As such, you will hear the terms sensitivity and specificity used in different healthcare contexts.

In epidemiological research, sensitivity refers to the proportion of subjects with a given disorder who test positive for a specified disease, exposure, or risk factor. Specificity represents the proportion of subjects without a given disorder who test negative for a specified disease, exposure, or risk factor. The concepts of sensitivity and specificity are also used with diagnostic medical research. The procedure for calculating sensitivity and specificity in epidemiological and diagnostic research is the same.

The calculation of sensitivity is depicted in the following *2 × 2 table* (**Table 7–1**). These tables are also referred to as *contingency tables*.

Table 7–1 Sensitivity and Specificity Contingency Table

	Has Condition	Does Not Have Condition
Test positive for disease, risk factor, or exposure	100 (*a*)	0 (*b*)
Test negative for disease, risk factor, or exposure	0 (*c*)	100 (*d*)

For example, based on 200 tests for a condition, the following would indicate 100% sensitivity and 100% specificity:

- Out of 100 people who have the condition, 100 of them test positive for the risk factor or exposure.
- Out of 100 people who do not have the condition, all 100 are free of the exposure or risk factor.

This finding would indicate to us that the diagnostic result, risk factor, or exposure of interest is perfectly associated with the condition.

$$\text{Sensitivity} = \frac{a}{a+c}$$

$$\text{Specificity} = \frac{d}{b+d}$$

However, this outcome is not realistic; there will always be some false positives and false negatives. Furthermore, it is exceedingly rare for a diagnostic result, risk factor, or exposure to be perfectly associated with a given condition.

Diagnostic screening tests are important tools in epidemiological research. These tests are used to determine the incidence and prevalence of a condition in a population. As such, the accuracy of screening tests is of a great importance. Inaccurate screening tests lead to incorrect information about the population. For example, the burden of disease in a given population is often relied upon as a key indicator of population health. In recent years, the proportion of individuals in the population who are overweight or obese is frequently referenced as a population health indicator.

In this case, the accuracy of body weight measurements would be of interest. It might seem that taking the weight of a patient is a highly accurate measure, but the accuracy of taking a person's body weight is dependent on a variety of factors, such as the ability of different scales to produce the same result, the types of scales used, whether the scales are calibrated, the consistency of the clinicians in taking body weights, and so on. It is not unusual for a person to weigh different amounts on different scales, including the scales used by healthcare providers. It is even possible for a person to step onto a scale, step off, and then back on and have two different results. If epidemiological researchers wish to use body mass as an indicator of obesity or overweight in the population, then the scales used must be accurate. They must be both sensitive and specific for body mass. According to the CDC, an adult with a BMI between 25 and 29.9 is considered overweight, and a person with a BMI of 30 or above is considered obese.[38]

Imagine a study in which the researchers evaluated the sensitivity and specificity of clinical body mass measures. The researchers select five clinics that all use the same scale for measuring body mass. The clinicians record the weight of the patient in pounds, the patient's height, and the patient's sex. They also mark on the patient's chart whether the patient meets the definition of obese or overweight according to the resulting body mass index (BMI) calculation. BMI is calculated with the following formula:[39]

$$\text{BMI} = \text{weight (lb)}/[\text{height (in)}]^2 \times 703$$

Additionally, the researchers measure the patients using a combination of two other measures that are known to be highly accurate. As such, the measures performed by the researchers are considered the reference standard, whereas the measures performed in the clinics are considered the experimental measures. **Table 7–2** shows the results of this hypothetical study:

In this hypothetical example, there were 2,000 patients, 1,000 of whom were not actually overweight and 1,000 of whom were overweight. When they were weighed at the clinic, out of the 1,000 overweight individuals 900 were identified correctly by the clinical measurements. This means that the test was 90% sensitive. Out of the 1,000 nonoverweight individuals, 800 were correctly identified. This means that the test was 80% specific. **Table 7–3** shows how the variables for the sensitivity and specificity calculations are placed in the contingency table:

The values for each of the variables in Table 7–3 were as follows: $a = 900$; $b = 200$; $c = 100$; $d = 800$. As such, **Table 7–4** shows the contingency table again, with the calculations for sensitivity and specificity.

Sensitivity and specificity are reported as percentages. As such, the sensitivity and specificity of the clinical body weight measurements were 90% and 80%, respectively. This means that 10% of individuals who were overweight were incorrectly identified as not overweight and 20% of individuals who were not overweight were incorrectly identified as overweight. In other words, the clinical body weight method had 10% false negatives and 20% false positives.

Even highly sensitive tests will have a small number of false negatives and highly specific tests will have a small number of false positives. As much as possible, screening tests should be both sensitive and specific. Both are important, depending on what is being measured. The more harmful the disease of interest, the more important it is that the diagnostic test has the characteristics of high sensitivity and high specificity. Tests with both high sensitivity and specificity are, however, somewhat rare.

Lastly, it is important to note that sensitivity and specificity can be influenced by the prevalence of the condition of interest. As prevalence increases, sensitivity increases, but specificity decreases. Conversely, as prevalence decreases, sensitivity decreases but specificity increases.

Table 7–2 BMI Research Results Contingency Table

	Actually Overweight (BMI 25.0–29.9)	Actually Not Overweight (BMI < 25)	Totals
Clinical BMI overweight	900	200	1,100
Clinical BMI not overweight	100	800	900
Totals	1,000	1,000	2,000

Table 7–3 Placement of Variables for BMI in the Contingency Table

	Actually Overweight (BMI 25.0–29.9)	Actually Not Overweight (BMI < 25)	Total
Clinical BMI overweight	a	b	$a + b$
Clinical BMI not overweight	c	d	$c + d$
Totals	$a + c$	$b + d$	$a + b + c + d$

Table 7–4 Sensitivity and Specificity of Clinical BMI Measurements

	Actually Overweight (BMI 25.0–29.9)	**Actually Not Overweight (BMI < 25)**	**Total**
Clinical BMI overweight	900	200	1,100
Clinical BMI not overweight	100	800	900
Totals	1,000	1,000	2,000

$$\text{Sensitivity} = \frac{a}{a+c} \qquad \text{Specificity} = \frac{d}{b+d}$$

$$= \frac{90}{90+10} \qquad\qquad = \frac{80}{80+20}$$

$$= 0.90 \qquad\qquad\qquad = 0.80$$

Positive Predictive Value and Negative Predictive Value

Positive predictive value (PPV) addresses how likely someone with a positive test result will actually have the disease, exposure, or risk factor. **Negative predictive value (NPV)** addresses how likely someone with a negative test result is to actually not have the disease, exposure, or risk factor. (See **Table 7–5**.) This is important in determining whether a test is useful for measuring a specific characteristic in a given population.

An Example of Sensitivity/Specificity and PPV/NPV from the Literature

Kontos, Wilson, and Fentiman[40] wanted to identify the sensitivity and specificity of digital infrared thermal imaging (DITI) among women receiving excision or core biopsy of breast lesions (benign and malignant) to determine the effectiveness of DITI in identifying primary cancers. DITI is a non-invasive diagnostic technique that allows visualization and quantification of changes in skin surface temperature. This can be done for certain cancers, deep vein thrombosis, and other conditions. The benefit is that it is noninvasive. Sixty-three symptomatic women were screened using DITI. Results found that the diagnostic test's sensitivity was 25%, specificity 85%, PPV 24%, and NPV 86%. **Table 7–6** demonstrates how the results were calculated. Note that among the 63 patients included in the study 126 lesions were tested with DITI (the experimental diagnostic tool) and with biopsy after surgical excision.

Table 7–5 Contingency Table for Positive and Negative Predictive Values

	Has Condition	**Does Not Have Condition**	
Test positive	True positive (a)	False positive (b)	Positive predictive value $= \dfrac{a}{a+b}$
Test negative	False negative (c)	True negative (d)	Negative predictive value $= \dfrac{d}{c+d}$

Table 7–6 Contingency Table for DITI Study

	Malignant Lesions	**Nonmalignant Lesions**	**Totals**
DITI positive test result	5	16	21
DITI negative test result	15	90	105
Totals	20	106	126

$$\text{Sensitivity} \left[\frac{a}{a+c}\right] : \frac{5}{5+15} = 0.250 \text{ (which is 25\%)}$$

$$\text{Specificity} \left[\frac{d}{b+d}\right] : \frac{90}{16+90} = 0.849 \text{ (which is 85\%)}$$

$$\text{PPV} \left[\frac{a}{a+b}\right] : \frac{5}{5+16} = 0.238 \text{ (which is 24\%)}$$

$$\text{NPV} \left[\frac{d}{c+d}\right] : \frac{90}{15+90} = 0.857 \text{ (which is 86\%)}$$

To restate each of the results shown in Table 7–6:

- *Sensitivity:* 25% of malignant breast lesions were correctly identified by the DITI test.
- *Specificity:* 85% of nonmalignant breast lesions were correctly identified by the DITI test.
- *PPV:* 24% of lesions identified by DITI as malignant were actually malignant.
- *NPV:* 86% of lesions identified by DITI as nonmalignant were actually nonmalignant.

Think about how often, using the DITI diagnostic test alone, you would be giving incorrect results to patients, leading to a delay in treatment or the provision of treatment to women who do not have malignancy. Because of the low sensitivity of this test for breast cancer, the researchers concluded that DITI is not suitable for primary screening of symptomatic patients and recommended that DITI not be used as a routine breast-screening test. It is worthwhile, however, to note the small sample size of this study, with only a total of 20 malignant lesions. More research involving larger sample sizes is needed.

It is important to note that this is an emerging area of investigation. As of the writing of this chapter, only five publications were listed in PubMed on this topic. A 2008 study by Arora et al.,[41] for example, which included 92 patients, reported 97% sensitivity, 44% specificity, 82% PPV, and 82% NPV.

In the Aroro et al. study, a total of 60 malignancies were evaluated using DITI and biopsy, making the study four times larger in terms of sample size than the more recent study. Even though the earlier study reported a higher level of sensitivity, the numbers were still not high enough to clinically recommend the use of this diagnostic tool for breast cancer screening.

Risk

The probability or chance that an individual will develop a disease or condition over a specified period of time is known as **risk**. You can think of risk as the cumulative incidence of a disease. If the incidence of oral cancer among white males of all ages is 15.7 per 100,000 men, this means that all white males have a 0.000006% risk of developing oral cancer. Of course, risk changes with age and with other factors, such as race, economic status, insurance status, comorbidities, and even geographic location. Risk applies not only to risk of disease, but also to characteristics associated with disease, which are known as risk factors. Some risk factors, such as diet and exercise, can be controlled (which makes them **modifiable risks**), whereas others, such as gender and ethnicity, cannot be controlled (which makes them **nonmodifiable risks**).

Risk of developing a disease or condition is dependent on dose, frequency, intensity of exposure, and duration of exposure period. When you are reading epidemiological research that summarizes data based on risk, you need to examine closely how the data are being reported and interpreted. In an observational study design, two of the most important measures of disease risk are the *relative risk* (RR) and the *odds ratio* (OR). Both compare the likelihood of an event occurring in at least two distinct groups; however, interpreting an OR is not as intuitive.

Relative Risk

Many epidemiological studies are designed to assess the strength of association between exposures and risk of developing a given disease, or RR. **Relative risk (RR)** is defined as the event rate among those exposed to a factor divided by the event rate among those not exposed to the same factor. The event rate is the proportion of the event of interest in the group. You could think of it as incidence or prevalence. RR provides us with a ratio of disease incidence among the population exposed to a risk factor versus the not exposed population, and so it can also be called the **risk ratio**.[42]

RR can only be calculated when using a cohort research design. A *cohort design* uses a large number of individuals who are followed over time (prospectively) to observe the development of a disease or condition while observing risk factors or exposures. EBP experts consider the RR to be more accurate than the OR, which is measured in retrospective (*case-controlled*) research studies that look for exposures in the histories of patients who have developed a given condition. A well-designed cohort study is superior to a case-controlled study.[43] A case-controlled study is a research design in which the researchers identify patients who have been diagnosed with or without a specific outcome (e.g., lung cancer) and they then look in the patients' histories for specific exposures or risk factors. They test for relationships between the exposures or risk factors and the outcome. This is a retrospective type of research, which generally has a greater risk of bias than prospective types of research.

To calculate RR, researchers first calculate the **exposed event rate** (EER) as well as the **control event rate (CER)**. Many epidemiologists use I_e to signify incidence in the exposed group and I_u to signify incidence in the unexposed group. We use CER and EER because the statistic of interest might be incidence or prevalence. Using a contingency table, these calculations would be as shown in **Figures 7-5** and **7-6**. The formula for EER is $a/(a + b)$. The formula for CER is $c/(c + d)$. Thus, the formula for calculating the RR is EER/CER, which can also be expressed as:

$$\frac{\frac{a}{a+b}}{\frac{c}{c+d}}$$

	Patients who develop the condition	Patients who do not develop the condition	Totals
Patients who have the exposure	**a**	b	**a + b**
Patients who do not have the exposure	c	d	c + d
Totals	a + c	b + d	a + b + c + d

Figure 7-5 EER Formula

	Patients who develop the condition	Patients who do not develop the condition	Totals
Patients who have the exposure	a	b	a + b
Patients who do not have the exposure	**c**	d	**c + d**
Totals	a + c	b + d	a + b + c + d

Figure 7-6 CER Formula

As a fictional example, let us consider a cohort study whose purpose is to determine the RR of heart attack among those with high triglycerides (> 200 mg/dL) compared to those with normal triglycerides (< 150 mg/dL). Out of 622 individuals (younger than age 60) who had normal triglycerides during a 5-year period, 35 had a heart attack. Over the same 5 years, there were another 690 individuals with triglyceride levels over 200 mg/dL, and 62 of these individuals had a heart attack. These variables can be placed into a **contingency table**.

Variable a is 62 (i.e., 62 individuals with *high* triglycerides who had heart attacks); variable c is 35 (i.e., 35 individuals with *normal* triglycerides had heart attacks). It also means that $a + b$ is 690, which is to say that 690 individuals had high triglycerides; $c + d$ is 622, which is to say that 622 individuals had normal triglycerides. Note that for purposes of clearly separating the exposed group from the unexposed group the researchers would not include in the study those who had triglycerides between 150 and 200 mg/dL. **Table 7–7** shows these numbers as a contingency table. Note that we do not need to know the values of b and c, though we could calculate them if we were interested in doing so.

To calculate the RR of having a heart attack when a patient's triglycerides are over 200 mg/dL, we would simply divide the incidence of heart attacks

$$EER = \frac{62}{690} = 0.089$$

$$CER = \frac{35}{622} = 0.056$$

$$RR = \frac{0.890}{0.056} = 1.59$$

An RR of 1.6 indicates that the risk of having a heart attack among people with triglyceride levels above 200 mg/dL is 1.6 times higher than people with triglyceride levels of 150 mg/dL or less. When calculating RR, we are assuming that the control population is representative of the population being studied. The following list provides ranges for considering the meaning of RR values in studies on exposures. **Table 7–8** provides the same information in simplified form:

- An RR of 1.0 indicates no association between exposure and disease.
- An RR greater than 1.0 represents an increased risk of disease among those who have been exposed.
- An RR less than 1.0 indicates a decreased risk of disease among those who have been exposed (this is referred to as a **protective factor**).

An RR of greater than 1.0 is often, but not always, considered clinically significant. The determination of clinical significance depends on the condition of

Table 7–7 Contingency Table for Relative Risk of Heart Attack for Those with High Triglycerides

	Patients Who Had a Heart Attack	Patients Who Did Not Have a Heart Attack	Totals
Patients with Tg > 200 mg/dL	62		690
Patients with Tg < 150 mg/dL	35		622
Totals			

among those individuals with high triglycerides (the EER) over the incidence among individuals with low triglycerides (the CER). Note that the exposed group is those individuals with high triglycerides and the control group is those individuals with normal triglycerides. Remember, RR = EER/CER:

Table 7–8 Interpretation of Relative Risk (RR) Scores in Studies on Exposures

RR < 1.0	RR = 1.0	RR > 1.0
Protective factor	Nonfactor	Risk factor

interest. For example, if living in a given area was associated with an RR of 1.5 for developing lung cancer, you might consider that to be clinically significant. However, if living in the same region was associated with a 1.5 RR for developing acne, you might not consider it clinically significant.

Also, clinical significance does not mean that when the RR is greater than 1.0 there is statistical significance associated with the RR value. Statistical significance must be calculated using an appropriate inferential statistic, such as chi square. When an RR value is reported the confidence interval (CI) should be provided so that readers can determine the accuracy of the measure.

Example of Relative Risk from the Literature

Gao, Chen, Schwarzschild, and Ascherio[44] prospectively examined bowel movement frequency at baseline in relation to future Parkinson's disease risk in two different studies, one with male patients and one with female patients. The data on male patients came from the Health Professionals Follow-up Study (HPFS) from 2000–2006 (33,901 men); the data on female patients came from the Nurses' Health Study (NHS) from 1982–2006. During the follow-up periods, the researchers identified 156 male Parkinson's disease cases (HPFS) and 402 female cases (NHS). In the HPFS, compared with men with daily bowel movements, men with a bowel movement every 3 days or more had a multivariate-adjusted relative risk of 4.98 (95% CI: 2.59–9.57) for developing Parkinson's disease in the next 6 years.

Note that the term *multivariate-adjusted relative risk* means that the researchers performed an adjustment to take into account other variables that influence risk, such as sex, age, smoking, and having a family member who had Parkinson's disease. They adjusted for these variables in order to be able to state the overall RR of Parkinson's. In the NHS, the corresponding RR was 2.15 (95% CI: 0.76–6.10). The researchers concluded that infrequent bowel movements may predate the onset of cardinal motor symptoms of Parkinson's

disease and could be beneficial in identifying populations with higher than average Parkinson's disease risk. In other words, the data show that infrequent bowel movements might be a risk factor for development of Parkinson's disease.

Odds Ratio

The **odds ratio** (OR) is the ratio of the odds of an event occurring in one group to the odds of an event occurring in another group. Similar to relative risk (RR), the OR is a measure of association that is calculated in case-control studies. To calculate an OR, researchers begin by calculating the odds of an event in each group (the exposed group and the unexposed group; that is, the control group). **Odds** are calculated by dividing the number subjects who have the condition by the number of subjects who do not have the condition. In the contingency table, this means the odds in the exposed group are $\frac{a}{b}$ and the odds in the control group are $\frac{c}{d}$:

- $\frac{a}{b}$ tells us the odds of having the condition for those who have the exposure.

- $\frac{c}{d}$ tells us the odds of having the condition for those who do not have the exposure.

Figure 7–7 displays the formulas for the odds of the condition in the exposed group and odds of the condition in the unexposed group.

	Have condition	Do not have condition	Totals
Had exposure	a	b	Exposed Group Odds $= \frac{a}{b}$
Did not have exposure	c	d	Unexposed Group Odds $= \frac{c}{d}$
Totals	$a + c$	$b + d$	$a + b + c + d$

Figure 7–7 Exposed Group and Unexposed Group Odds Formulas in Contingency Table

The odds formula tells us for each person with the condition how many people do not have the condition. Let's look at a contingency table with numbers related to automobile accident deaths among those who did not wear seatbelts versus those who did wear seatbelts in the United States in 2011. In this example, not wearing a seatbelt is the exposure. It is the exposure because not wearing a seatbelt is believed to be the factor associated with harm. The numbers used in this example are based on data from the U.S. Census Bureau's *2012 Statistical Abstract.*[45] The proportions in this table are the same as the U.S. Census Bureau numbers, but the whole numbers have been reduced by a factor of 100 for simplification. **Table 7–9** displays the contingency table for death and survival in automobile accidents distributed by seatbelt usage.

Among the exposed group, the odds of death were 271/21,528, which is 0.013 (1.3%) odds of death. Among the unexposed group, the odds of death were 88/86,113, which is 0.001 (0.1%) odds of death. These odds may seem acceptable until we compare them to one another.

The odds ratio formula, therefore, is $\frac{a}{b} \div \frac{c}{d}$, which tells us the relative odds of having the condition for those with the exposure compared to those without the exposure. You will find with a little algebra that the odds ratio is a cross-product multiplication, meaning that the formula can be expressed more simply as *ad/bc*. **Figure 7–8** shows how this works.

In our seatbelt example, the odds ratio calculation would be 0.0123/0.001, which produces an odds ratio of 12.3. This means that the odds of death in a motor vehicle accident are 12.3 times greater for those who do not wear seatbelts compared to those who do.

Table 7–9 Contingency Table for Death and Survival in Automobile Accidents

	Died	**Survived**	**Totals**
Did not wear seatbelt	271	21,528	21,799
Wore seatbelt	88	86,113	86,201
Totals	359	107,641	108,000

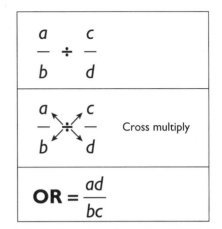

Figure 7–8 Algebraic Transformation of Odds Ratio

Odds ratios are used exclusively in retrospective research to determine if individuals with a given condition have a specific exposure in common. This type of research is referred to as case-control research. A researcher performing a *case-control study* starts by gathering participants who have the outcome of interest (cases) as well as participants who do not have the outcome of interest (controls). The researcher then assesses whether the cases and controls have been exposed to the risk factor under study. (A case-control study is, therefore, retrospective in nature because the researchers look into previous exposures in the patients' histories, rather than following patients forward in time to watch for outcomes.) The OR is then calculated to determine the rate of disease or condition and its relationship to the risk factor exposure.[46]

One More Odds Ratio Calculation

Because the odds ratio tends to be a little more abstract compared to the other biostatistics we have discussed, we are including another example demonstrating how an odds ratio is calculated. Let us consider a hypothetical case-control study aimed at examining the prevalence of breast cancer among 112 women 70 years of age who used hormone replacement therapy (HRT) for a minimum of 5 years. These participants were matched, based on ethnicity, with 112 women 70 years of age who never used HRT. Of the 112 women who used HRT, 10 were diagnosed with breast cancer. Among the

112 women who had not used HRT, 2 were diagnosed with breast cancer. To calculate the odds of developing breast cancer among the women who used HRT, you take the number of women on HRT who by age 70 developed breast cancer (10) and divide it by the number on HRT who did not develop breast cancer (102). **Table 7–10** displays the data from this hypothetical study.

In this example, the odds of developing breast cancer if you used HRT for at least 5 years were 0.10 (rounded to the nearest hundredth). The odds for the unexposed group were 0.02. The odds ratio is the ratio of these two odds, which is 0.10 divided by 0.02, or 5.39:

$$OR = \frac{0.10}{0.02} = 5.39$$

In other words, in this hypothetical study the odds for developing breast cancer among women 70 years of age who used HRT for a minimum of 5 years were 5.4 times the odds compared to women 70 years of age who did not use HRT. This should *not* be interpreted as women 70 years of age who used HRT for a minimum of 5 years are 5.4 times *more likely* to develop breast cancer than women 70 years of age who did not use HRT. This is a common mistake made by people when they are interpreting research results in

a study that reports an OR. An altogether different statistic, the likelihood ratio, is used to calculate the relative likelihood of an outcome between two groups. An odds ratio is based on the odds in each group, whereas a likelihood ratio is based on the percentage in each group with the exposure.

The OR is interpreted on the same scale as RR; the higher the number, the stronger the association between the disease or condition and having had exposure to the risk factor. An OR of 1.0 indicates that the odds are equivalent. An OR greater than 1.0 means that the odds are greater in the exposed group. An OR of less than 1.0 means that the odds are less in the exposed group. **Table 7–11** shows how to interpret odds ratios.

As previously stated, the OR often provides a good approximation of the RR, but the reader needs to interpret the results with caution because a case-control study is retrospective in nature, with only one period of observation. However, compared to cohort studies, case-control studies are less expensive, do not take as long to complete, and the logistics of the research design are usually easier to manage. It is not unusual in the progression of research on a particular question that retrospective studies are performed initially to determine if the expense of cohort studies is warranted. This leads to two critiquing tips we have for you when reading studies that report odds ratios. First, verify that the study was retrospective, or at least that the OR is reported on retrospective data. Second, when you come across OR results in a study that are relevant to the clinical question you are attempting to answer, expand your literature search for more recent cohort studies, randomized control trials, or meta-analyses.

Table 7–10 Contingency Table for Breast Cancer and HRT Usage

	Developed Breast Cancer	Did Not Develop Breast Cancer	Totals
Used HRT	10	102	112
Did not use HRT	2	110	112
Totals	12	212	224

Exposed group odds $= \frac{a}{b}$; $\frac{10}{102} = 0.098$

Unexposed group odds $= \frac{c}{d}$; $\frac{2}{110} = 0.018$

Table 7–11 Interpretation of OR Scores in Studies on Exposures

OR < 1.0	OR = 1.0	OR > 1.0
Protective factor	Non-factor	Risk factor

Example of an Odds Ratio from the Literature

Burton et al.[47] implemented a study to define the prevalence and risk factors for behavioral disorders in children with epilepsy from a rural district in Tanzania. Two hundred two children 6 to 14 years of age were identified through a cross-sectional survey. The comparison group of children without epilepsy was matched based on age and gender to the case group of children with epilepsy. The Rutter questionnaire,[48] a valid and reliable tool, was used to measure behavior. Behavioral disorders were diagnosed in 68 of the 103 children with epilepsy (66%) and in 19 of the 99 controls (19%). Behavior disorders were significantly more common in children with epilepsy as compared to the control group (univariate odds ratio 8.2; 95% CI: 4.3–15.6; *p* < 0.001). To reduce the burden of behavior disorders in this setting, the researchers recommended behavior assessment along with behavior intervention programs for children with epilepsy. Note that in this analysis the researchers included only one variable, epilepsy. They did not account for other variables, such as age and sex. Had they included multiple variables, then they would have produced a multivariate odds ratio.

Attributable Risk Measures

Attributable risk (AR) is the incidence of a disease or condition in the exposed (or at risk) population that would be eliminated if the exposure (or risk) were removed. In other words, it is the difference between the exposed (or experimental) event rate and the unexposed (or control) event rate. It is considered a measure of impact, because AR measures the proportion of disease cases related or linked to an exposure within a given population.[49] In other words, it determines how much risk is attributed to getting a disease or condition based on a person's exposure to something. AR is calculated (see **Figure 7–9**) by subtracting the incidence in the unexposed population (CER) from the incidence in the exposed population (EER). **Table 7–12** is an example of an attributable risk contingency table from a hypothetical study of the effect of exposure to vitamin C and D supplements in terms of rate of bone fractures.

To calculate the incidence in the exposed group (EER), you would use the following formula:

$$\frac{a}{a+b} = EER; \text{ or } \frac{78}{1,639} = 0.048.$$

To calculate a rate per 100 persons, you would multiply 0.048 by 100 to obtain 4.8 bone fracture

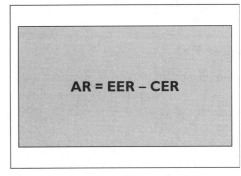

AR = EER – CER

Figure 7–9 Attributable Risk Formula

Table 7–12 Example of an Attributable Risk Contingency Table

Taking Vitamin C and D Supplement	Cases of Bone Fracture	No Cases of Bone Fracture	Total
Never taken supplements (*exposed to the risk*)	78	1,561	1,639
Daily supplements (*not exposed to the risk*)	22	775	797
Total	100	2,336	2,436

cases per 100 persons. (We multiply by 100 in order to express the rate as a more understandable number. However, we could calculate AR with the 0.048 value if we chose to do so.)

The calculation for the incidence in the unexposed (CER) is:

$$\frac{c}{c+d} = CER; \text{ or } \frac{22}{797} = 0.028$$

or a rate of 2.8 bone fracture cases per 100 persons. The formula for calculating the AR in this instance is: 4.8 − 2.8 = 2.0.

The results of these calculations indicate that if individuals who reported not taking vitamin C and D supplements would change and begin daily supplements, their incidence of bone fractures could decrease by 2 per 100 persons.

You will see AR reported in the literature, as well as one of its variants, ARR (absolute risk reduction) or ARI (absolute risk increase). You may see the term absolute risk also abbreviated AR, which can be confusing, because absolute risk differs from attributable risk. You will need to read carefully when you see the abbreviation AR.

Absolute Risk

Absolute risk is another way of stating the event rate or incidence rate of a group. For example, if the incidence of a given condition was 2.5% in 2011 for a specific population, then the absolute risk for the condition is 2.5%. In epidemiological research, the event rate in the control group is the absolute risk of the condition for that group. Similarly, the event rate in the exposed group is the absolute risk of the condition for that group. Absolute risk for each group is used to calculate attributable risk.

Absolute Risk Reduction/Increase

Attributable risk is also referred to as **absolute risk reduction** or **absolute risk increase**. Some researchers prefer these terms because they indicate how an exposure affected the groups. Exposures can affect groups in three ways, producing either an increase or a reduction in risk:

1. Being exposed might increase risk of a bad outcome. *Example:* Having a parent who died of heart disease at an early age increases the patient's risk of heart disease.
2. Being exposed might decrease risk of a bad outcome. *Example:* Having consistent exercise habits decreases the patient's risk of glucose intolerance.
3. Being exposed might increase risk of a good outcome. *Example:* Having healthy nutrition habits increases the patient's longevity (living 5 years longer) than average.

You might be tempted to consider a fourth alternative, being exposed might decrease risk of a good outcome. However, this alternative is rarely, if ever, researched.

In each case, a proportion of the risk can be attributed to the exposure. When an exposure reduces risk, it is referred to as *absolute risk reduction*. When an exposure increases risk, it is referred to as *absolute risk increase*. Whichever type of attributable risk is present, the calculation is the same. However, you might have to think through which type of attributable risk is present. It is possible for the formula CER − EER to produce a negative number. For this reason, ARR and ARI are treated as absolute values. **Table 7–13** demonstrates the three types of attributable risk results. Examples 1 and 3 demonstrate why attributable risk needs to be treated as an absolute value.

Attributable Risk Percent

We can also calculate **the attributable risk percent (AR%)**. Whereas AR is simply the difference between the two groups, the AR% is the percent of the incidence of a disease in the exposed population that is due to the exposure (lack of vitamin supplements). In other words, it is the *percent* of the incidence of a disease in the exposed that would be eliminated if the risk factor (lack of daily vitamin C and D supplement) was removed. The AR% is calculated by dividing the AR by the EER and then multiplying the product by 100 to obtain a percentage. For our example, the calculation would be:

$$AR\% = \left(\frac{AR}{EER}\right) \times 100 = \left(\frac{2.0}{4.8}\right) \times 100 = 41.7$$

Table 7–13   Examples of the Three Forms of Attributable Risk

	Example 1: ARI	**Example 2: ARR**	**Example 3: ARI**
Exposed group	Has a parent who died of heart disease at early age.	Exercises 60 minutes per day at target heart rate.	Maintains healthy nutrition habits.
Nonexposed (control) group	No heart disease in parents or grandparents.	Leads a sedentary lifestyle with little to no exercise.	Maintains unhealthy nutrition habits.
Outcome	Patients develop heart disease.	Patients develop glucose intolerance.	Greater longevity (living 5 years longer) than average.
EER (exposed group event rate)	3%	0.5%	45%
CER (control group event rate)	1%	15%	20%
AR (attributable risk: EER – CER)	= 3% – 1% = |2%|	= 0.5% – 15% = |14.5%|	= 45% – 20% = |25%|
Explanation	There is a 2% difference in incidence of heart disease between those who had a parent die early of heart disease and those whose parents did not have heart disease.	There is a 14.5% difference in incidence of glucose intolerance between those who lead a sedentary lifestyle and those who have a daily exercise habit.	There is a 25% difference in incidence of 5-year longevity between those who maintain healthy nutrition habits and those with unhealthy nutrition habits.

This result indicates that there would be a 41.7% reduction in bone fracture incidence if the exposed group included a daily vitamin C and D supplement. This concept applies not only to removing a risk factor, but also to removing an exposure or to adding a risk factor or exposure.

Population Attributable Risk and Population Attributable Risk Percent

Our final calculations related to AR are the **population attributable risk (PAR)** and **population attributable risk percent (PAR%)**. PAR represents the proportion of disease cases among the population, both exposed and not exposed. It is the reduction in incidence of a disease in the population if the exposure were eliminated. The PAR is calculated by subtracting the incidence in the unexposed (CER) from the incidence in the population (exposed and unexposed groups) PER (Population Event Rate). Note that the abbreviation I_p

is often used to signify incidence in the population. We use PER instead because the statistic of interest could be incidence or prevalence in the population. We already calculated the CER, which was 0.028, or 2.8 bone fractures per 100 persons. To calculate the PER, we use the following formula:

$$PER: 22 + \frac{22}{2,436} = 0.041, \text{ or } 4.1 \text{ per } 100 \text{ persons}$$

Now we can calculate the PAR, which is 4.1 – 2.8 = 1.3; that is to say, 1.3 cases per 100 persons. This result indicates that a reduction of 1.3 bone fracture cases per 100 persons (exposed and unexposed) is expected if everyone consumes a daily vitamin C and D supplement.

PAR% represents the *percent* of the incidence of a disease in the population (exposed and unexposed) that is due to exposure. It is the percent reduction in incidence of disease in the population if the exposure were eliminated. Dividing the PAR by the incidence in the total population and then multiplying the results by 100 to obtain a percentage will give you the PAR $\% \left(\dfrac{1.3}{4.1} \times 100 = 31.7\% \right)$. This result indicates that if everyone in the population took a daily vitamin C and D supplement, there would be a 31.7% reduction in the number of bone fractures.

When attempting to understand and explain variation in disease burden within geographic areas or populations, attributable risk (AR) can be helpful.[50] When setting public health priorities, AR is often used when a number of possible risk factors are contributing to the incidence of disease but a decision about where and when to intervene must be made. AR is also helpful in determining the risk related to dangerous behaviors, such as driving a motorcycle without a helmet or a car without a seatbelt.

Example of an Attributable Risk Measure from the Literature

Guy et al.[51] undertook an analysis of the potential population impact and cost savings that would likely result from modifying key HIV risk factors among men who have sex with men (MSM) in Sydney, Australia. The researchers recruited 1,426 men with negative HIV status between 2001 and 2004 and followed them to mid-2007. During the study period, the participants were tested for HIV annually and detailed information about sexual risk behavior was collected every 6 months. The use of PAR allowed the researchers to estimate the number of HIV infections in the population that were associated with specific risk behaviors, such as unprotected anal intercourse and casual sex partners. The PAR associated with unprotected anal intercourse was 34%, which means that 34% of the risk of HIV could be removed by avoiding unprotected anal intercourse. These findings can be used to identify targeted health promotion and risk reduction activities that could reduce the HIV transmission rate among MSM.

Confidence Intervals

The importance of correctly interpreting confidence intervals cannot be overstated. Many journals require

that research reports include three key statistical indices: the point estimate, the associated p-value, and its confidence interval.[52] Epidemiologists consider the confidence interval (CI) to be more meaningful than a **point estimate** (a single number such as a sample mean or incidence rate) or the p-value (statistical significance). The CI provides you with a range of values that is likely to contain the true population parameter being measured and describes the amount of uncertainty associated with a sample estimate of the population parameter.[53,54]

The CI is important when appraising the evidence and precision of epidemiological studies. It is often constructed around indices of risk, such as an OR or RR. The confidence interval has three components: the upper limit boundary, the lower limit boundary, and the confidence level. The most commonly used confidence levels are 95% and 99%. Researchers choose the confidence level. If they choose a 95% confidence level, they are saying that the interval represents the range of values within which you can be 95% sure that the true value for the population parameter can be found. In other words, if you sample a population 100 different times, the CI will contain the population parameter under study 95 times. This also means that you have a 5% chance of error or a 5% chance that the value for the true population parameter will not be within the CI. Most researchers are comfortable with this level of error.

One factor that affects the width of the CI is the level of confidence selected. A 99% CI is wider than a 95% CI. The difference between the upper and lower limit numbers in a CI represents data precision; however, variability in the data as well as the sample size can influence this precision. A narrow CI suggests greater precision and usually results from having more data points or a larger sample size. In contrast, if the CI is relatively wide, it could mean a relatively imprecise measurement. For example, if the RR is 2.5 and the 95% CI is 2.1–2.9, we would be more confident that we have a precise measurement compared to an RR of 2.5 with a 95% CI that is between 0.6 and 4.4. We would say that the second measure had more variability.

As consumers of epidemiological research, it is important that you read study findings carefully and have an understanding of the statistical measures reported before drawing conclusions about the results and making a decision to use them as evidence to support healthcare practices. Consider the confidence interval reported with the statistic of interest. Is it a wide interval or a narrow interval?

It is reasonable to assume that the true population parameter can fall anywhere within the range of the confidence interval. In the prior example of an RR of 2.5 with a 95% CI of 2.1–2.9, it is reasonable for us to assume the true RR value is 2.1. It is also reasonable for us to assume the true RR value is 2.9. The question for you to ask yourself is whether this would change your clinical decision. Consider another example where the RR of developing a disease was 10.6 with a 95% CI of 1.0–20.2. This means that the true RR could be as low as 1.0 or as high as 20.2. If the true RR is 1.0, this means there is no increased risk of developing the disease. This is a wide confidence interval.

The point estimate of RR = 10.6 by itself is misleading. If you had only the 10.6 RR number to go on, you might be highly motivated to take steps to eliminate the exposure associated with this high level of relative risk. However, when you take into account the confidence interval, you can see that an RR of 1.0 indicates no increased risk associated with the exposure. Alternately, the confidence interval also indicates a significantly higher RR of 20.2. This wide range of possibilities means that you, as the clinician, need more information because the RR measure is simply not precise enough.

Example of Confidence Intervals from the Literature

Andersen et al.[55] described the trends in cerebral palsy (CP) among 903 European children who were born moderately preterm (MPT; gestational age 32 to 36 weeks) between 1980 and 1998. The overall prevalence of CP of children born MPT varied between 12.2 (95% CI = 8.5–17.1) per 1,000 live births in 1983 and 4.5 (95% CI = 3.2–6.3) per 1,000 in 1997. The researchers concluded that the decreasing trend in the prevalence of CP among

children born MPT could be related to improvements in perinatal and neonatal care. In this study, the CIs for each point estimate were narrow and did not overlap.

STUDIES OF PROGNOSIS

In health-related disciplines, *prognosis* is defined as predicting or estimating the probability of future conditions or outcomes. *Prognostic research* uses multiple variables to predict health outcomes in specific populations. *Prognostic predicators* include factors such as age, gender, ethnicity, family history, stage of disease, treatment, comorbidities, and test results. However, it is also important to consider psychosocial and environmental factors as prognostic predictors. The findings from prognosis studies are typically used as evidence by healthcare providers to inform patients about the future course of an illness and to guide people in making informed clinical decisions about their health or treatment options.[56] For example, a patient might be told that based on the current evidence, he or she has a 75% chance of surviving for at least 5 years after receiving a particular treatment for a disease.

Prognosis research is not limited to disease or illness. Prognostication can be used to predict the future in seemingly healthy individuals. For example, the Framingham Risk Score is used to predict future heart disease. Genetic testing in women is used to predict the probability of developing breast cancer.[56] The vast majority of screening tests are used to predict outcomes. These tests are based on prognosis research. These types of prognostic tools are important to healthcare professionals; if we are able to identify individuals who might possibly develop an illness, we can implement appropriate evidence-based interventions to prevent the development or advancement of disease and thereby keep healthcare spending costs down, improve longevity, and improve quality of life.[57]

Systematic reviews of prognosis studies are relatively new to prognosis research, but increasing in areas such as cancer, low back pain, and cardiovascular disease. (A systematic review is used to synthesize and combine multiple primary research findings in a specific topic area.) Challenges have been reported in the literature regarding the use of systematic reviews for prognosis research. These challenges include, but are not limited to, variation in research design, inconsistent outcome reporting, and differences in the selection of predictor variables.[58–60]

In 2008, the Cochrane Collaboration Prognosis Methods Group was established with the purpose of facilitating and improving the quality of systematic reviews in prognosis research. This group is now part of the Cochrane Collaboration, an international network of more than 28,000 individuals from over 100 countries that was founded in 1993. The goal of the Cochrane Collaboration is to help people make informed decisions about health care based on preparing, maintaining, and ensuring accessibility to quality systematic reviews. The establishment of this group is an important step in prognosis research because quality systematic reviews are instrumental in providing healthcare professionals with the latest medical evidence.

Example of a Prognosis Study from the Literature

Messer, Griffiths, and Baudouin[61] conducted an integrative review of the literature to determine whether clinical variables available at the time of an intensive care unit (ICU) admission were predictive of intermediate-term mortality among patients with an acute exacerbation of chronic obstructive pulmonary disease (AECOPD). The integrative literature review identified 28 studies assessing prognostic variables within the ICU.

The prognostic variables associated with intermediate-term mortality reflected the underlying severity of disease prior to the ICU admission. Low Glasgow Coma Scale (GCS) score, cardiorespiratory arrest, cardiac dysrhythmia, and length of current hospital stay were associated with immediate-term mortality from AECOPD. Age, BMI, functional capacity, pulmonary function tests, prior hospital or ICU admissions, and long-term oxygen therapy were not found to be associated with intermediate-term mortality or with the cause of the AECOPD. In other words, ICU patients with any of the

prognostic factors had a higher risk of immediate mortality from AECOPD. Low GCS, cardiorespiratory arrest, cardiac dysrhythmia, and/or a long hospital stay are indications of a poor prognosis for ICU patients.

LOCATING EPIDEMIOLOGICAL INFORMATION

Accessing quality, current epidemiological information is fairly easy today because of the Internet and other electronic resources. When searching for information, you can use a variety of different approaches. Your approach will depend on what you need; for example, peer-reviewed research articles versus incidence or prevalence data. However, because there is so much epidemiological information available to you, critical attention in using what you find and making comparisons is imperative.

You can perform a single-field search or an advanced search on the Internet or through a library's literature databases to find epidemiological information. Literature databases are computer databases that contain bibliographic reference information from journals, newspapers, books, dissertations, audiovisuals, conference proceedings, and other printed material. Some databases include full-text journal articles, books, and newspapers. These databases are convenient because they provide comprehensive, scholarly information. The premier literature databases used by healthcare professionals are PubMed, EMBASE, the Cumulative Index to Nursing and Allied Health Literature (CINAHL), and OVID.

When using search engines on the Internet, such as Google, you must be discerning in appraising the quality of the epidemiological information you retrieve. You may discover papers, blogs, and PowerPoint presentations on a topic that you are interested in exploring, but remember that the information might not be valid or that it could be outdated. Conversely, through the Internet you can access high-quality websites such as those of the National Library of Medicine (NLM), the National Institutes of Health (NIH), the CDC, the National Center for Health Statistics (NCHS), and the World Health Organization (WHO). These websites can provide you with specific epidemiological information about a disease or health issue, such as HIV or heart disease. The WHO website is particularly important when you are looking for global epidemiological data and not just data from the United States.

Other resources for epidemiological information include organizations that target a specific health issue, such as the American Cancer Society and the American Heart Association. Organizations that address a major health issue or topic will have websites where national disease incidence and prevalence data can often be found. If you are interested in finding epidemiological information specific to a geographic region, accessing the county or state public health website or contacting the local epidemiologist can be advantageous. Major universities that have a School of Public Health often have websites where epidemiological information can be found along with faculty who are experts in epidemiology or a specific health topic.

Searching for epidemiological information can be challenging because at times you might become overwhelmed with the volume of information or frustrated because you cannot find what you need. Unfortunately, not every health issue or disease is reportable by law. For example, HIV infection is a reportable disease, but asthma is not. So how do we know how many people have really been diagnosed with asthma? These data are often extrapolated based on hospitalizations or insurance records. Nevertheless, even when a disease is reportable by law, the data you find are only as good as what are collected and reported by laboratories and healthcare professionals.

CRITIQUING EPIDEMIOLOGICAL RESEARCH

The strategies for critiquing an epidemiological study are the same as critiquing other types of research. Furthermore, it is important that you critique epidemiological publications as thoroughly as any other type of publication. The data reported by researchers on risk factors, prognosis, incidence/prevalence, and so on must be considered carefully before you accept them and base clinical decisions on them.

When reading an epidemiological study, consider the level of evidence. A systematic review is likely to be more reliable than a single cohort study, for example. Consider the source of the publication. There have been examples in the literature of certain organizations publishing epidemiological research that supports their product. The funding of a study is usually an indication of possible bias of the authors.

When reading the statistics presented in an epidemiological study, consider whether the authors used the appropriate statistical tests for the type of data presented. Also, look for statements about the shape of the distribution and the satisfaction of assumptions associated with the statistical tests employed. Read the confidence intervals carefully and determine for yourself if their ranges are too wide.

Lastly, think in general terms about the findings of the study in the context of the overall body of literature on the topic. Are the presented findings consistent with the other publications, or is there a difference? If so, what do the authors say about the difference? Different findings need to be acknowledged and explained.

CHAPTER SUMMARY

Determining the relationship between the occurrence of disease (incidence and prevalence) and environmental, occupational, or lifestyle risk factors as well as genetic traits is the major aim of epidemiological research. Based on evidence, we can use that information in developing, implementing, and evaluating public health interventions or control measures. Being able to predict the impact of removing a particular risk exposure based on evidence-based interventions or control measures is an important public health consideration. It is also important for developing a complete differential diagnosis.

Results of epidemiological research help clinicians determine the likelihood of a disease, a risk factor, or an exposure according to factors such as medical geography, age, gender, family history, race/ethnicity, and so on. Epidemiology also provides information about disease outbreaks, including common-source and point-source outbreaks, as well as syndemic diseases. Furthermore, epidemiology provides information on prognosis.

Key concepts of epidemiology with which you need to be familiar include:

- Incidence and prevalence
- Risk factors
- Screening
- Sensitivity and specificity
- Exposed event rate (EER) and control event rate (CER)
- Positive predictive value and negative predictive value
- Relative risk
- Odds (exposed group odds and unexposed group odds) and the odds ratio
- Attributable risk (absolute risk reduction/absolute risk increase)
- Attributable risk percent
- Absolute risk
- Population attributable risk and population attributable risk percent

Many of these concepts are statistics calculated through the use of a 2 × 2 table, which is also known as a contingency table. A contingency table is used with dichotomous results, such as positive for diagnosis versus negative for diagnosis, positive for risk factor versus negative for risk factor, or positive for exposure versus negative for exposure. Many of the concepts employed in epidemiology are also applied in other areas of healthcare research, such as studies on diagnosis, treatment, patient education, prognosis, and harm.

Many sources of epidemiological research are available, including literature databases, the CDC, the WHO, and the NCHS. Epidemiological research must be critically appraised by readers in the same manner as other healthcare research publications. One important skill to apply when critiquing the statistics presented in an epidemiological publications is interpretation of the confidence intervals presented. Well-written publications will include confidence intervals for the primary statistical results. These confidence intervals will be sufficiently narrow such that the results are precise,

without overlap between experimental and control groups.

EXERCISES

1. Researchers were interested in the accuracy of a new HIV screening test in order to determine if the new test should be used instead of the current test. They performed a study comparing the New HIV Screening Test to the current standard screening test. Consider how a contingency table would be constructed for such a study and answer the following questions.

   a. In the following New HIV Screening Test contingency table, fill in the labels that go in the highlighted cells.

New HIV Screening Test			

   b. Identify the test result represented by each of the four values: *a, b, c,* and *d.*

New HIV Screening Test			
	a	*b*	
	c	*d*	

   c. For each of the following formulas, identify the statistic calculated.

      i. $\dfrac{a}{a+c}$

      ii. $\dfrac{a}{b}$

      iii. $\dfrac{d}{c+d}$

      iv. $\dfrac{d}{b+d}$

v. $\dfrac{a}{b}$

vi. $\dfrac{a}{a+b}$

2. Small Town, USA, had a population of 28,000 persons 18 years of age and older at the end of 2011. In October, November, and December of that year, Small Town had the following new HIV cases among persons 18 years of age and older:
   - October: 25 cases
   - November: 20 cases
   - December: 10 cases
   Previously 1,200 people 18 years of age and older had been diagnosed with HIV prior to 2011.

   a. What was the incidence of HIV among persons 18 years of age and older during the month of December?
   b. What was the prevalence of HIV for 2011 among persons 18 years of age and older?

3. Clinicians working in primary care observed a trend among their adult male patients with colon cancer (CC). Nearly 30% of their patients with CC had a first-degree relative who had Crohn's disease. Several of these clinicians co-authored articles explaining the trend they had observed in their practice. The publication drew the attention of cancer center researchers and a nationwide, case-control study was performed in an attempt to determine if having a first-degree relative with Crohn's disease was associated with a patient developing CC. The results of the study are included in the following contingency table. (Note that this is a fictional study, not a real one.)

CC Familial Risk Factors	Had CC	Did Not Have CC
First-degree relative had Crohn's	10	2,050
First-degree relative did not have Crohn's	445	112,600

a. Based on the data provided, calculate the following statistics:
   i. EER
   ii. CER
   iii. AR (attributable risk).
b. What is the clinical take-away from the results?

REFERENCES

1. Rakel RE, Rakel DP. *Textbook of family medicine.* 8th ed. Philadelphia: Saunders; 2011.
2. Friis R, Sellers T. *Epidemiology for public health practice.* 4th ed. Sudbury, MA: Jones & Bartlett; 2009.
3. Kleinbum DG, Sullivan KM, Barker ND. *A pocket guide to epidemiology.* New York: Springer Science; 2007.
4. Valanis B. *Epidemiology in health care.* 3rd ed. Stamford, CT: Appleton & Lange; 1999.
5. Dever GE. *Managerial epidemiology: Practice, methods, and concepts.* Sudbury, MA: Jones & Bartlett; 2006.
6. Lilienfeld DE, Stolley PD. *Foundations of epidemiology.* 3rd ed. New York: Oxford; 1994.
7. Gerstman BB. *Epidemiology kept simple: An introduction to traditional and modern epidemiology.* 2nd ed. Hoboken, NJ: Wiley-Liss; 2003.
8. Merrill RM. *Introduction to epidemiology.* 5th ed. Sudbury, MA: Jones & Bartlett; 2010.
9. Hill AB. The environment and disease: Association or causation? *Proc Royal Soc Med.* 1965;58:295–300.
10. Friedman GD. *Primer of epidemiology.* 5th ed. New York: McGraw-Hill; 2004.
11. U.S. Department of Health and Human Services. *Healthy people.* [Website]. Available at: www.healthypeople.gov. Accessed March 15, 2012.
12. Dicker R. A brief review of the basic principles of epidemiology. In Gregg M (Ed.). *Field epidemiology.* 3rd ed. (pp. 16–37). New York: Oxford; 2008.
13. Dworkin M. How an outbreak is investigated. In Dworkin M (Ed.). *Outbreak investigations around the world: Case studies in infectious disease field epidemiology* (pp. 1–18). Sudbury, MA: Jones & Bartlett; 2010.
14. Centers for Disease Control and Prevention. Current trends update on acquired immune deficiency syndrome. *MMRW.* 1982;31(37):507–508.
15. Greenberg R, Daniels S, Flanders W, Eley J, Boring J. *Medical epidemiology.* 4th ed. New York: Lange Medical Books/McGraw-Hill; 2005.
16. Susser E, Bresnahan M. Origins of epidemiology. *Ann NY Acad Sci.* 2001;964:6–18.

17. Missouri Department of Health and Senior Services. *Introduction epidemiological methods.* 2004. Available at: http://bioterrorism.slu.edu/bt/products /bio_epi/scripts/mod4.pdf. Accessed March 3, 2012.

18. Bonita R, Beaglehole R, Kjellstrom T. *Basic epidemiology.* 2nd ed. Geneva, Switzerland: World Health Organization; 2006.

19. Fletcher R, Fletcher S. *Clinical epidemiology: The essentials.* 4th ed. Philadelphia: Lippincott, Williams, and Wilkins; 2005.

20. Centers for Disease Control and Prevention. Syndemic Prevention Network. Definition: Syndemic. Updated January 30, 2008. Available at: www.cdc.gov /syndemics/definition.htm. Accessed March 3, 2012.

21. Centers for Disease Control and Prevention. Social determinates of health. Updated January 20, 2012. Available at: www.cdc.gov/socialdeterminants. Accessed March 3, 2012.

22. Sandra R, Harper S. Data systems linking social determinants of health outcomes: Advancing public goods to support research and evidence-based policy and programs. *Public Health Reports.* 2011;126:6–13.

23. Trostle JA. Cultural epidemiology. In Killewo J, Heggenhougen HK, Quah SR (Eds.). *Epidemiology and demography in public health* (pp. 258–266). Amsterdam, The Netherlands: Elsevier; 2010.

24. Kohrt B, Hadley C, Hruschka D. Culture and epidemiology special issue: Towards an integrated study of culture and population health. *Ann Human Biol.* 2009;36(3):229–234.

25. Glass GE. Update: Spatial aspects of epidemiology: The interface with medical geography. *Epidem Rev.* 2000;22:136–139.

26. Centers for Disease Control and Prevention. 150th anniversary of John Snow and the pump handle. *MMWR.* 2004;53:783.

27. Miettinen S. Demography, epidemiology and public health. In Killewo J, Heggenhougen HK, Quah SR (Eds.). *Epidemiology and demography in public health* (pp. 364–367). Amsterdam, The Netherlands: Elsevier; 2010.

28. Wallace RB. Bridging epidemiology and demography: Theories and themes. *Ann NY Acad Sci.* 2001;954:63–75.

29. Hibbard R, Elwood LS, Galovski T. Risk and protective factors for posttraumatic stress disorder, prolonged grief, and depression in survivors of the violent death of a loved one. *J Loss Trauma.* 2010;15:426–447.

30. Schaal S, Dusingizemungu J, Jacob N, Neuner F, Elbert T. Associations between prolonged grief disorder, depression, posttraumatic stress disorder and anxiety in Rwandan genocide survivors. *Death Studies.* 2012;36:97–119.

31. Centers for Disease Control. *Lung cancer risk factors.* Updated December 14, 2011. Available at: www.cdc.gov/cancer/lung/basic_info/risk_factors. htm. Accessed March 4, 2012.

32. U.S. Department of Health and Human Services, Centers for Disease Control and Prevention. *The health consequences of smoking: A report of the Surgeon General.* Washington, DC: National Center for Chronic Disease and Health Promotion, Office of Smoking and Health; 2004.

33. National Heart, Lung, and Blood Institute. *What are coronary heart disease risk factors?* 2011. Available at: www.nhlbi.nih.gov/health/health-topics/topics /hd/. Accessed September 12, 2012.

34. Oleseke D. *Epidemiology and the delivery of health care services: Methods and applications.* 3rd ed. New York: Springer; 2009.

35. American Cancer Society. *Cancer prevention and early detection facts and figures, 2011.* Atlanta, GA: Author; 2011.

36. Tests and Measures. Cameron P. Denver Developmental Screening Test II. Test information and article review. 2012. Available at: http://blogs .elon.edu/ptkids/2011/03/16/p-cameron-denver -developmental-screening-test-ii-test-information -and-article-review/. Accessed September 12, 2012.

37. Olsen J, Christensen K, Murray J, Ekbom A. *An introduction to epidemiology for health professionals.* New York: Springer; 2010.

38. Centers for Disease Control and Prevention. *Defining overweight and obesity.* Updated June 21, 2010. Available at: www.cdc.gov/obesity/defining .html. Accessed March 3, 2012.

39. Centers for Disease Control and Prevention. *About BMI for adults.* Updated September 13, 2011. Available at: www.cdc.gov/healthyweight/assessing /bmi/adult_bmi/index.html#Interpreted. Accessed March 3, 2012.

40. Kontos M, Wilson R, Fentiman I. Digital infrared thermal imaging (DITI) of breast lesions: Sensitivity and specificity of detection of primary breast cancers. *Clinical Radiology.* 2011;66(6):536–539.

41. Arora N, Martins D, Ruggerio D, Tousimis E, Swistel AJ, Osborne MP, et al. Effectiveness of a noninvasive digital infrared thermal imaging system in the detection of breast cancer. *Am J Surg.* 2008;196(4):523–526.

42. Spitalnic S. Risk assessment: Relative risk and absolute risk reduction. *Hospital Physician.* 2005;41(10):43–46.

43. Kier KL. Biostatistical applications in epidemiology. *Pharmacotherapy.* 2011;31(1):9–22.

44. Gao S, Chen H, Schwarzschild MA, Ascherio A. A prospective study of bowel movement frequency and risk of Parkinson's disease. *Am J Epidemiol.* 2011;174(5):546–551.

45. U.S. Census Bureau. Motor vehicle accidents and fatalities. *2012 Statistical Abstract.* Available at: www.census

.gov/compendia/statab/cats/transportation/motor
_vehicle_accidents_and_fatalities.html. Accessed
March 3, 2012.

46. Spitalnic S. Risk assessment II: Odds ratio. *Hospital Physician.* 2006;42(1):23–26.

47. Burton K, Rogathe J, Hunter E, Burton M, Swai M, Todd J. et al. Behavioural comorbidity in Tanzanian children with epilepsy: A community-based case-control study. *Dev Med Child Neurol.* 2011;53(12): 1135–1142.

48. Rutter M. A children's behaviour questionnaire for completion by teachers: Preliminary findings. *J Child Psychol Psychiatry.* 1967;8(1):1–11.

49. Kaelin MA, Bayona M. *Attributable risk applications in epidemiology.* 2004. Available at: www.collegeboard.com/prod_downloads/yes/4297_MODULE_17.pdf. Accessed September 12, 2012.

50. Yiannakoulias N. Using population attributable risk to understand geographic disease clusters. *Health Place.* 2009:15;1142–1148.

51. Guy RJ, Wand H, Wilson DP, Prestage G, Jin F, Templeton et al. Using population attributable risk to choose HIV prevention strategies in men who have sex with men. *BioMed Central Pub Health.* 2011;11(247).

52. Hirji KF, Fagerland MW. Calculating unreported confidence intervals for paired data. *BioMed Central Med Res Method.* 2011;11(66).

53. Dorey FJ. Confidence intervals: What is the real result in the target population? *Clin Orthopaedics Related Res.* 2010;468:3137–3138.

54. Wang EW, Ghogomu N, Voelker CJ, Phil D, Rich JT, Paniello RC, et al. A practical guide for understanding confidence intervals and *P* values. *Otolaryngol Head Neck Surg.* 2009;140(6):794–799.

55. Andersen GL, Romundstad P, Cruz J, Himmelmann K., Sellier E, Cans C., et al. Cerebral palsy among children born moderately preterm or at moderately low birthweight between 1980 and 1998: A European register-based study. *Dev Med Child Neurol.* 2011;53(10):913–919.

56. Moons KG, Royston P, Vergouwe Y, Grobbee DE, Altman DG. Prognosis and prognostic research: What, why, and how? *Br Med J.* 2009;338:3117–1320.

57. Vogenberg FR. Predictive and prognostic models. Implications for healthcare decision-making in a modern recession. *Am Drug Health Benefits.* 2009;2(6):218–222.

58. Altman DG, Riley RD. Primer: An evidence-based approach to prognostic markers. *Nature.* 2005;2(9):466–472.

59. Hayden JA, Cote P, Bombardier C. Evaluation of the quality of prognosis studies in systematic reviews. *Ann Int Med.* 2006;144:427–437.

60. Hemingway H, Riley RD, Altman DG. Ten steps towards improving prognosis research. *Br Med J.* 2009;339.

61. Messer B, Griffiths J, Baudouin SV. The prognostic variables predictive of mortality in patients with an exacerbation of COPD admitted to the ICU: An integrative review. *QJM.* 2011;105(2):115–126.

ANSWERS TO EXERCISES

1a.

New HIV Screening Test	Have HIV	Do Not Have HIV	
Tested positive for HIV			
Tested negative for HIV			

1b. a = true positives b = false positives c = false negatives d = true negatives

1c. i. sensitivity
ii. odds ratio
iii. negative predictive value
iv. specificity
v. exposed group odds
vi. positive predictive value

2a. There were 10 new cases in December; therefore the numerator is 10. In computing the denominator, you must ask yourself the following question: Who in the population is at risk of becoming HIV infected as of December 1, 2011? Remember, the 1,200 people previously diagnosed cannot be part of the denominator. Forty-five persons were diagnosed in October and November; they are *not* new cases in December. Therefore, the denominator is 28,000 minus 1,200 (prior to October diagnoses), minus 45 cases in October and November, which equals 26,755 for the population at risk.

$$\frac{10}{26,755} = 0.0037$$

To change the result into a rate, multiply by 10,000. This equals 3.7 cases per 10,000. Remember, creating a rate allows you to make comparisons across populations.

Incidence:

Number of the defined group of people with newly acquired diagnosis or exposure
Number of people in the defined group during a specified period of time

Figure 7–10

Prevalence:

Number of the defined group of people with a given diagnosis or exposure
Number of people in the defined group during a specified period of time

Figure 7–11

In the month of December 2010, the number of new HIV infections (incidence) among person 18 years of age and older was 3.7 cases per 10,000 persons.

2b. Prior to October 2011, there were 1,200 cases of HIV infection among persons 18 years of age and older in Small Town, USA. In the last quarter of the year, October, November, and December, 55 new cases were identified. When you add the 55 new cases of HIV to the 1,200 existing cases of persons living with HIV, the numerator now represents a total of 1,255 people living with HIV. The denominator represents everyone who is 18 years of age and older who is at risk for HIV infection, which is 28,000 minus 1,255, which is now 26,745.

$$\frac{1,255}{26,745} = 0.047$$

To change the result into a rate, multiply by 10,000. This equals 470 cases per 10,000.

In 2011, the number of people living with HIV (prevalence) was 470 cases per 10,000 persons.

3a.

i. $EER = \dfrac{a}{a+b} = \dfrac{10}{10+2,050} = 0.485\%$

   $(0.485\% \times 100,000 = 485\, \text{per}\, 100,000)$

5 per 1,000 adult males who had a first-degree relative with Crohn's had CC.

ii. $CER = \dfrac{c}{c+d} = \dfrac{445}{445+112,600} = 0.394\%$

   $(0.394\% \times 100,000 = 394\, \text{cases per}\, 100,000)$

92 per 100,000 adult males who had a first-degree relative with Crohn's had CC.

iii. AR (attributable risk) = [EER − CER] = [0.485% − 0.394%] = 0.092%

   0.092% of the risk of CC can be attributed to having a first-degree relative with Crohn's disease. Out of 100,000 patients, 92 more cases of CC occur among those who have first-degree relatives with Crohn's disease than among those who do not.

3b. This case-control study indicates that little of the risk of colon cancer (CC) is attributable to having a first-degree relative who has been diagnosed with Crohn's disease. This could indicate that it is not necessary when taking a patient's history to ask if he has a first-degree relative with Crohn's. It is important to note that this was a one-time study and it was *retrospective* in nature. The results rely upon several important factors. First, that the researchers were successful in identifying information on the first-degree relatives of the participants in the study. Second, the relatives were evaluated for Crohn's. Crohn's disease is difficult to diagnose, because its signs and symptoms are difficult to distinguish from other causes of abdominal pain and digestive problems. Advanced imaging techniques must be used to diagnose Crohn's disease. Also, in this study, the researchers were relying on data collected in patient charts. It is difficult to determine if the charts were accurate and complete. We do not know how the information about family members was gathered. More than likely it was collected by asking the patients if they knew whether any of their first-degree relatives (mother, father, siblings, or children) had been di-agnosed with Crohn's. Patient memory is a notoriously biased source of data. Lastly, the data were collected in cancer treatment centers, meaning the results might be skewed. It is common for patients who have been diagnosed with a serious disease to recall exposures to a greater degree than people without the diagnosis. This means the true event rates could be even closer to one another than found in the research. This does not, however, mean that the question has been resolved. The type of research performed in this case indicates a need for further research to be performed.

Evidence-Based Practice in Assessment and Diagnosis

Bernadette Howlett, PhD

INTRODUCTION

The terms *diagnosis* and *assessment* are sometimes used interchangeably, but we will distinguish these words here. Furthermore, the terms have varying definitions across health professions. As such we will offer several definitions of the term diagnosis, although by no means an exhaustive list, as well as definitions of the term assessment. You might find it helpful when searching for information related to diagnosis and assessment to use both terms in your searches.

Diagnosis, according to the National Library of Medicine (NLM) is, "The determination of the nature of a disease or condition, or the distinguishing of one disease or condition from another."[1] The National Institute on Alcohol Abuse and Alcoholism offers this definition: "A mechanism for classifying or categorizing individuals who are afflicted with a particular disorder based on the kinds and severity of problems or symptoms that are associated with that disorder."[2] NANDA International, which is an organization that focuses on diagnosis in nursing, defines **nursing diagnosis** as, "a clinical judgment about actual or potential individual, family,

or community experiences/responses to health problems/life processes. A nursing diagnosis provides the basis for selection of nursing interventions to achieve outcomes for which the nurse has accountability."[3] Additionally, **oral diagnosis** is defined as: "Examination of the mouth and teeth toward the identification and diagnosis of intra-oral disease or manifestation of non-oral conditions."[4]

As we said earlier, diagnosis differs from assessment, which is another term with multiple definitions. In fact, the word *assessment* has fewer formal definitions than the word *diagnosis*, adding to the inconsistent uses of the two terms. The word assessment does not appear in the MeSH database in PubMed, indicating there is not an accepted definition of the term. In the MeSH database there are multiple forms of assessment related to different disciplines, such as nursing assessment, self-assessment, geriatric assessment, personality assessment, and nutrition assessment. There are many more examples of assessment, so we provide just one of the associated definitions as well as our own definition for purposes of this chapter. The term **nursing assessment**, is defined by the NLM as, "Evaluation of the nature and extent of nursing problems presented by a patient for the purpose of patient care planning."[5]

Due to the lack of agreement on the definition of assessment, we offer the following: **Assessment** is collecting the data upon which a diagnosis can be based. Assessment is the process of identifying the signs and symptoms of disease and recording the associated data for the purpose of informing a diagnosis. An assessment is not a diagnosis; it is a process of data collection and the collected data itself. For example, the presence of calculus on teeth can be observed and noted through a clinical assessment but the diagnosis of periodontal disease would require additional information.

While we are on the subject of definitions of diagnosis and assessment, a term that is closely related to the term *diagnosis* is the term **differential diagnosis**, which is, according to the NLM, "the determination of which one of two or more diseases or conditions a patient is suffering from by systematically comparing and contrasting results of diagnostic measures."[6] Here, however, we are focused on evidence-based practice (EBP) related to diagnosis and assessment.

Diagnosis and assessment are interactive processes that involve determining the health problem, based on findings from the history and physical exam. Diagnostic and assessment procedures are selected and utilized to determine the final diagnosis. The assessment and diagnosis process includes, not necessarily in this order, the chief complaint (or reason for the clinical encounter), the patient's history, initial assessment (which includes the presenting signs and symptoms), establishment of a differential diagnosis, diagnostic procedures, and identification of a final diagnosis (or diagnoses). The selection of a diagnosis is an official decision that is usually entered into the patient record and assigned a code such as an ICD (International Classification of Diseases). There are legal and financial considerations involved with diagnosis. For example, insurance coverage varies for different diagnoses.

Each health professional has a different role with regard to assessment and diagnosis that is determined by scope of practice. As such, it is essential for clinicians to remain within the legal confines of practice laws and regulations established at the federal, state, and local level. Practice regulations and laws vary from state to state with regard to the roles and services of each type of healthcare professional. Generally, assessments are performed by most health professionals, but formulation of the diagnosis is reserved for specific professionals (physicians, dentists, psychiatrists, physician assistants, nurse practitioners). Even though there are, in some professions, strict guidelines about who formulates the official diagnosis, the process of diagnosis is most often an interprofessional, team effort.

The assessment and diagnosis processes are not only interprofessional, but are multidimensional for individual clinicians. During the assessment and diagnostic processes the interdependency between your fund of scientific and health-related knowledge, the patient's needs and preferences, and current evidence will be highly apparent... and crucial. After all, medicine (we use the term here to refer to all types of health care) is a *practice* rather than a science. It is informed by more than information that can be objectively observed and quantified. Kathryn Montgomery, who spent years studying physicians in their practice settings, explains:[7]

> There is no question that medicine is scientific or that the benefits of biomedicine are enormous . . . . Yet medicine is not itself a science. Although scientific and technological advances refine clinical problems and provide solutions, physicians still work in situations of inescapable uncertainty.
>
> . . .
>
> Useful information is available in overwhelming quantities, and physicians have the daily task of sorting through it and deciding how some part applies to the individual patient in a given circumstance.
>
> . . .
>
> Scientific information reduces but does not eliminate medicine's uncertainty.
>
> . . .
>
> Despite its reliance on a well-stocked fund of scientific knowledge and its use of technology, [medicine] is still a practice: the care of sick people and the prevention of disease. The recent emphasis on evidence-based medicine grounds that practice more firmly in clinical research and aims to refine and extend clinical judgment, but it will not alter the character of medicine or it rationality . . . [sic] Medicine's success relies on the physicians' capacity for

clinical judgment. It is neither a science nor a technical skill (although it puts both to use) but the ability to work out how general rules—scientific principles, clinical guidelines— apply to one particular patient. This is—to use Aristotle's word—phronesis, or practical reasoning.[1]

Her observations apply equally to all types of healthcare providers. For this reason, we feel it is important to frame the incorporation of evidence in clinical decision making as a practice; hence the term *evidence-based practice.*

Perhaps the single most important decision made by clinicians is the diagnosis and its associated differential. When applying EBP to assessment and diagnosis, you will employ concurrent, retrospective, and prospective approaches. The general steps for EBP (**Figure 8–1**) during the diagnostic process are the same as for other processes (i.e., treatment, prevention, and epidemiology), but the information need relates to selecting and interpreting the best diagnostic procedure. The central evidence-based question in diagnosis is: Which diagnostic procedure is most appropriate for an individual situation? For example, which lab test is the most accurate for diagnosing HIV? Or, when is history and physical exam alone (without an x-ray) sufficient for diagnosing a sprained ankle?

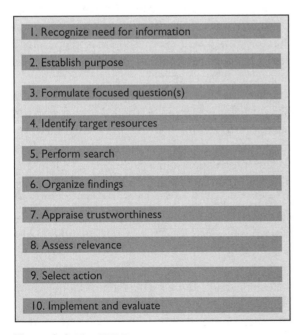

1. Recognize need for information

2. Establish purpose

3. Formulate focused question(s)

4. Identify target resources

5. Perform search

6. Organize findings

7. Appraise trustworthiness

8. Assess relevance

9. Select action

10. Implement and evaluate

Figure 8–1 The EBP Process

TYPES OF DIAGNOSTIC PROCEDURES

The three major categories of diagnostic procedures are (1) history and physical exam, (2) laboratory tests, and, (3) imaging. With some diseases and disorders, you use all three types. In many cases, you have the option to choose from among them. Sometimes the history and physical exam alone is sufficient to arrive at an accurate diagnosis. Other times more invasive tests are needed, such as blood draws, spinal taps, and biopsies. And still other times it is necessary to have an image taken, such as an x-ray, a **CT (computed tomography)** scan, an **MRI (magnetic resonance imaging)** scan, a nuclear medicine study, a PET (positron emission tomography) scan, or an ultrasound. One of the challenges in diagnosis is determining which procedures to use in light of the differential, the available resources, the degree of invasiveness, the patient's preferences, and accuracy of the diagnostic procedure options.

This is especially true in the United States today, where we tend to expect more testing, laboring under the belief that labs and images provide better evidence than history and physical exam alone. As documented by Smith-Bindman et al., in recent years the use of imaging procedures has increased significantly.[8] CT examinations nearly tripled from 52 per 1,000 cases in 1996 to 149 per 1,000 cases in 2010. Similarly, MRI use increased from 17 per 1,000 to 65 per 1,000, which was more than a 380% increase. All types of imaging increased over the 15-year period studied, except nuclear medicine. In addition to a belief in the superior accuracy of imaging, another reason suggested for the significant increase in imaging is **defensive medical practice**; that is, the excessive use of diagnostic procedures to avoid lawsuits by showing that every available measure was employed. Another motive suggested has been that of pure financial gain. However, the research showed that profit motives were not a likely explanation for overuse of diagnostic imaging, because the rate of increase among HMOs was similar to that of fee-for-service organizations. In HMOs, there is no profit motive for performing such tests.

The point of this discussion about the increase in use of imaging procedures is to underscore the need for evidence-based diagnosis. The selection of diagnostic tools should be based on patient-centered outcomes rather than fear of lawsuits. Some diagnostic procedures are invasive and carry risk of harm to patients. The potential risk of harm from a lab test or an image must be weighed against the inherent bias associated with history and physical exam procedures. Lab tests tend to be invasive, and imaging often exposes patients to radiation and/or chemicals. Although these tests might produce more information, they might or might not be more accurate than the history and physical exam. In fact, in many cases (certainly not all cases), diagnosis can be reliably based on history and physical exam more than any other source. Your skills and experiences as a clinician greatly influence the accuracy of the history and physical exam results.

The purposes of developing new diagnostic procedures can be to reduce invasiveness or discomfort, lower cost, speed up the diagnostic process, decrease the number of patient encounters needed for the purpose of diagnosis, or increase the accuracy of diagnostic options. When assessing a diagnostic procedure consider the purpose of having a new diagnostic tool. Will the new tool achieve one of the purposes we just listed? Is the current standard of care meeting the needs of your patients, or is there sufficient room for improvement to justify the potential cost associated with a new diagnostic procedure? Often new diagnostic procedures involve purchasing equipment, which can be very expensive; buying supplies; and obtaining additional training (possibly certification or licensing). There might be financial pressure from organizations to recuperate the cost of the new diagnostic capability. There might even be motivation to use the new capability even when the current diagnostic procedure is sufficient simply because it is new and interesting.

History and Physical Exam

The history and physical exam includes a set of skills and procedures. They are based on the clinical team's ability to elicit information from the patient as well as information on the patient's family. Often the history and physical exam involves several people, including the first person who speaks to the patient when he or she either calls or presents to the service, the person who collects the initial information (perhaps on an admission form or during a medical severity exam), the person who formulates the working diagnosis, and the person who determines the final diagnosis. Perhaps all of these communications happen with just one person, but more than likely there are four or five members of the healthcare team involved in gathering the patient's history and performing the physical exam. Certain redundancies in collection of history and physical exam information are intentional, in fact, in order to ensure that mistakes are avoided.

From the moment a patient contacts your practice or service, the team is gathering information. First, there is the reason for being seen. In an emergency department, the reason might be an injury from a car crash. In a women's health clinic, the reason might be that the patient thinks she's pregnant. In a family practice, the reason might be the patient needs an employment physical. For that matter, a patient might show up at any one of these places for any one of these reasons. But we digress. The reason for the visit is often the first piece of information gathered. Sometimes the reason given for a visit turns out not to be the actual issue or just one of several issues the patient is facing.

Several protocols are available for collecting a patient history. Generally, there are two types of patient histories: the focused history and the complete history. A **focused history** is designed to collect information about a specific problem and differentiate between critical and noncritical causes. A focused history covers only the relevant body systems, past medical/surgical history, medications, family, and social history. On the other hand, a **complete history** covers *all* body systems and collects information on the patient's entire health status, including items such as (but not limited to): past medical/surgical history, medications, family, and social history. The selection of a focused or a complete history depends on the nature of the encounter, the severity of the problem, the amount of time available, patient preferences, and the cost of care.

The patient history not only provides important information about the patient's health, but it also helps engender the patient's trust in you and the clinical team. The manner in which the patient history is gathered greatly influences the patient's willingness to participate in the healthcare encounter. The more a patient trusts you, the better the information you will get. The same is true for the physical exam. Patients must cooperate with each physical exam procedure in order for you to get accurate information.

Clinicians use a countless number of physical exam procedures. Dental hygienists perform intra- and extraoral exams, for example, to look for signs of oral cancer. A nurse will examine a patient's abdomen with visual inspection, auscultation of bowel sounds, and palpation to test for abnormal masses. Physical therapists and athletic trainers use the Hoover test to look for nonorganic etiology of back pain. An ophthalmologist will perform a visual acuity exam. We could fill several libraries just listing all of the types of physical exam procedures.

For both the history and the physical exam, research can help you determine which items will more consistently provide the most helpful information. Much greater research effort tends to be focused on diagnostic lab tests and radiologic procedures than on history and physical exam procedures. This is most likely because there is minimal regulation of history and physical exam procedures compared to laboratory and imaging equipment. Additionally, history and physical exam procedures are typically less invasive and lower risk than labs and imaging, not to mention the lack of a profit motive associated with history and physical exam. There simply is less opportunity to make money on selling products associated with history and physical exam procedures compared to selling imaging and laboratory equipment. In many cases manufacturers fund the research performed on diagnostic devices and supplies.

In terms of evidence, epidemiological research is highly relevant to diagnosis. Epidemiological research provides information on the risk factors associated with disease and the incidence and prevalence of a disease. Epidemiological information helps you determine how to prioritize the differential diagnosis by giving you the likelihood of each diagnosis in the differential. Epidemiology helps you determine the importance of family history and social history risk factors.

For example, according to the Mayo Clinic[9] up to 90% of people with migraines have a family history of migraine attacks. Also, most patients will have their first migraine by the time they are 40 years old. In adulthood, women are three times more likely to have migraines than men, whereas in childhood boys are more often affected than girls. This information is useful in diagnosing a patient who presents with headache. If the patient has family members who have migraine and the patient is an adult female younger than age 40, the research indicates a greater likelihood for migraine. This is not to say that her headache might not be caused by a brain tumor, aneurysm, muscle contraction (tension), genetic malformation, drugs, infection, underlying disease, or injury. However, it does mean that migraine will be high on the differential diagnosis if the physical signs and symptoms do not point to one of the other items in the differential for headache.

When a patient presents with headache, in addition to collecting history information, you will perform a physical examination. It is likely in this case that you would perform a focused clinical exam. According to the American Academy of Family Physicians (AAFP),[10] a complete neurological exam should be performed when an adult presents with acute headache and "the general physical examination should include vital signs, funduscopic and cardiovascular assessment, and palpation of the head and face." Regarding the neurological examination, the AAFP states:

> A complete neurologic examination is essential, and the findings must be documented. The examination should include mental status, level of consciousness, cranial nerve testing, pupillary responses, motor strength testing, deep tendon reflexes, sensation, pathologic reflexes (e.g., Babinski's sign), cerebellar function and gait testing, and signs of meningeal

irritation (Kernig's and Brudzinski's signs). Particular attention should be given to detecting problems related to the optic, oculomotor, trochlear, and abducens nerves (cranial nerves II, III, IV, and VI, respectively).[10]

However, according to the AAFP most patients with headache have normal neurological and general physical examinations. These normal findings are important pertinent negatives for diagnosis of headache. **Pertinent negatives** are findings that are pertinent to other diagnoses (such as aneurysm), and they are negative for the diagnosis of interest (migraine in this case). Pertinent negatives help you rule out items in the differential.

Laboratory Tests

Laboratory tests are essential tools for diagnosis. New types of tests emerge daily, ranging from blood tests, to biopsies, to tests of excretions (such as urine, stool, and saliva). Some lab tests can be performed in the clinic, whereas others have to be sent to the laboratory. More information is available in the literature about lab tests than about history and physical exam procedures. Research questions associated with lab tests include sensitivity/specificity, positive and negative predictive value, complications, discomfort, cost, indications/contraindications, and relative efficacy according to population. Sensitivity/specificity (S/S) and positive/negative predictive values (PPV/NPV) are important characteristics of any diagnostic procedure. It is rare for these characteristics to be researched with history and physical exam procedures. However, S/S and PPV/NPV data should be accessible on the lab tests used.

Locating S/S and PPV/NPV information might be challenging, however. We recommend looking in the packaging materials that come with the equipment as well as searching the usual research databases and the manufacturer's website. If you cannot find the information, we encourage you to contact the manufacturer. Many devices require FDA approval, and it is likely that research is available.

Knowing about the accuracy of lab tests is important in deciding your approach to each patient. For example, should otherwise healthy adult males

receive the prostate-specific antigen (PSA) test at a certain age? (The **PSA test** has been used to test for prostate cancer.) Should all adult women receive a mammogram every year? Your answers to these questions will depend, in part, on the S/S and PPV/NPV for these tests. (We will discuss other statistical values for diagnostic tests later in the chapter.)

It is important not only to consider the statistical accuracy of the lab tests you use, but also the discomfort, cost, complications, and indications/contraindications of the tests. It is very worthwhile to look up research about these topics as part of your evidence-based diagnosis activities. For example, the results of a PSA test might indicate further testing, namely a prostate biopsy. Although the PSA test itself is only minimally invasive (it requires just a blood draw), the prostate biopsy is a much more invasive and expensive procedure.

The first step we recommend you to take is to look up pictures of prostate biopsy procedures. (Be aware that the pictures are likely to show exposed rectums and possibly testicles. Do not look this up if seeing such images will be distressing to you.) We suggest looking up these images to help you conceptualize the experience your patients will have if they receive this procedure. The point is that you might reconsider using the PSA test if the results are not accurate enough to justify the discomfort and cost of the prostate biopsy.

In fact, as of May 2012, the AAFP is recommending against performing PSA screening for asymptomatic men in the general population, regardless of age.[11] According to the AAFP, most men who are found to be positive for prostate cancer with the PSA test did not benefit, because biopsy later showed the tumors to be nonaggressive. Nonetheless, oftentimes the patients receive aggressive disease treatments. According to the AAFP, United States Preventive Services Task Force (USPSTF) research found that:

PSA testing often produces false-positive results (about 80% of PSA test results are false-positive when a PSA threshold between 2.5 micrograms per liter and 4.0 micrograms per liter is used). Such results are associated with negative psychological effects, as well as additional, unnecessary testing.

[Furthermore], nearly 90% of U.S. men with PSA-detected prostate cancer are treated with surgery, radiation or androgen deprivation. As many as 5 in 1,000 men who are treated surgically will die within 1 month of the procedure and between 10 and 70 of these men will have serious complications from surgery. In addition, of men treated with radiotherapy or surgery, 200–300 in 1,000 will suffer long-term problems, including urinary incontinence, impotence or both.[11]

By no means does the recommendation from the AAFP and the USPSTF indicate that PSA testing should be withheld. The decision to utilize any given lab test should be based on the complete clinical picture with each individual patient, and the patient should be involved in the decision. The AAFP article quotes AAFP President Glen Stream, MD, MBI, as saying "When it comes down to individual doctors and their individual patients, they may still do the testing, but it needs to be done using all the information available. Having that discussion, and knowing the test may do more harm than good, is important."

Imaging

Another important category of diagnostic tests is imaging. There are many types of diagnostic images, ranging from x-ray, to US, CT, MRI, and others. As we mentioned earlier, there are risks associated with imaging tests, such as radiation exposure, adverse reactions to contrast media, and psychological harm (such as claustrophobia). Furthermore, imaging procedures can be quite expensive, especially functional images. Functional images are images that show not only the structures in the imaged area, but how the tissue is functioning, such as blood flow. Some functional images are live-action, showing function in real time. Not surprisingly, functional imaging tends to be even more expensive, but also has the potential to be more informative.

As we already mentioned, it is important to consider the costs, side effects, and benefits from the information provided by images. When considering an imaging test, ask yourself if having the image confirm the diagnosis would change the course of treatment. If treatment would be the same with or without the image, then it might not be necessary to perform the test. And, as with other types of diagnostic testing, consider S/S, PPV/NPV, patient preference, access, time, and indications/contraindications. We will discuss the list of considerations with regard to assessment and diagnostic procedures in a later section of this chapter.

Reference Standards

One important consideration in evaluating an assessment or diagnostic procedure is the **reference standard test**. The reference standard test is the current standard, or the **gold standard**. It is the test that is normally used or the test that has been shown to be the most accurate. New diagnostic procedures should be tested in side-by-side comparison to the current reference standard. For example, the combination of history, physical exam, and biopsy is the most accurate method for diagnosis of prostate cancer. If a new type of lab test, or a new version of the PSA test, were developed, the new test should be compared against the gold standard for prostate cancer diagnosis among a known population of patients. (The gold standard being history/physical exam/prostate biopsy.) The known population should include those with the diagnosis and those who are free of the diagnosis.

One way for you to evaluate the research on a given diagnostic procedure is to look up the statistics on the reference standard. If the reference standard is a highly accurate and reliable test (such as the HIV ELISA test; ELISA stands for enzyme-linked immunosorbent assay) then the new diagnostic tool should be more accurate or at least equally accurate with some other advantage (less invasive, less costly, less time to result, more accessible, etc.). If, however, the reference standard has a low level of accuracy, then the comparison must be reported carefully. For example, if one test is 70% sensitive and another test is 80% sensitive, the researchers might present the difference as statistically significant, as it may well be. They could state that the new test represents a 14.3% relative improvement in sensitivity. It is a matter of whether they use an absolute difference (80 –70) or a relative difference $\left(\frac{80-70}{70}\right)$. Consider the following possible way of presenting these results:

New Cool Diagnostic Procedure (NCDP) showed a 143% relative improvement (n = 477; p = 0.003) in sensitivity (80%) compared to Old Uncool Diagnostic Procedure (OUDP). The sensitivity of OUDP was 70%.

Such a statement could be misleading. It is important to look for the actual statistics for each diagnostic procedure and determine if the accuracy and reliability of each one is sufficient for clinical purposes. In summary, every diagnostic procedure should be compared to a known reference standard, preferably the gold standard. The researchers should report the accuracy and other important characteristics of each test studied (cost, time, invasiveness, complications, etc.), and they should present the results in terms of clinical relevance. The researchers should demonstrate how outcomes that matter will be sufficiently improved in comparison to the current standard or the gold standard to justify the use of the new diagnostic procedure.

DIAGNOSTIC TOOL SELECTION FACTORS

As evidenced by the discussion thus far, numerous considerations must be taken into account when selecting a diagnostic procedure. It is worthwhile to look for research related to each of these considerations (when time allows and the circumstances warrant it).

Cost

The cost of a diagnostic procedure needs to be considered from several perspectives: first is the cost for the diagnostic equipment, supplies, training, and maintenance; second is the cost incurred by patients, depending on whether the diagnostic procedure is covered by insurance; third is the cost to insurance companies (or the government) for the diagnostic procedure. Each form of cost has different results and implications. It can be challenging

to obtain some of this information. You might perform a general literature search. Some organizations might have a financial motive for making this kind of information difficult to locate. However, more frequently questions of cost are being investigated and reported, especially for health care that is funded through Medicare and Medicaid.

Access

Issues of access are in part related to cost (some procedures are too expensive for some healthcare organizations or for patients), but there are other access issues. For example, new technologies take time to progress from the early adoption phase to widespread use. Organizations take a certain amount of risk in adopting new diagnostic procedures. Little support might be available for the product if something malfunctions. The clinicians and staff who use the equipment might not have access to a technical support resource based on their hours of operation. Parts and supplies might be difficult to access. Equipment and software can quickly become outdated, and manufacturers can go out of business due to competition. Smaller organizations and practices with more limited resources are slower to adopt new technologies and diagnostic procedures due to the risk and cost involved. It is important for researchers to examine and discuss issues of access in publications related to assessment and diagnostic procedures.

Practitioner Experience

Another essential consideration is the level of experience practitioners have with a given diagnostic procedure. When a modified procedure is developed that is similar to a procedure that is familiar to clinicians, then it is easier to understand the research and consider its implications. However, when a new type of diagnostic procedure is introduced, more cognitive effort is required for understanding the research and the implications of the new option. Furthermore, the level of experience of the practitioners who administered the diagnostic procedure during the research is pivotal.

Publications related to diagnostic procedures should explain the experience of the clinicians who participated in the research that compared the diagnostic procedures. The research clinicians should have significant expertise in all diagnostic procedures used in the study. The researchers should describe any relevant certifications and licenses.

Patient Preference

Diagnostic procedure issues involving patient preferences (such as travel distances for tests available in limited locations, length of time to get results, and fear or discomfort with the procedure) should also be studied and described. For example, one of the reasons that imaging has increased so dramatically is that patients prefer noninvasive procedures and tend to believe that imaging provides more complete and accurate information.[8] There is a tendency, in other words, for patients (and perhaps healthcare professionals) to view technology as superior to or less biased than human senses and to perceive the discomfort of an invasive procedure (such as a biopsy or blood test) as a greater problem than the risk of exposure or harm from radiation or the chemicals (such as contrast media) used with some imaging studies. Perhaps this is because discomfort is experienced immediately with invasive procedures but harm from radiation is not guaranteed and will not be experienced until sometime in the future.

Interestingly, it is easy to forget that imaging technologies also rely on humans to operate them and to interpret the data they produce. As such, imaging techniques are prone to human error but perceived as less so than history and physical exam procedures. Research on various types of imaging techniques has shown an inconsistency in results as interpreted by different radiologists and clinicians. An increasing body of research is also examining the necessity of imaging. For example, a study by Tocci et al.[12] compared the decision to use MRI for evaluation of foot and ankle injuries. The study included 201 patients who did not have fractures. Among foot and ankle specialists, who are highly skilled in performing a focused history

and physical exam related to foot and ankle injuries, only 5.9% would have performed an MRI. Of those 5.9%, in all cases the MRI ordered by the foot and ankle specialist provided information that was helpful in the treatment of the injury. In contrast, 15.4% of the patients had an MRI performed by an outside source prior to being seen by the specialist. Eighty-seven percent of the prereferral MRIs were found to be unnecessary.

That is not to say that patient preference should be trumped by evidence. If a patient with a foot/ankle injury requests an imaging study, that request needs to be considered. The relative merits of the procedure as well as the risks and costs need to be discussed with the patient. Additionally, the patient should be advised to consider the possibility that insurance might not cover the test if it is later deemed to have been unnecessary. (The clinician needs to also consider the possibility, because your organization might get stuck with the bill.) If the indication for the use of an imaging study is equivocal, it is the patient's preference to have it done, and if the patient is able to pay for it, then you might decide to go forward with the test in order to relieve the patient's worry. Imagine, for example, that the patient is a figure skater, runner, or avid hiker. It is important to keep in mind that there are many variables that go into every decision and that there are rarely, if ever, definitive rules that fit with every case.

Invasiveness

We have mentioned the issue of invasiveness as a consideration in terms of patient discomfort. It is also a consideration for you as the clinician. Invasive procedures often have increased risks of harm, including injury, infection, and emotional trauma. For example, consider those children who experienced unnecessary spinal taps at the hands of Arthur Howard Wentworth (a physician who administered unnecessary lumbar punctures to children in order to determine if the procedure had unfavorable results. He deemed the procedure harmless, despite the pain it caused.).[13] The pain experienced by those children might have led to a lifelong fear of health care or of needles. It might have resulted in distrust of healthcare providers that inhibited their ability to seek care when needed later in life.

In addition to the potential harm caused by invasive procedures, clinicians need to consider their ability to perform the procedure. Accurate diagnostic results depend on your ability to perform the procedure correctly and to adapt to the unique anatomy and physiology of each patient. Diagnostic research publications should explain the role of the clinicians' ability to perform the procedure. This is important in terms of the clinicians who performed the procedure for the study as well as for clinicians who will perform the procedure in standard practice. Researchers should report the effect that skill and experience have on the outcome of the procedure. If a procedure is particularly difficult, the publication should say so. It should also explain what mistakes are most commonly made and what complications most commonly occur as a result.

Time

Time is an important issue from many perspectives in health care. It includes the amount of time the clinician has to discuss diagnostic options with the patient before selecting one, the amount of time it takes to perform a diagnostic procedure, the amount of time it takes to get the results from the procedure, and the amount of time it takes for patients to travel to the location where the procedure is available. For example, patients experiencing ST segment elevation myocardial infarction (STEMI) have a 90-minute target window for percutaneous coronary intervention (PCI).[14] PCI is a diagnostic tool that can also be used for intervention. Blockages in coronary arteries can be identified and treated during the same procedure. The golden 90-minute window is often referred to as *door-to-balloon* time. Patients treated within this window have better outcomes in terms of mortality than patients who receive the intervention after 90 minutes have passed.

The research performed to determine the time element associated with STEMI is an excellent example of time as a research question in EBP.

The evidence supporting this recommendation is strong. It can be somewhat challenging to find details related to time. You need to be fairly creative in how you form your search question. Sometimes you may not know what kind of time information is relevant. One strategy is to simply keep an eye out for time information associated with the diagnostic procedure of interest. Another strategy is to begin by looking at the information provided by the manufacturer or to contact your lab and ask if they have that information. The challenge is in locating research on which the time information is based. The better your knowledge of the diagnostic procedure, the better your ability to locate research related to it, if any has been published.

Indications/Contraindications, Side Effects, Complications

In addition to time, invasiveness, patient preference, practitioner experience, access, and cost, diagnostic research should also provide information on the indications, contraindications, and side effects of diagnostic procedures. During a clinical trial, researchers should (and usually do) keep track of many variables for each patient. A particular diagnostic procedure might not work well with a certain type of patient. Severity of disease, age, sex, ethnicity, socioeconomic status, and comorbidities (as well as other variables) can all be important influencing variables in terms of the accuracy of a diagnostic test. Researchers should track and report on all such variables. In many cases, this tracking of variables leads to identification of indications and contraindications.

For example, PCI is indicated for patients with suspected STEMI (assuming the clinical presentation and early lab tests support it). However, PCI has absolute as well as relative contraindications. According to the *Merck Manual*, one absolute contraindication for PCI is "significant obstruction of the left main coronary artery without a nonobstructed bypass graft to the left anterior descending or left circumflex arteries."[15] Relative contraindications include coagulopathy, hypercoagulable states, diffusely diseased vessels without focal stenosis, a single diseased vessel providing all perfusion to the myocardium, total occlusion of a coronary artery, and stenosis of less than 50%. These contraindications have been determined both through understanding of coronary as well as circulatory anatomy and physiology as well as research on PCI.

Diagnostic research should also report side effects associated with the procedure. For example, contrast-induced nephropathy (CIN) is a risk associated with PCI.[16] CIN is a type of kidney injury that can occur with procedures that utilize iodinated contrast material. It results in a hazardous increase in serum creatinine concentration and significantly increases the risk of cardiac morbidity and mortality. In fact, of all angiographic procedures, according to the *Merck Manual*, PCI has the highest risk of CIN.[15] We should caution with this discussion that, according to Palevsky,[16] despite the significant number of studies that have reported adverse clinical outcomes associated with CIN, the evidence is not sufficient to definitively support a causal relationship.

It is generally not too difficult to locate information on indications, contraindications, and side effects. A search that combines the name of the treatment with the terms *indications*, *contraindications*, *side effects*, and *complications* will often yield the information needed. In the case of PCI, we performed this search using a general Internet search engine, and within the first few hits was a link to the Medscape page on PCI. The site included links for background information, indications, contraindications, outcomes, and complications. The information included descriptions of the research as well as links to the references. The levels and types of studies were described. We were then able to look up the references and evaluate the quality of the information provided by this site.

DIAGNOSTIC GUIDELINES, ALGORITHMS, AND STANDARDS OF CARE

An important tool in diagnosis is the diagnostic guideline, algorithm, and standard of care. A *diagnostic*

guideline provides recommendations about diagnostic criteria, staging of disease severity, and differentiating subtypes of a disease. A *diagnostic algorithm* offers a standardized set of steps and criteria for guiding diagnosis. Diagnostic algorithms provide the sequence of diagnostic tests to perform. Many diagnostic guidelines include an algorithm. It is important to remember that guidelines and algorithms cannot replace your clinical judgment and the insight you have with individual patients. They are additional tools to inform your practice. Guidelines and algorithms can help you avoid missing a step or failing to consider an alternative diagnosis. They cannot give you, however, any information about the patient in front of you.

Another source that informs your diagnostic strategy is the local **standard of care**. The standard of care is the *usual practice* utilized by other clinicians and experts in the region. Standards of care tend to vary geographically and are significantly influenced by the history in a region and the experiences of clinicians working near one another. Medicine has historically been a journeyman-style practice in which masters have passed down their craft to subsequent generations. As such, that craft has formed somewhat differently from one area to the next. To a certain degree EBP has been viewed as the polar opposite to standard of care. Such dichotomies are neither accurate nor helpful, because there is clearly a valuable role for both in formulating the most likely diagnosis.

DIAGNOSTIC BIOSTATISTICS

Now we arrive at the main event for this chapter, diagnostic biostatistics. In this section we discuss the concepts of sensitivity/specificity and positive predictive value/negative predictive value, and we introduce the concepts of **AUC (area under the curve)** and the **ROC (receiver operating characteristic)** curve as well as the likelihood ratio, pre-test odds, and post-test odds.

Sensitivity and Specificity

With regard to diagnostic testing, *sensitivity* is the ability of a diagnostic test to be positive given the person tested has the disease/problem; *specificity* is the ability of the test to be negative given that the person does not have the disease/problem.[17] Sensitivity and specificity tell you the accuracy of the diagnostic tools you use. Sensitivity and specificity can be calculated on lab tests, imaging studies, guidelines, and clinical exam techniques. Sensitivity and specificity research is used when a new diagnostic test is developed. New diagnostic tests are most often developed when the current tests available are too expensive or too invasive. They are also developed when no test has previously existed or current tests are known to be of low sensitivity and/or specificity.

When there is not an existing gold standard test to use for comparison, the selection of the sample patients in the study is of even greater importance. Whatever the situation, researchers must explain how the study sample was selected and how they were determined to have or not have the diagnosis. Most often sensitivity and specificity research is performed on lab tests and imaging studies, with little attention paid to guidelines and even less effort spent on clinical exam techniques. Additionally, more resources are expended on research involving diagnostic studies used for diseases with greater morbidity and mortality.

It is important that you evaluate the accuracy of the diagnostic tests you use in your practice by looking for research on the sensitivity and specificity of the tests. This is depicted in the following *2 × 2 table* (**Table 8–1**); such tables are also referred to as *contingency tables*.

To calculate sensitivity, researchers divide the number of true positives (*a*) by the total number of patients with the condition (*a* + *c*). That is to say that sensitivity is the proportion of true positives out of all who have the condition. Similarly,

to calculate specificity, researchers divide the number of patients who tested negative (*d*) by the total number of patients who do not have the condition (*b* + *d*), which is to say that specificity is the proportion of true negatives out of all who do not have the condition. Thus, the formulas to calculate sensitivity and specificity are as follows:

$$\text{Sensitivity } \frac{a}{(a+c)}$$
$$\text{Specificity } \frac{d}{(b+d)}$$

A visual way to think about the formulas for sensitivity and specificity is to see them as vertical arrows over the contingency table. Note that if a total row is added below the contingency table, this row creates a cell for the denominators in the two formulas (as shown in **Figures 8–2** and **8–3**). The denominator for sensitivity is *a* + *c* and the denominator for specificity is *b* + *d*.

At this point, you might be asking how researchers know the total number of patients who have the disease or the total number of patients who do not have the disease. In order to evaluate the sensitivity and specificity of diagnostic tests, researchers

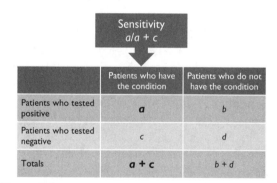

Figure 8–2 Visual Way to Think of the Sensitivity Formula

Table 8–1 Sensitivity and Specificity Contingency Table

	Patients Who Have the Condition	Patients Who Do Not Have the Condition
Patients who tested positive	*a*	*b*
Patients who tested negative	*c*	*d*

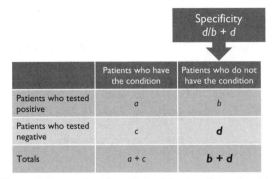

Figure 8–3 Visual Way to Think of the Specificity Formula

begin with a population of patients who are already known to have the disease through prior testing as well as positive clinical signs and symptoms. As we discussed earlier, the prior clinical test used for such research is often referred to as the *reference standard* or the *gold standard*.

Based on 100 test results, the contingency table shown in **Table 8–2** indicates 100% sensitivity and 100% specificity.

To state sensitivity and specificity, we would say, "100% of those with the condition tested positive" (for 100% sensitivity) or "100% of those without the condition tested negative" (for 100% specificity).

A study published in 2011 by Boppana et al.[18] evaluated the sensitivity and specificity of two PCR (polymerase chain reaction) saliva screening tests to test newborns for cytomegalovirus (CMV). One test was a liquid-saliva test and the other was a dry-saliva test. The advantage of the liquid-saliva test is that the test can be performed without having

to wait for the specimen to dry. The current assay used for testing for CMV (rapid culture) cannot be automated, meaning that the test takes more time because the culture requires time to grow.

CMV is a type of herpesvirus infection that is often asymptomatic at birth but can lead to hearing loss if not treated early. It is a common infection that is usually harmless. However, it can cause serious disease in infants who are infected before birth (congenital CMV). According to the Centers for Disease Control and Prevention (CDC),[19] about 1 in 150 infants are born with congenital CMV. Of those with congenital CMV, 1 in 5 develops permanent problems as a result of the infection.

The researchers in the CMV diagnostic study identified 85 newborns who tested positive for CMV on the current reference standard test (rapid culture performed on saliva specimens).[18] The goal of the study was to determine if an automated test using PCR on dried or liquid saliva would produce results as accurate as the rapid culture but in less time. In other words, the rapid culture is the *gold standard* used in this study, and the PCR saliva test is the experimental diagnostic procedure. **Table 8–3** shows the results for the liquid-saliva PCR assay.

In this study by Boppana et al.,[18] the number of patients in the liquid-saliva group (n = 17,654) who had the condition (based on positive rapid culture) was 85. Hence, the value that represents $a + c$ is 85. Of the 85 subjects with CMV, all of them tested positive via the liquid-saliva PCR test, producing a sensitivity of 100%. There were zero false-negative

Table 8–2 Contingency Table with 100% Sensitivity and 100% Specificity

	Patients Who Have the Condition	Patients Who Do Not Have the Condition
Patients who tested positive	100	0
Patients who tested negative	0	100
Totals	100	100
	Sensitivity = $a/a+c$ Sensitivity = $100/100$ Sensitivity = 100%*	Specificity = $d/b+d$ Specificity = $100/100$ Specificity = 100%*

* Note that sensitivity and specificity are expressed as percentages.

Table 8–3 Contingency Table for Liquid-Saliva PCR Test (n = 17,654)

	Patients Who Have the Condition	**Patients Who Do Not Have the Condition**
Patients who tested positive	**85**	17
Patients who tested negative	0	**17,552**
Totals	**85**	**17,569**

$$\text{Sensitivity} = \frac{a}{(a+c)} \qquad \text{Specificity} = \frac{d}{(b+d)}$$

$$\text{Sensitivity} = \frac{100}{100+0} \qquad \text{Specificity} = \frac{17,552}{17+17,552}$$

$$\text{Sensitivity} = \frac{100}{100} \qquad \text{Specificity} = \frac{17,552}{17,569}$$

$$\text{Sensitivity} = 100\% \qquad \text{Specificity} = 99.9\%$$

results ($c = 0$). A total of 17,569 newborns were identified who did not have CMV according to the rapid culture test. Of these newborns without CMV, 17,552 tested negative on the liquid-saliva PCR test, producing a specificity of 99.9%. There were 17 false-positive results ($b = 17$).

For the dry-saliva group, the authors found that the dry-saliva test had 97.4% sensitivity and 99.9% specificity after screening 17,327 newborns. Of the dry-saliva group, 76 were positive for CMV and 17,251 were negative for CMV on rapid culture. Based on these values of 97.4% sensitivity and 99.9% specificity for the dry-saliva test, what are the values for a, b, c, and d in the contingency table (**Table 8–4**)?

We know that 76 subjects had CMV and 17,251 subjects did not have CMV. Knowing these numbers, as well as the sensitivity (97.4%) and specificity (99.9%), we can calculate the number of true positives (a) and the number of true negatives (d) as well as the number of false positives (c) and false negatives (b). The number of true positives can be calculated by multiplying sensitivity (SN) by the total number of patients who are positive for the condition (*TotDxPos*). The abbreviation **Dx** means *diagnosis*. (Also, while we are on the topic of medical abbreviations, **Tx** stands for *treatment*, and *Sx* stands for *symptoms* or for *surgery*.)

Total Dx Positives (*TotDxPos*) were 76. Similarly, we can calculate false positives by multiplying

Table 8–4 Contingency Table for Dry-Saliva PCR Test (n = 17,327)

	Patients Who Have the Condition	**Patients Who Do Not Have the Condition**
Patients who tested positive		
Patients who tested negative		
Totals	**76**	**17,251**

$$\text{Sensitivity} = \frac{a}{a+c} \qquad \text{Specificity} = \frac{d}{b+d}$$

specificity (SP) by the total number of patients who are negative for the condition (*TotDxNeg*). *TotDxNeg* were 17,251. **Table 8–5** shows the formulas.

Note that there is some rounding required to get to the values of 74 for true positives and 17,234 for true negatives. The values for both must be whole numbers because the number represents a count of the number of infants. There cannot be a partial infant.

Now that we know *a* (true positives) and *d* (true negatives) it is a simple matter of subtraction to calculate *c* (false positives) and *b* (false negatives). To calculate false positives (*c*), we subtract the true positives (*a*) from the *TotDxPos*. To calculate the false negatives (*b*), we subtract the true negatives (*d*) from *TotDxNeg*. **Table 8–6** shows these formulas.

The complete contingency table, therefore, is as shown in **Table 8–7**.

Before we discuss the meaning of the results, we want to present a version of the contingency table (**Table 8–8**) that shows each of the cells with its semantic abbreviation.

Table 8–9 presents one more way to present this table.

Thus, based on the results of this study,[18] the liquid-saliva PCR test is a little more sensitive than the dry-saliva PCR test and the two tests are equally specific. Furthermore, both tests are sufficiently sensitive and specific to warrant consideration as utilization for a first-line test, and rapid culture can be reserved as a second-line test to be used to confirm a positive result or as an alternative when the PCR results are in question.

Table 8–5 Formulas to Calculate True Positives (*a*) and True Negatives (*d*)

True Positives (*a*)	True Negatives (*d*)
$a = SN \times TotDxPos$	$d = SP \times TotDxNeg$
$a = .974 \times 76$	$d = .999 \times 17{,}251$
$a = 74$	$d = 17{,}234$

Table 8–6 Formulas to Calculate False Positives (*c*) and False Negatives (*b*)

False Positives (*c*)	False Negatives (*b*)
$c = TotDxPos - a$	$b = TotDxNeg - d$
$c = 76 - 74$	$b = 17{,}251 - 17{,}234$
$c = 2$	$b = 17$

Table 8–8 Contingency Table with Each of the Cells with Its Semantic Abbreviation

	DxPos	DxNeg	Totals
TestPos	TruePos	FalseNeg	TotTestPos
TestNeg	FalsePos	TrueNeg	TotTestNeg
Totals	TotDxPos	TotDxNeg	Sample Size

Table 8–9 Contingency Table with Each of the Cells with Its Symbols

	Dx+	Dx–	Totals
Test+	T+	F–	TotTest+
Test–	F+	T–	TotTest–
Totals	TotDx+	TotDx–	Sample size

Table 8–7 Contingency Table for Dry-Saliva PCR Test

	Patients Who Have the Condition	Patients Who Do Not Have the Condition
Patients who tested positive	74	17
Patients who tested negative	2	17,234
Totals	**76**	**17,251**

The results of the study mean that the liquid-saliva PCR assay could be a slightly better choice based on accuracy and time alone. Advantages of both the liquid- and dry-saliva PCR tests, according to the authors,[18] include the fact that they are less invasive than rapid culture and the procedure is more simplified for clinicians to collect the samples, as is storage and transportation of samples. Additionally, the tests are considerably less expensive than rapid culture, which requires extraction of DNA. The data from the study indicate that either the liquid-saliva PCR or the dry-saliva PCR can be used as a screening or diagnostic tool for CMV with newborns.

The dry-saliva method had one additional advantage; it is easier to maintain the sample in a form that is ready for testing. A liquid-saliva sample must be kept in liquid form, whereas the dry-saliva sample can be kept at room temperature without affecting the sample. In summary, the dry-saliva sample ends up being preferable because of the simplified handling and lower cost along with the nearly equivalent sensitivity and specificity of the method. Note: this is an academic discussion about the PCR study and not a recommendation. Usage of the dry- or wet-saliva test should not be based on the information we provided in this discussion.

As much as possible, diagnostic procedures should be both sensitive and specific. Both are important. The more harmful the disease of interest, the more important it is that the diagnostic test has characteristics of high sensitivity and high specificity. Even when a test has been shown to be highly sensitive and specific, like the test in the CMV study, clinicians must always consider the potential harm from an incorrect result. Even a test that shows 100% sensitivity can produce an erroneous result or be incorrectly handled. The specimen could be labeled incorrectly when it is taken. The equipment in the lab might not be set correctly. Laboratory conditions might alter the characteristics of a specimen. Any number of errors can, and do, happen in the handling of biomedical specimens. Labs and hospitals track their error rates. It is important for you to be aware of these rates as well as aware of your own potential to make a mistake.

If an infant were to be deemed free of CMV due to a false-negative result, the lack of timely treatment can lead to hearing loss. Similarly, if an infant is diagnosed with CMV when he or she actually does not have it, the infant might be exposed to antiviral medication therapy and risk the harm associated with that treatment. Antiviral medications can have serious side effects.

Confidence Intervals with Sensitivity and Specificity

It is important that researchers include confidence intervals associated with the sensitivity and specificity values they report. The confidence interval (CI) tells you the accuracy of the authors' estimation of sensitivity and specificity. With inferential statistics, the best researchers can do is to estimate the true value (the population parameter) based on the results of a sample. The CI gives you a range, based on the sample, in which the population parameter can most likely be found. In this discussion the population parameters of interest are sensitivity and specificity. At best, researchers can estimate these values and report the likely range in which true sensitivity and specificity can be found.

In the study by Boppana et al.,[18] the authors stated, "The sensitivity and specificity of the liquid-saliva PCR assay were 100% (95% CI, 95.8 to 100) and 99.9% (95% CI, 99.9 to 100), respectively." Thus, the population parameter for sensitivity is between 95.8% and 100%. If the study was performed repeatedly, the result for sensitivity would range between 95.8% and 100%. This means that the sensitivity of the liquid-saliva PCR test could be as low as 95.8%. There is also a 5% chance that the true value for sensitivity is outside the range of 95.8% and 100%. It is possible that the sensitivity value could be lower than reported. This is why the range is referred to as a 95% confidence interval.

The population parameter for specificity is between 99.9% and 100%. Note that although sensitivity was reported as 100%, it is a less accurate estimate of the parameter than the result for specificity. The range for specificity was only a distance of 0.1%. If the study were performed repeatedly, the result for specificity would fall between 99.9% and 100% in 95 out of 100 experiments. We could interpret these CIs as telling us that specificity is slightly more trustworthy than sensitivity. The CI for sensitivity also tells us that we should not think of the liquid-saliva PCR test as 100% sensitive. It is reasonable to think of it as 95.8% sensitive.

Online and Other Electronic Calculators for Sensitivity and Specificity

One last item we want to share regarding sensitivity and specificity is that they can be determined through the use of calculators. Some of these calculators are available for free online; others are part of software you can download or a database you can pay for a license to use. Be aware that these calculators can also have flaws and that it is worth your time to check the values they produce by performing your own calculation.

Positive Predictive Value/Negative Predictive Value

In addition to sensitivity and specificity, positive and negative predictive values can help determine if a given test is accurate. *Positive predictive value* (PPV) is the proportion of people with a positive test result who actually have the diagnosis or exposure. *Negative predictive value* (NPV) is the proportion of people with a negative test result who do not actually have the diagnosis. PPV and NPV are particularly helpful in determining whether a test is useful for measuring a specific characteristic in a given population. However, they can also be used with diagnostic procedures. **Table 8–10** shows the contingency table for positive and negative predictive values.

The formulas for PPV and NPV are as follows:

$$PPV = \frac{a}{a+b}$$
$$NPV = \frac{d}{c+d}$$

It may be helpful to think of PPV and NPV in visual terms. Whereas sensitivity and specificity can be thought of as vertical calculations on the contingency table, PPV and NPV can be thought of as horizontal calculations. **Figures 8–4** and **8–5** provide a visual way to think about PPV and NPV.

The authors of the CMV study[18] also calculated PPV and NPV. They tested 17,327 infants with dry-saliva PCR. On the rapid culture test, 76 infants were identified with CMV. On the dry-saliva PCR test, 74 infants were identified. The following table (**Table 8–11**) presents the values for *a*, *b*, *c*, and *d* for the dry-saliva test.

The calculation for PPV is as follows:

$$PPV = \frac{74}{74+17} = 81.3\%$$

This means that 81.3% of infants with a positive test result for the dry-saliva PCR test actually have

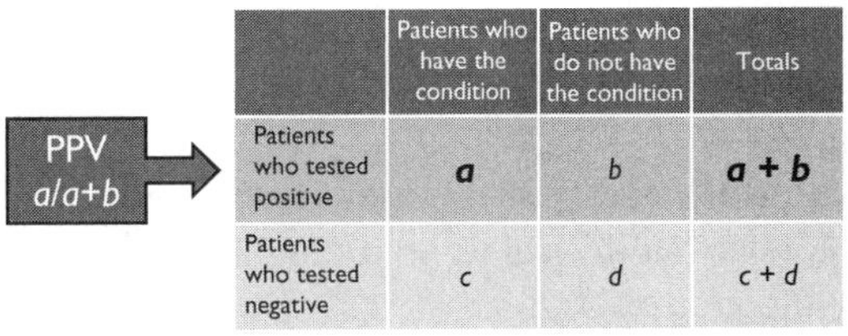

Figure 8–4 Visual Way to Think of PPV Formula

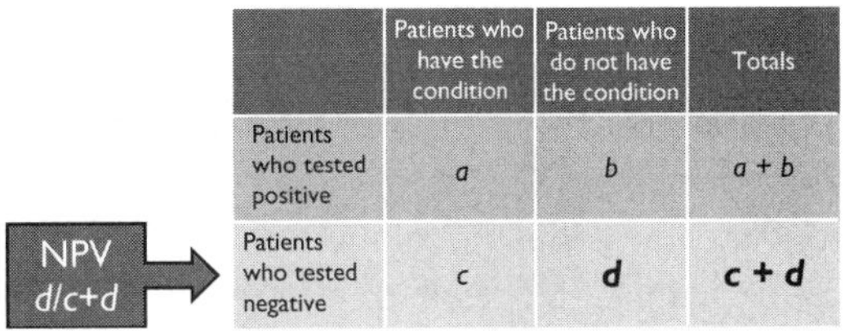

Figure 8–5 Visual Way to Think of NPV Formula

Table 8–10 Contingency Table for Positive and Negative Predictive Values

	Patients Who Have the Condition	Patients Who Do Not Have the Condition
Patients who tested positive	a	b
Patients who tested negative	c	d

Table 8–11 Contingency Table for Dry-Saliva PCR Testing

	Patients Who Have the Condition	Patients Who Do Not Have the Condition
Patients who tested positive	74	17
Patients who tested negative	2	17,234
Total	**76**	**17,251**

the condition. The calculation for NPV is as follows:

$$NPV = \frac{17,234}{2 + 17,234} = 100.0\%$$

This means that 100.0% (rounded to nearest 0.1%) of infants with a negative result for the dry-saliva PCR test actually do not have the condition.

This improves our understanding of the dry-saliva PCR test. Although it has 97.4% sensitivity (meaning 97.4% of those with the disorder will have a positive test result), it has a 81.3% positive predictive value (meaning 81.3% of those who have a positive result actually have the disorder). This information is helpful in terms of using the test to rule in the diagnosis. The test is perhaps not as strong for ruling in a diagnosis as it is for ruling out the diagnosis, because the PPV is fairly low. The specificity of the test was 99.9% (meaning 99.9% of infants who do not have the disorder will have a negative test result), and the NPV was 100% (meaning 100% of infants who have a negative test result do not in fact have the disorder).

Looking at it from this perspective tells us that a negative result on the dry-saliva PCR test is a strong indicator that the infant does not have CMV. However, a positive result on dry-saliva PCR likely indicates a need to follow up with another test, most likely the rapid culture. The question then remains as to whether to begin antiviral treatment while awaiting the result of the culture. We will not enter into a discussion of this as it is beyond the scope of our purpose here. The message here is that if you look for data on sensitivity, specificity, PPV, and NPV you can get a complete picture of the trustworthiness of a given diagnostic test and add that information to your clinical judgment. You will need to take into account the standard of care, any guidelines available on the next step to take, available resources, the patient's clinical picture, and the preferences of the infant's parents. We recommend that you pay close attention to what you learn from your instructors on the topic of CMV as well as reading current literature on the topic.

Prevalence and PPV/NPV

PPV and NPV are affected by the prevalence of the disease among the population being tested. In some studies, the sample has a high prevalence of the disorder, which will change the PPV and NPV values compared to the population in general. It is important that studies involving assessment of diagnostic procedures select a sample that represents a level of prevalence that is similar to that of the population for whom the test is intended. Let's consider the following hypothetical scenario.

A lab test for lung cancer has a sensitivity and specificity of 95%. In the general population, the prevalence of lung cancer is approximately 0.1% (including all adults in the United States as of January 2009). Now, imagine a clinical trial that includes only smokers. Among this group, the prevalence of lung cancer was 2.0%. The contingency tables in **Tables 8–12** and **8–13**) show the values for sensitivity and specificity for these two groups:

You can calculate prevalence in the general population sample by dividing the total number of subjects who have lung cancer by the total number of subjects in the study: $\frac{1,000}{1,000,000} = 0.001$, or 0.1%.

Table 8–12 Lung Cancer Contingency Table for Prevalence of 0.1% in the General Population

	Lung CA+	Lung CA–	Total
Test+	950	49,950	
Test–	50	949,050	
Total	1,000	999,000	1,000,000

Table 8–13 Lung Cancer Contingency Table for Prevalence of 2.0% in a Study with Smokers

	Lung CA+	Lung CA–	Total
Test+	19,000	49,000	
Test–	1,000	931,000	
Total	20,000	980,000	1,000,000

You can calculate prevalence in the sample of smokers by dividing the total number of subjects who have lung cancer by the total number of subjects in the study: $\frac{20,000}{1,000,000} = 0.02$, or 2.0%. You can see that sensitivity and specificity are identical between these two groups (**Table 8–14**). And, the sample size is also identical (1 million).

Now, let us look at PPV and NPV. First, we need to calculate the total number of patients who test positive ($a + b$) and the total who test negative ($c + d$) (**Table 8–15**).

Hence, the complete contingency table for the general population is shown in **Table 8–16**.

Table 8–14 Sensitivity and Specificity

	General Population	Study with Smokers
Sensitivity	$\frac{950}{1,000} = 0.95$	$\frac{19,000}{20,000} = 0.95$
Specificity	$\frac{949,050}{999,000} = 0.95$	$\frac{931,000}{980,000} = 0.95$

Next, we calculate *TotTestPos* and *TotTestNeg* for the sample of smokers, filling in the indicated cells in **Table 8–17**.

Hence, the complete contingency table for lung cancer among smokers is as shown in **Table 8–18**.

Now we have all of the information needed to calculate PPV and NPV. We can then see the difference in PPV and NPV that occurs due to changes in prevalence alone (**Table 8–19**).

As you can see, PPV increases significantly as prevalence increases. The PPV of the hypothetical lung cancer test in this example is 19% among the general population, which has a 0.1% prevalence

Table 8–15 Lung Cancer Contingency Table for Prevalence of 0.1% in the General Population

	Lung CA+	Lung CA–	Total
Test+	950	49,950	*TotTestPos*
Test–	50	949,050	*TotTestNeg*
Total	1,000	999,000	1,000,000

$TotTestPos = a + b = 950 + 49,950 = 50,900$
$TotTestNeg = c + d = 50 + 949,050 = 949,100$

Table 8–16 Complete Contingency Table for General Population

	Lung CA+	Lung CA–	Total
Test+	950	49,950	50,900
Test–	50	949,050	949,100
Total	1,000	999,000	1,000,000

Table 8–17 Lung Cancer Contingency Table for Prevalence of 2.0% in a Study with Smokers

	Lung CA+	Lung CA–	Total
Test+	19,000	49,000	*TotTestPos*
Test–	1,000	931,000	*TotTestNeg*
Total	20,000	980,000	1,000,000

$TotTestPos = a + b = 19,000 + 49,000 = 68,000$
$TotTestNeg = c + d = 1,000 + 931,000 = 932,000$

Table 8–18 Complete Contingency Table for Smokers

	Lung CA+	Lung CA–	Total
Test+	19,000	49,000	68,000
Test–	1,000	931,000	932,000
Total	20,000	980,000	1,000,000

Table 8–19 PPV and NPV in General Population vs. Smokers Showing Influence of Prevalence

	General Population	Study with Smokers
PPV	$\dfrac{950}{50,900} = 0.019$	$\dfrac{49,000}{68,000} = 0.28$
NPV	$\dfrac{949,050}{949,100} = 1.00$	$\dfrac{931,000}{932,000} = 0.99$

of lung cancer. The PPV among the smoking population is 28%. The smoking population has a lung cancer prevalence of 2.0%. The effect on NPV is the opposite: The higher the prevalence, the lower the NPV. In this example, the difference is only 0.01%. However, note that the sample size is identical between the two groups and that the sensitivity and specificity are identical. The greater the difference in prevalence between the study sample and the population, the greater the effect on both PPV and NPV. In short, what you need to remember is that increased prevalence leads to increased PPV and decreased NPV.

Online and Electronic Calculators of PPV and NPV

As we discussed in an earlier section on sensitivity and specificity, online calculators are available that will produce PPV and NPV values. If you read an article that provides enough data, you can calculate these values yourself. It is useful to perform these calculations not only to double-check the values reported in an article, but also if an article fails to present all of the values. It is not uncommon for an article to pro-

vide only sensitivity and specificity but not provide PPV and NPV. There is even some disagreement as to the applicability of PPV and NPV to diagnostic procedures. But, as we demonstrated earlier, you might find it useful to determine PPV and NPV in order to develop a full understanding of the accuracy of a diagnostic procedure.

Confidence Interval

We have said this multiple times, and perhaps you do not need to hear it again, but it is helpful if statistics are reported with confidence intervals. In the CMV diagnosis study, the authors reported the following details about PPV and NPV: "The positive and negative predictive values for the dried-saliva PCR assay were 90.2% (95% CI, 81.7 to 95.7) and 99.9% (95% CI, 99.9 to 100), respectively (based on 74 of 82 infants and 17,243 of 17,245 infants, respectively)."[18] As you can see, the population parameter for PPV most likely falls between 81.7% and 95.7% and the population parameter for NPV falls between 99.9% and 100%. As with sensitivity and specificity for the dry-saliva PCR test, the confidence interval for NPV is much narrower than the confidence interval for PPV. It is possible that the true PPV is as low as 81.7% and the true NPV is as low as 99.9%. This again reinforces the notion that the dry-saliva PCR test is a stronger test for ruling out the disease than for ruling it in. As we have said before, you must determine the implications of this for clinical practice. Research in this area of investigation continues, and it will be worth your time to look for more recent studies and for higher level studies, such as meta-analyses.

Likelihood Ratio

The **likelihood ratio (LR)** is another way to examine the accuracy of a diagnostic test. The two types of LR tests are the positive LR (**LR +**) and the negative LR (**LR–**):

$$LR+ = \frac{Sensitivity}{1 - Specificity}$$

$$LR- = \frac{1 - Sensitivity}{Specificity}$$

Before we talk about the reason behind having both a positive and a negative form of the LR test, let's calculate them. We will return to the dry-saliva PCR research we discussed earlier. **Table 8–20** presents the full contingency table for the data.

We know from our earlier calculations that sensitivity was 97.4% and specificity was 99.9%. The calculations for LR + and LR– would be as shown in **Table 8–21**.

The **positive likelihood ratio (PLR)** tells us the relative likelihood of having the disease if the infant has a positive test result. In this case, infants with a positive test result on the dry-saliva assay have a 988 times greater likelihood of having the disease. The **negative likelihood ratio (NLR)** tells us the relative likelihood of having the disease if the infant tests negative on the dry-saliva PCR test. In this case, infants with a negative test result have 0.26 times lesser likelihood of having the disease. It is 'lesser' because it is less than 1.0. A positive or negative LR of greater than 1.0 indicates the test result is associated with having the disease. So, it makes sense in this case that the positive LR is well

above 1.0 and the negative LR is well below 1.0. The closer that LR + and LR– are to 1.0, the less accurate the diagnostic test.

AUC and ROC Curve

The final diagnostic biostatistics we will discuss are the AUC (area under the curve) and the ROC (receiver operating characteristic). These two pieces of information are associated with one another and provide more detail about a diagnostic test. The ROC is presented as a plot that compares the true positive rate to the false positive rate. The greater the true positive rate compared to the false positive rate, the stronger the diagnostic test. The ratio of the false positive rate to the true positive rate produces a proportion called the *area under the curve* (AUC). An AUC of 0.50 (50%) means that the diagnostic test is no better than chance. An AUC of 1.0 (100%) means that the diagnostic test is perfectly accurate. The ROC curve is a visual representation of the AUC statistic.

Figure 8–6 shows what an ROC curve would look like for a study comparing a new diagnostic protocol to the standard diagnostic protocol. The AUC value for the New Protocol represented here would be 0.78 and the AUC value for the Standard Protocol would be 0.73. This means that the ratio of true positives to false positives is 78% for the New Protocol and 73% for the Standard Protocol. This tells us that the New Protocol is somewhat better than the Standard Protocol.

Table 8–20 Complete Contingency Table for Dry-Saliva PCR Assay

	CMV+	CMV–	Totals
Test+	74	17	91
Test–	2	17,234	17,236
	76	17,251	17,327

Table 8–21 Calculation of LR+ and LR– for Dry-Saliva PCR Assay

	LR+	LR–
Formula	$\dfrac{Sensitivity}{1-Specificity}$	$\dfrac{1-Sensitivity}{Specificity}$
Formula with values	$\dfrac{0.974}{1-.999}$	$\dfrac{1-0.974}{0.999}$
Results	2,100	0.026

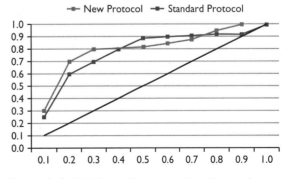

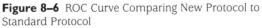

Figure 8–6 ROC Curve Comparing New Protocol to Standard Protocol

CHAPTER SUMMARY

In general, the three categories of diagnostic procedures are history and physical exam, laboratory tests, and imaging. All types of diagnostic procedures can be researched, although there tends to be more research related to lab tests and imaging tests due to their invasiveness, side effects, and costs. Diagnostic procedure studies need to utilize a reference standard that is the most accurate test available in order to produce valid results regarding the diagnostic procedure of interest.

Many issues must be considered in determining if a given diagnostic procedure is the best choice in an individual clinical situation. Considerations include cost, access, practitioner experience, patient preference, invasiveness, time, indications, contraindications, and accuracy. In performing diagnostic procedure research, authors should collect and present data related to each of these topics as well as discuss the results. Alas, if authors did everything we have said they *should* do, articles would become books.

The diagnosis biostatistics we presented in this chapter—sensitivity, specificity, PPV, NPV, LR+, LR–, AUC, and the ROC curve (which technically isn't a statistic but a visual presentation of AUC)—are only a sampling of the statistics you will encounter in reading studies on diagnostic procedures. We selected some of the most commonly reported biostatistics for diagnostic procedure research as well as statistics whose calculations were, for the most part, straightforward.

You will encounter other statistics when reading articles and other information sources related to diagnostic procedures. We encourage you to have a colleague you can approach as well as several reference books related to both diagnostic procedures as well as biostatistics. Just as health care is itself a team sport, so is evidence-based diagnostic practice.

EXERCISES

1. In a hypothetical study comparing clinical diagnostic procedures for broken nose to CT imaging, a sample of 22,000 patients who presented to emergency departments with nose injuries that were suspicious for broken nose were evaluated with clinical criteria, including epistaxis, periorbital and/or perinasal ecchymosis, nasal wound or laceration, airway obstruction, nasal inflammation, lateral deviation, irregular nasal dorsum, and acute septal injury. Clinicians recorded an assessment of either broken or not broken and then the patients were provided a CT. Not all patients who had a nose injury were indicated for CT, and not all of them wanted the CT to be performed. The present results include only those patients who had the CT.

The present study was undertaken in order to determine the accuracy of clinical diagnostic criteria alone for achieving a correct diagnosis of broken nose. CT scans are the most sensitive and specific tests for broken nose, but they are very expensive, they expose patients to radiation, and they add significant time to a patient's emergency department visit. Furthermore, CT is not available in all hospitals. Due to access limitations, CT might not be an option for some patients. X-ray is the most common diagnostic tool utilized for evaluation of nose injuries. However, like CT, x-rays are more expensive than a clinical exam. They also expose patients to radiation and they take more time. We selected CT as the reference standard for this comparison study. If clinical exam techniques can approach the accuracy of CT then it might be possible to reduce usage of both CT and x-ray in diagnosis of nose injuries. In the present study, each individual clinical sign was compared to CT and each pair of clinical signs was compared to CT. The most accurate clinical exam strategy was the combination of epistaxis and nasal wound.

The following contingency table presents the values associated with the combination of epistaxis and nasal wound for diagnosis of a broken nose.

Contingency Table with the Values Associated with the Combination of Epistaxis and Nasal Wound for Diagnosis Broken Nose

	Fracture+	Fracture–	Total
Test+	5,050	1	5,051
Test–	11,650	5,299	16,949
Total	16,700	5,300	22,000

Based on the information presented, calculate the following:

    a. Sensitivity

    b. Specificity

    c. PPV

    d. NPV

    e. LR+

    f. LR–

2. Based on the results of your calculations for Exercise 1 and the explanation of the research, evaluate the use of clinical criteria as the only diagnostic procedure for evaluating a nose injury. Write a one- to two-paragraph explanation you would give to a colleague about your decision. Be sure to address all of the issues discussed in this chapter (cost, access, practitioner experience, patient preference, invasiveness, time, indications, contraindications, accuracy) and any others you feel are relevant.

REFERENCES

1. U.S. Library of Medicine. Medical Subject Heading Database in PubMed. [Online database]. ND. Available at: www.ncbi.nlm.nih.gov.libpublic3 .library.isu.edu/mesh?term = diagnosis. Accessed September 6, 2012.
2. National Institute on Alcohol Abuse and Alcoholism. *Module 5: Diagnosis and Assessment of Alcohol Use Disorders.*
3. NANDA International. NANDA-1 Nursing Diagnosis Resources. [Website]. 2012. Available at: www .nanda.org/NursingDiagnosisFAQ.aspx. Accessed September 6, 2012.
4. U.S. Library of Medicine. Medical Subject Heading Database in PubMed. 1965. Available at: www.ncbi.nlm.nih.gov.libpublic3.library.isu .edu/mesh?term = oral%20diagnosis. Accessed September 6, 2012.
5. U.S. Library of Medicine. Medical Subject Heading Database in PubMed. [Online database]. 1987. Available at: www.ncbi.nlm.nih.gov.libpublic3 .library.isu.edu/mesh. Accessed September 6, 2012.
6. U.S. Library of Medicine. Medical Subject Headings Database in PubMed. [Online database]. ND. Available at: www.ncbi.nlm.nih.gov.libpublic3 .library.isu.edu/mesh?term = differential%20 diagnosis. Accessed September 6, 2012.
7. Montgomery K. *How doctors think: Clinical judgment and the practice of medicine.* Oxford, England: Oxford University Press; 2006.
8. Smith-Bindman R, Miglioretti DL, Johnson E, Lee C, Spencer Feigelson H, Kruger RT, et al. Use of diagnostic imaging studies and associated radiation exposure for patients enrolled in large integrated health care systems, 1996–2010. *JAMA.* 2012;307(22).
9. Mayo Clinic Staff. *Migraine risk factors.* Updated June 4, 2011. Available at: www.mayoclinic.com /health/migraine-headache/ds00120/dsection = risk-factors. Accessed May 15, 2012.
10. Clinch CR. Evaluation of acute headache in adults. *Am Fam Physician.* 2001;63(4):685–693.
11. Brown M. AAFP, USPSTF issue final recommendation against routine PSA-based screening for prostate cancer: Evidence simply does not support test's benefit, says task force co-chair. May 22, 2012. Available at: www.aafp.org. Accessed May 28, 2012.
12. Tocci SL, Madom IA, Bradley MP, Langer PR, DiGiovanni CW. The diagnostic value of MRI in foot and ankle surgery. *Foot Ankle Int.* 2007;28(2):166–168.
13. Grodin MA, Glantz LH (eds). *Children as research subjects: Science, ethics, and law.* Oxford, England: Oxford University Press; 1994.
14. American College of Cardiology and American Heart Association. ACC/AHA guidelines for the management of patients with ST-elevation myocardial infarction. *Circulation.* 2004;110:588–636.
15. *Merck Manual.* Percutaneous coronary interventions (PCI). Last full review/revision May 2009 by Michael J. Shea, MD. Available at: www.merckmanuals .com/. Accessed May 20, 2012.
16. Palevsky P. Defining contrast-induced nephropathy. *Clin J Am Soc Nephrol.* 2009;4(7):1151–1153.
17. Olsen J, Christensen K, Murray J, Ekbom A. *An introduction to epidemiology for health professionals.* New York: Springer; 2010.
18. Boppana SB, Ross SA, Shimamura M, Palmer AL, Ahmed A, Michaels MG. Saliva polymerase-chain-reaction assay for cytomegalovirus screening in newborns. *N Engl J Med.* 2011;364(22):2111–2118.
19. Centers for Disease Control and Prevention. Cytomegalovirus (CMV) and congenital CMV infection. December 6, 2010. Available at: www.cdc.gov /cmv/overview.html. Accessed February 26, 2012.

ANSWERS TO EXERCISES

1. (a) 30.24%; (b) 99.98%; (c) 99.98%; (d) 31.26%; (e) 1603; (f) 0.7
2. There is not necessarily a *correct* answer, but we will discuss our thoughts about each of the issues requested in the exercise:
   - *Cost:* The abstract from the article gave a believable explanation about the value of identifying an accurate clinical exam technique to potentially reduce usage

of CT and x-ray. However, no numbers were provided regarding the actual cost of each approach.

- *Access:* The abstract discusses issues of access, especially with regard to CT. The concern makes sense. The abstract does not include exact numbers about access to CT and x-ray.
- *Practitioner experience:* The topic is not raised in the abstract. It is not clear if practitioner experience with the clinical examination of a nose injury affects the accuracy of the results. In the full article, it would be important to look for information about this topic.
- *Patient preference:* The authors did mention that some patients chose not to have the CT performed and that for some patients CT was not appropriate. They did not give reasons for either. It is not clear how many patients chose not to have the CT and for how many it was contraindicated.
- *Invasiveness:* The nose exam is more invasive than CT. It would be important to know how to perform each of the exams listed in the study in order to have an opinion about the invasiveness of each procedure. The authors do not discuss this issue.
- *Time:* Time is an important consideration mentioned in the abstract. The authors discuss in the abstract the time required to perform a CT or an x-ray. The actual amounts of time are not presented. It is not possible to determine from the abstract if the authors measured the amount of time needed for the CTs. More information about this question is needed.
- *Indications:* The only indication for CT in the abstract is that a patient presented with a nose injury that was suspicious for a broken nose. More information about this topic is needed and might be presented in the article.
- *Contraindications:* The authors provide no details in the abstract about contraindications. More information about this topic is needed and might be presented in the article.
- *Accuracy:* The abstract reported that the best combination of clinical exam procedures was epistaxis and nasal wound. The calculations you completed for accuracy revealed this combination had 30% sensitivity, 100% specificity, 100% PPV, and 31% NPV. These values indicate that clinical exam alone may not be sufficient for definitively diagnosing a broken nose. It would be worthwhile to look for additional research on this question to see if other studies have had different results.

Evidence-Based Practice in Treatment, Harm, and Prevention

Bernadette Howlett, PhD

INTRODUCTION

Studies on treatment, harm, and prevention comprise major areas of interest in research and in clinical practice. *Treatment* is a word with many definitions and uses as well as synonyms. Oftentimes, the preferred term is a synonym for treatment, **therapeutics**, which is defined as: "Procedures concerned with the remedial treatment or prevention of diseases."[1] This definition fits with our use of the term *treatment*, but the word *therapeutics* itself might not fit with the wide array of treatments available across the many different healthcare fields. We use the term *treatment* rather than *therapeutics* in this chapter because of the broad, interprofessional lens in which we apply evidence-based practice (EBP).

For purposes of this discussion, we differentiate **studies of treatment**, **harm**, and **prevention** by the characteristics presented in **Table 9–1**.

From an interprofessional perspective, treatment procedures include a range of activities that achieve the objective of *remedial treatment* or *prevention of disease*. Treatment is remedial when it is utilized to intervene in an existing disease process or condition. Examples of remedial or preventive treatment include activities such as informing patients about their condition; administering and prescribing medications/vaccinations; developing nutritional plans; educating patients on prevention activities; explaining how to take medications; or performing physical therapy, occupational therapy, surgery, radiotherapy, wound care, and so on. Based on the previous definition of therapeutics, we might not consider certain activities—such as informing a patient of his or her diagnosis—as therapeutics. Informing and educating patients on their condition might serve as a first step in a treatment plan, or it might comprise the entirety of a treatment plan.

For example, an entire treatment plan might be to inform a patient who has signs and symptoms of an upper respiratory infection that the cause is a common virus and no medication treatment is required. In many instances, the mere act of telling a patient the cause of his or her symptoms is

Table 9–1 Characteristics of Treatment, Harm, and Prevention Studies

Type of Study	Characteristics
Studies of treatment	• Interventional, prospective studies with the purpose of treating a diagnosed condition (e.g., case studies, case series, control trials, randomized controlled trials [RCTs], cohort studies). • Observational, prospective studies with the purpose of determining outcomes of patients with a diagnosed condition who are already receiving a specific treatment (e.g., cohort studies, systematic reviews, meta-analyses).
Studies of harm	• Observational, retrospective studies with the purpose of identifying harmful exposures (e.g., case-control studies). • Observational, prospective studies with the purpose of identifying harmful exposures (e.g., cohort studies, systematic reviews, meta-analyses).
Studies of prevention	• Interventional, prospective studies with the purpose of preventing patients from developing a condition (e.g., case studies, case series, control trials, RCTs, cohort studies). • Observational, prospective studies with the purpose of determining whether patients develop a given condition (e.g., case studies, case series, cohort studies, systematic reviews, meta-analyses).

a form of treatment, because the information can relieve anxiety and help the patient move forward. As such, we prefer the term *treatment* to the term *therapeutics* for this chapter.

Studies on *harm* explore adverse consequences of treatment or the natural progression of disease, as well as harm caused by complications from interactions between treatments. Later in this chapter we will discuss various types of harm research as well as considerations in locating and evaluating harm research.

Studies on *prevention* explore questions such as identification of prevention strategies, evaluation of prevention strategies and programs, efficacy of screening modalities, and the necessity for population screening. The U.S. Preventive Services Task Force (USPSTF) is an organization that performs a significant number of these types of studies. We will explore resources for literature on prevention, treatment, and harm later in this chapter. We will also examine biostatistics frequently found in studies of treatment, harm, and prevention.

TREATMENT RESEARCH

Research into treatment modalities explores many types of questions related to an array of issues, including efficacy of treatment, interactions between treatments, factors that influence treatment adherence or treatment discontinuation, cost of treatment, patient preferences, and access to treatment. You can employ EBP to inform yourself and your patients about the relative merits of treatment alternatives and help the patient (and often the patient's family) select a treatment plan (although in some situations the patient does not make the choice, such as when he or she is unconscious).

At times, patients ask providers to choose the treatment for them. This is appropriate in some situations, whereas in others it is preferable for the patient to choose the treatment plan. Additionally, treatment decisions are often collaborative between the patient and the provider, with inclusion of family members, as appropriate. Engaging in collaborative treatment decisions presents clinicians with one of the greatest challenges in EBP—explaining the results of research findings to patients. The population's educational experiences related to research (and to health care for that matter) vary considerably, with some patients having minimal health or research literacy.

Nonetheless, the clinical and research knowledge you possess can be invaluable in helping patients and their family members choose a course of treatment. In this chapter, we will help you with your fund of knowledge related to interpreting and evaluating treatment, harm, and prevention information in order to strengthen your ability to communicate with patients about evidence. We will also examine several of the more common biostatistics presented in treatment research publications.

Treatment is arguably the category of EBP with the greatest amount of published information. Significantly more resources are expended on pharmaceutical research, for example, that on other types of health-related research. This is most likely linked to the extensive usage of medications to treat diseases and symptoms as well as the immense profits generated from manufacturing and selling medications. Furthermore, medications are more closely regulated and monitored than other types of treatments, although medical devices also face considerable regulation. Regulation leads to a greater amount of research and more stringent standards for treatments to become legal.

Research publications on treatment should justify the need for the research in terms of epidemiological data as well as gaps in current knowledge. There should be sufficient cause for the research to be performed in terms of potential improvement in outcomes that matter (e.g., reduced morbidity, mortality, cost, discomfort, side effects, and so on.) Authors should describe the existing body of literature on the topic, showing how the current study fits into the larger body of knowledge. The researchers should also describe the population affected by the condition of interest and explain how well the sample in the study represents the population.

All treatment modalities employed in the study should be explained sufficiently for clinical readers to be able to replicate the treatment. Lastly, authors should present the limitations of their research as well as recommendations for further research and implications to clinical practice from the present study. As readers, we should be able to draw a line from the problem that the research is intended to help solve, through the methods employed in the study and the end points evaluated, to clinical practices that improve health outcomes for relevant populations.

TREATMENT SELECTION

The primary objective of treatment research is to provide information to assist you and your patients with the selection of a treatment. Publications related to treatments should include complete explanations of treatment-selection issues, such as efficacy, indications, contraindications, side effects, interactions, adherence, cost, access, and temporal considerations (e.g., how long it takes for the treatment to take effect). In the best of situations, every treatment study would address all of these topics. However, most often only a few of the topics are considered in any individual study, and some topics might not be examined at all. In order to gain a complete understanding of a treatment modality, it will likely be necessary for you to perform several searches using different combinations of search terms. Information on each of these factors will influence the decision to select a given treatment.

> One of the most straightforward techniques for evaluating an article is to simply ask what problem the study is intended to help solve and whether the methods and results actually address the problem.

We will walk through the various treatment-selection factors discussed above in the context of several specific publications.

Efficacy

Efficacy is "the ability of an intervention to produce the desired beneficial effect."[2] In order to achieve efficacy, each treatment should have its intended effect, to a meaningful degree, in order to prevent a disease, eliminate a disease, or reduce symptoms of disease. For example, a vaccination for varicella (the virus that causes chickenpox) should prevent people from contracting chickenpox. The vaccine should (optimally) be 100% effective in preventing any form of varicella. The Centers for Disease Control and Prevention (CDC), however, reported that one dose of the single-antigen varicella vaccine is 70–90% effective for preventing any form of the virus and more than 95% effective against moderate and severe forms.[3] The CDC also reported that efficacy increases with a second dose, such that 88–98% of any form of varicella infection is prevented (based on postlicensure studies).

Efficacy information is most helpful when derived from head-to-head comparative studies. Many studies either offer no comparison or comparison with just a placebo. The information produced by such studies will provide foundational knowledge, but will offer little insight into the relative efficacy of the study treatment compared to the current standard or other available treatments. Optimally, each new treatment would be tested against all other available treatments. This sort of study is rare, however, due to the cost and complexity of conducting such research. For this reason, meta-analyses and systematic reviews are helpful, because they summarize multiple studies.

Outcome Measures

Clinical trials often select one or more end points related to safety and/or efficacy, such as pain, quality of life, disease progression, or death. These end points are often referred to as primary or secondary outcome measures. **Primary outcome measures** are end points that are intended to be directly impacted by the intervention. **Secondary outcome measures** are additional end points that are evaluated but that are not the specific focus of the intervention. The end points of a trial should be clearly identified, and the method for measuring them should be thoroughly explained and validated.

Minimal Clinically Important Differences

Effect size is an important consideration in health-related research. If an intervention is intended to reduce pain, how much pain reduction is meaningful? How much difference between the treatment and control groups in pain reduction is meaningful? Whatever the measure of efficacy, the absolute difference in effect is a critical consideration. It is possible for a statistically significant difference to be found in data where the absolute or clinical difference is essentially meaningless. The minimum threshold for treatment effects is referred to as **minimal clinically important differences (MCIDs)** or **minimal clinically significant differences (MCSDs)**, the terms are used interchangeably. An MCID (or MCSD) is the smallest difference in score in an outcome of interest to patients that is perceived as beneficial and would mandate a change in treatment.[4]

For some conditions, research has been performed to determine the MCIDs to be achieved in treatment studies. For example, the **Western Ontario and McMaster Universities Osteoarthritis (WOMAC) scale** is used to measure pain, stiffness, and physical function in hip or knee osteoarthritis (OA). A study was performed to determine the MCID for the WOMAC scale among patients with knee and hip OA. The researchers utilized a visual analog version of the WOMAC scale (with a range of 0 to 100 mm). The MCID they reported was a range of –7.9 mm to –32.6 mm. This means that the score selected by the patient must be 7.9 mm to 32.6 mm points lower in order for the improvement to be deemed clinically meaningful. **Figure 9–1** illustrates a –7.9 mm improvement.[5]

Figure 9–1 is a hypothetical diagram based on the findings reported in the study. The column on the left shows an average WOMAC score of 90 mm prior to treatment; the column on the right shows an average WOMAC score of 82 mm after treatment. The average score posttreatment is 8 mm lower than at pretreatment. This amount

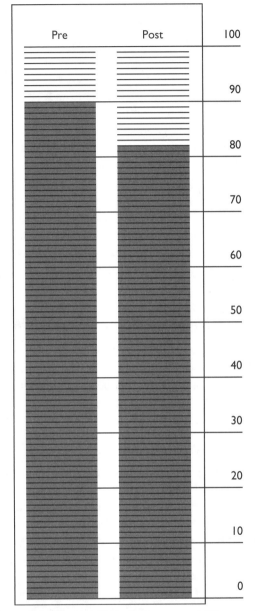

Figure 9–1 Minimal Clinically Important Difference in WOMAC Score

for a given assessment tool. Nonetheless, another way you can evaluate the quality of a treatment publication is to look for MCID/MCSD information in the article. At a minimum, the authors should mention whether any prior MCID/MCSD research was available. They should also explain how they determined the level of efficacy they utilized to represent a clinically important difference among their study sample when no MCID/MCSD studies have been published. In the case of the WOMAC scale, multiple MCID/MCSD studies have been performed.

On a final note, MCID/MCSD data can also be valuable from a clinical standpoint, because they indicate the amount of change that patients and clinicians perceive to be associated with quality of life and health status. In addition to using MCID/MCSD data in a treatment study, you can reference that information to assess the efficacy of treatments you administer (being careful to ensure that your patient fits with the patients in the MCID/MCSD study).

Example: Efficacy of Massage Therapy

A randomized control trial by Perlman et al.[6] evaluated the efficacy of massage therapy for OA of the knee. The study is an example of a head-to-head comparison between the usual care provided for OA of the knee and four regimens of massage therapy for OA. The authors assessed the following four efficacy outcome measures: WOMAC scale, visual analog pain scale, range of motion, and time to walk 50 feet. These measures were taken at baseline and at 8, 16, and 24 weeks. The control group received usual care for OA.

The study was a follow-up to earlier research that had demonstrated the feasibility, safety, and potential efficacy with a duration of 8 weeks subsequent to treatment.[7] The researchers enrolled 125 adults with diagnosed OA of the knee.

of improvement in pain would be considered clinically important according to the study.[5]

Treatment studies should reference any existing MCID/MCSD research and compare their efficacy results to the existing MCID/MCSD criteria. The concepts of MCID and MCSD are fairly new; therefore, existing research might not be available

In what phase would you categorize the study based on what you have read about it so far? If you retrieve the article, you can find the answer in the Introduction section of the article.

Explanation of the Efficacy Outcome Measures

The study protocol included both primary and secondary outcome measures. The primary outcome measure was the WOMAC Osteoarthritis Index. Secondary measures included pain (as reported by patients on a **visual analog scale [VAS]**), joint flexibility (measured by range of motion), and time needed to walk 50 feet. Each outcome measurement tool or procedure was described in the protocol with references to original literature and explanations about the validity of at least one of the assessment tools (the VAS).

In the trial, WOMAC VAS scores improved 24 points (95% CI: 15.3–32.7) among the 60-minute massage group compared to a 6.3-point (95% CI: 0.1–12.8) improvement in the usual care group. This difference in WOMAC VAS scores between the experimental groups and the control group was statistically significant. The authors of the massage therapy study reported two MCID references. In one reference,[8] an 18% improvement from baseline was found to be clinically important, whereas the other study[9] reported an improvement of 15 points as clinically important. In the OA study, a change of 24 points represented an improvement of 41.5% from baseline, so in terms of the first reference the amount of improvement between the two 60-minute massage therapy groups was clinically important. A 24-point improvement is considered clinically important according to the other MCID study.

The final question, then, is the amount of change in WOMAC score in the control group. It is possible that the control group also had a clinically important change in WOMAC score. The control group, which received usual care, improved by 6.3 points (95% CI: 0.1–12.8). Even if we consider the high end of the confidence interval (12.8 points), the improvement in WOMAC score among the control group would not be clinically important.

In terms of efficacy, the authors of this study have met their obligation to provide the information we need. They reported the amount of the effect, with confidence intervals, as well as two reference standards that define the MCID. Based on what we have discussed about this article thus far, we might consider recommending 60 minutes of massage therapy for patients with OA of the knee, in whom the treatment is not contraindicated. Furthermore, if this treatment is utilized we would most likely look for an improvement of at least 15 points on the WOMAC scale as the basis for determining if the treatment is sufficient. This would require administering the WOMAC scale to the patient prior to and subsequent to treatment. Of course, feedback from the patient during a follow-up interview might be a more efficient way to determine if the patient deems the massage therapy to be sufficiently efficacious.

Description of the Treatment Modality

The researchers in this example provided a link to the study protocol that described the massage treatments utilized but did not detail the usual care protocol followed. Presumably, usual care involved medication to treat pain and inflammation. Four 8-week regimens of a standardized Swedish massage therapy (30 or 60 minutes weekly or biweekly) were evaluated. The article also included a table that detailed the amount of time spent on each region of the body for each of the two time periods (30 or 60 minutes). Thus, there were four experimental treatments compared to the control treatment: (1) 30 minutes of massage therapy weekly; (2) 30 minutes of massage therapy biweekly; (3) 60 minutes of massage therapy weekly; and (4) 60 minutes of massage therapy biweekly.

With regard to pain, the study reported a significant improvement for both groups receiving the 60-minute treatments. The visual analog WOMAC Pain Subscale includes response options from 0 to 100 for each of five questions related to pain.[5] This scale provides a range of 0 to 500 points for the pain subscale. The higher the WOMAC Pain Subscale score, the worse the pain.

Protection of Human Subjects

We think we should point out here that the authors of this study described their IRB approval as follows:

The study protocol, consent form and all recruitment materials were approved by the Institutional Review Boards of the University of Medicine and Dentistry of New Jersey (Newark, NJ), Griffin Hospital (Derby, CT), and the Saint Barnabas Medical Center (Livingston, NJ). The study was conducted in accordance with the Declaration of Helsinki.

Indications and Contraindications

Indications and contraindications are the circumstances in which a given treatment should be used (**indications**) and should not be used (**contraindications**) because there is risk of harm to the patient. For example, the varicella vaccination is indicated for children 12 months of age and older, without evidence of immunity; adults without evidence of immunity; healthcare personnel and caretakers of immunocompromised persons; and those at risk for exposure/transmission.[10] The varicella vaccine is contraindicated under the following circumstances:

- Hypersensitivity to gelatin, neomycin
- Pregnancy
- HIV: CD4 + count < 200 cells/μL
- Other immunosuppression (excluding meditions and radiation)
- Active tuberculosis
- Methotrexate: risk of infection with live virus

Indications and contraindications are studied throughout preclinical trials as well as clinical trials. Generally, information on indications and contraindications can be readily located (even through simple Internet searches). However, it can be challenging to locate the evidence on which the lists of indications and contraindications are based. We recommend utilizing trustworthy general information sources to locate indications and contraindications and then checking the references they provide. These references will give you insight into the underlying research and help you develop search terms to locate further research with information on indications and contraindications.

One way to locate information on contraindications is to locate the MeSH for the treatment modality in PubMed and select the "contraindications" option. With regard to the study of OA and massage, we used the Search Builder tool to look for information on contraindications of massage therapy in this manner. The Search Builder produced the following search string: "Massage/contraindications"[Mesh]. This search resulted in 18 articles ranging from 1991 to 2009 related to several different conditions, including pregnancy and malignant lymphedema. Articles also discussed the risk of dislodging plaque, which could cause a coronary event or stroke. Unfortunately, none of the articles addressed contraindications of Swedish massage in general or specifically with OA of the knee. We would need to expand our search to other resources in order to locate information on contraindications.

Note that PubMed does not have a subheading for indications. It would be necessary to use a combination of keywords to perform that search. Additionally, the same search strategy used in PubMed could be used in other sources. You might also find a general textbook on Swedish massage to be helpful in terms of identifying the indications for this treatment modality. Generally, more research is focused on contraindications than indications.

Side Effects and Complications

Treatments nearly always have side effects or complications. **Side effects** are unintended symptoms from treatment, prevention, diagnostic, or screening procedures.[11] **Complications** are unintended adverse events, such as injury or death. Not all side effects are harmful, but, generally, complications are considered harmful. Researchers identify expected side effects and complications as part of the development of a treatment and then carefully monitor both animal subjects and human subjects throughout preclinical and clinical trials. During clinical trials, side effects are referred to as **adverse events (AE**s). Complications are referred to as *serious adverse events* (SAEs) and *adverse events of special interest* (AESIs). An AE is "any undesirable experience associated with the use of a medical product in a patient."[12] An AE becomes an SAE under the following circumstances:

- Death
- Life-threatening circumstances
- Hospitalization
- Disability or permanent change
- Congenital anomaly/birth defect
- Required intervention to prevent permanent impairment or damage
- Other serious events that may jeopardize the patient or that may require medical or surgical intervention (treatment) to prevent one of the other outcomes.

AESIs are those events that have been identified as potentially associated with a given treatment. AESIs are closely monitored and reported. For example, according to a listing on ClinicalTrials.gov, a multicenter study on lenalidomide plus dexamethasone (used for treating multiple myeloma) included two AESIs: peripheral neuropathy up to 124 weeks after treatment and venous thromboembolic events within 124 weeks after treatment.[13] Multiple myeloma is a form of cancer that starts in the plasma cells in bone marrow.[14]

During clinical trials on drugs and biological products, researchers must report all AEs to the FDA. While we are on the topic, **biologics** are defined by the FDA as follows:

> Biological products, like other drugs, are used for the treatment, prevention, or cure of disease in humans. In contrast to chemically synthesized small molecular weight drugs, which have a well-defined structure and can be thoroughly characterized, biological products are generally derived from living material—human, animal, or microorganism—are complex in structure, and thus are usually not fully characterized.[15]

The FDA maintains an online database where adverse events are reported called the FDA **Adverse Event Reporting System (AERS)**. It is currently located at www.fda.gov/Drugs /GuidanceComplianceRegulatoryInformation /Surveillance/AdverseDrugEffects/default.htm. The data reported to AERS are available to the public either online or through Freedom of Information Act requests.

Search terms you can use to locate information on side effects include:

- Side effects (or side-effects)
- Complications
- Adverse events
- Serious adverse events
- Safety

Example: Side Effects of Varicella Vaccination

We performed a search for side effects on the varicella vaccination by using a general Internet search engine, entering the terms "side effects" and "varicella vaccination." The second hit in the list was the CDC's vaccine information site. On that page was a link to "Information for Health Care Professionals." One of the links on this page was entitled, "Vaccine Safety and Monitoring." This link brought us to the page with the information we sought. The webpage included the name of the medication and the following statistics on adverse events:

> Since Varivax was licensed, it has been very safe. From March 1995 to December 2005, almost 48 million doses have been given to people in the United States. During that time, there were 25,306 adverse events reported to the Vaccine Adverse Event Reporting System (VAERS). The most common events were rash, fever, or pain, redness, or soreness at the injection site.[16]

The CDC webpage also had links to the references that supported the information provided on the page. As such, it is possible to evaluate the statement in two ways: (1) by checking the references provided and (2) by performing a separate search (if you still have questions about the side effects of the treatment).

Interactions

The term **interaction**, in the context of healthcare provision, is defined as "mutual or reciprocal action or influence."[17] It means that the treatment is having a reciprocal action or influence with something else, such as another treatment. The most common type of interaction addressed in research is drug–drug interaction. However, interactions are possible between other types of treatments as well as between treatments and other healthcare interventions (e.g., diagnostic procedures, screening tests, prevention activities, and even activities of daily living).

Interactions can increase the effect of a treatment (positive interaction) or reduce the effect of a treatment (negative interaction). Furthermore, positive and negative interactions can lead to adverse events. For example, a given treatment might increase the efficacy of a medication, leading to harmful side effects from overdosing the medication. If an interaction is known to increase the efficacy of a treatment, then the **dose** of that treatment might be reduced in order to compensate for the interaction effect. For instance, according to MD Consult, there is a positive interaction between ascorbic acid (vitamin C) and iron supplements:

> Ascorbic acid, by maintaining iron in the ferrous state, can enhance the absorption of oral iron; however, the magnitude of this increase is in the range of 10% and only occurs with doses of ascorbic acid, vitamin C, of 500 mg or greater. Healthy individuals usually absorb iron supplements (e.g., iron salts or polysaccharide–iron complex) adequately from the GI tract, but some patients may benefit from receiving supplemental ascorbic acid with each oral iron dose.[18]

The positive interaction could be utilized to improve iron absorption, making the iron supplementation therapy more effective. However, an adverse event can also be associated with the interaction. For example, patients who have iron overload often become vitamin C deficient, most likely due to iron's oxidizing effect on vitamin C. Also, higher doses of vitamin C can lead to iron deposition, in heart tissue particularly, resulting in cardiac decompensation. MD Consult explains the interaction as follows:

> In patients with severe chronic iron overload, the concomitant use of deferoxamine with > 500 mg/day PO of vitamin C in adults has led to impairment of cardiac function; the dysfunction was reversible when vitamin C was discontinued. The manufacturer of deferoxamine recommends certain precautions for the coadministration of vitamin C with deferoxamine.[18]

The same publication references a small study that identified an adverse interaction between vitamin C and a medication called propranolol (which is often used to treat hypertension):

> In a small, crossover study, coadministration of 2 g ascorbic acid, vitamin C substantially reduced propranolol AUC and also diminished the bradycardic action of propranolol. Since there were decreased amounts of propranolol metabolites recovered in the urine after pretreatment with ascorbic acid, it was postulated that ascorbic acid reduces the oral bioavailability of propranolol.[5942] Until more data are available, clinicians should advise patients against taking large doses of ascorbic acid with doses of propranolol. Taking ascorbic acid at least 1 hour prior to doses of oral propranolol may alleviate this problem; however, further study is necessary to confirm this.[18]

Medication interactions are of sufficient concern, in fact, that a whole field of health care has emerged (at least in part) to contend with it: medication reconciliation. According to the Joint Commission, *medication reconciliation* is:

> [T]he process of comparing a patient's medication orders to all of the medications that the patient has been taking. This reconciliation is done to avoid medication errors such as omissions, duplications, dosing errors, or drug interactions [emphasis added]. It should be done at every transition of care in which

new medications are ordered or existing orders are rewritten. Transitions in care include changes in setting, service, practitioner, or level of care. This process comprises five steps: (1) develop a list of current medications; (2) develop a list of medications to be prescribed; (3) compare the medications on the two lists; (4) make clinical decisions based on the comparison; and (5) communicate the new list to appropriate caregivers and to the patient.[19]

Furthermore, FDA regulations are in place regarding the study of drug–drug interactions. The FDA has a website where the public can look up information on drug safety (available at www.fda.gov/Drugs/DrugSafety/ucm199082.htm, as of the writing of this chapter). Many other sources of information on drug interactions are also available. Note, however, that less information is available on interactions related to nondrug treatments. Once again, this might be a function of the preponderance of drugs used for treatment, the profits available from pharmaceutical sales to fund such research, and the regulations requiring it.

Other factors can influence treatment interactions, such as a patient's age and health status. For example, treatment interactions can be more pronounced, or of higher risk, among geriatric patients. According to Cassel:

Older adults experience a variety of age-related changes in pharmacokinetics and pharmacodynamics, resulting in a need to modify drug dosing regimens from those used in a study. Comorbid conditions and their treatments result in novel drug–drug and drug–disease interactions that are not detected during phase III trials because of the stringent inclusion and exclusion criteria and the relatively small numbers of subjects tested.[20]

In other words, individual patients might have interactions that have not occurred in previous clinical trials. This is a reminder that data produced in controlled studies are likely to represent a segment of the patient population and that each patient is a separate study in him- or herself.

One final thought regarding interactions, even if you work, or will work, in a profession that does not prescribe or administer medications, the treatments you administer might interact with medications, making it worthwhile for you to know about drug interactions and how to find information on them. Additionally, you might be able to direct patients to information about drug interactions that could help them in making treatment decisions. You might also, because of your ability to locate and evaluate information about drug interactions, be a resource to colleagues who are seeking information on the subject.

Administration and Dosage

We touched earlier on the importance of treatment publications describing the method of administering the treatment as well as the dosage. Variations in treatment can significantly alter treatment outcomes. For example, in the study on massage therapy for OA of the knee, a single method of administration was utilized and four dosages were tested. The two 60-minute doses were found to be significantly effective, whereas the two 30-minute doses were not.[6]

Administration of treatment includes the issues of mode, method, and dosage. The **mode** (or route) **of administration** is how the treatment reaches its target location (e.g., absorption through the skin). The **method of administration** is the technique for performing the treatment (e.g., holding an instrument at a specific angle, using a specific amount of pressure, at a particular location), as well as who will administer the treatment (the patient or a clinician). The **dosage** is the amount and frequency.

Many different modes for administering treatments are possible, with varying levels of invasiveness. Examples include drops in the eyes; ointments on the skin; injections into skin, muscles, or blood vessels; oral medications; inhalation (such as nebulized substances); and rectal or vaginal insertion. Even a therapy that is not physically invasive, such as cognitive behavioral therapy (CBT), has a mode of administration. In this case, the ears might be deemed the primary mode of administration, at least among hearing patients. Of course, treatments can have multiple modes of administration, as in the case of CBT, which might also proceed through visual as well as auditory and even integumentary (the skin) routes. Each mode of administration has risks associated with it, such as infection or injury.

When seeking approval for clinical trials researchers must disclose any such risks and provide methods for reducing the risks, strategies for dealing with associated adverse events, and justification for the risks in light of the expected benefits of the research. The mode of administration should also be carefully explained to research participants and again in resulting publications. As we mentioned earlier, the explanation should be sufficient that when you read it you could reproduce the treatment via the described mode of administration.

With regard to methods of administration, the possibilities are almost limitless. The methods of treatment administration must be studied and carefully described in publications, although it is challenging to adequately describe many administration methods using a medium such as text. Imagine for a moment trying to describe how to tie your shoes using just the written word. Some treatments have a common language that is used to explain methods of administration, which can help. Your basic and ongoing clinical training will generally provide you with the fund of knowledge necessary to interpret explanations of administration methods. Furthermore, other media, such as video and photographs, can be much more effective than text for demonstrating administration methods. Currently, few publications provide multiple media to document the methods of administration in treatment studies. Perhaps this situation will improve with time.

In addition to the mode and method of administration, the dosage should be similarly approved for research, justified in terms of risk/benefit, and thoroughly explained. Dosage has to do with frequency of administration and quantity of treatment per dose. Dosages can be studied during Phase I, II, III, or IV clinical trials. Well-designed studies should compare the various doses that are available for the target population and disorder, preferably in head-to-head comparisons with the various applicable doses of the usual treatment(s).

Dosage can influence both efficacy and safety. In many instances, researchers (as well as clinicians) seek a balance between efficacy and safety. Higher doses of some treatments might increase the efficacy of the treatment, but they might also increase the severity of side effects. Furthermore, the dosage that works in a clinical trial might not work as effectively or be as safe when administered to an individual patient. In general, researchers are interested in finding the lowest effective dose for a given treatment. This practice cannot only reduce the risk of adverse events, but it can also reduce the cost of the treatment.

Another important area of consideration related to administration and dosage is patient instructions. If a patient will self-administer the treatment, the mode, method, and dosage need to be carefully explained and demonstrated. Another area of investigation for researchers is the efficacy of patient instructions. The better the instructions and education, the greater the level of adherence (which happens to be our next topic). Procedures for patient instructions can include verbal information from a clinician, written materials (such as a pamphlet or instructions on a prescription bottle), a video, a website, or a demonstration. It would be terrific if various methods of informing/educating patients as well as different combinations of them were studied and compared. However, little of this type of research has been performed. Nonetheless, even if researchers do not specifically study different patient information/education procedures, a well-written publication will include a statement about how patients were informed or educated during the clinical trial.

Adherence

The term **adherence** means the degree to which patients are able to sustain a treatment regimen according to how it was prescribed. Another word often used to mean the same thing is **compliance**. However, there has been some debate regarding the two terms, suggesting a distinction between them. Consider the following definitions of adherence and compliance:

Adherence:[21]
- To stick to or hold fast
- To be devoted
- To follow closely or exactly

Compliance:[22]
- The act of conforming, acquiescing, or yielding
- A tendency to yield readily to others
- Cooperation or obedience

According to the debate over these two terms, the distinction between them has to do with locus of control. We *choose* to adhere, but we can be *forced* to comply. When we comply, we are being subjected to an external authority. When we adhere, we have authority over ourselves. The *American Heritage Medical Dictionary*[23] makes the following distinction between the terms:

> *Adherence [emphasis added] is the extent to which the patient continues the agreed-upon mode of treatment under limited supervision when faced with conflicting demands, as distinguished from compliance or maintenance.*

> *Compliance [emphasis added] is the degree of constancy and accuracy with which a patient follows a prescribed regimen, as distinguished from adherence or maintenance.*

One author explained the difference between the two terms succinctly: "the distinction between adherence and compliance is the action of the patient. Compliance implies passive obedience, and adherence implies active decision-making."[24] The concept of adherence is in alignment with patient-centered practice, as it recognizes the autonomy and self-determination of the patient.

You will find both adherence and compliance used in publications to mean essentially the same thing: the degree to which patients are able to sustain a treatment regimen according to how it was prescribed. Although the semantics we have discussed might well be very important to how you approach and think about patients, the specific use of each term is often not defined by authors, and the distinction might not be important to your search for relevant treatment information. We

recommend that you use both terms when searching for information on how well patients were able to sustain a treatment.

Adherence is not only an issue for patients, but also for providers. Many treatments are administered by providers. Treatments can range from relatively simple to highly complex and from relatively easy to extremely difficult. All treatments require attention to detail. Some treatments require precise technical skills. Treatment publications should discuss the degree of provider adherence to the treatment protocol and describe issues that influence provider adherence. For instance, in the study on massage therapy for OA of the knee, the authors described provider adherence as follows:

> *Each study therapist was taught and agreed to the protocol and signed a form attesting to adherence to the study protocol after each massage session. Study personnel reviewed adherence to the protocol at regular intervals throughout the study period. No deviations from the manualized massage protocol occurred.*[6]

Patient adherence can be influenced by many factors, including side effects, ability to afford the treatment, time, access, sociocultural issues, readiness to change, values, health literacy, level of physical activity, nutrition, and other patient needs/preferences. Publications on treatments should provide information on patient adherence as well as factors associated with it. In the massage therapy article, the researchers tracked patient adherence by counting the number of massage visits that subjects completed and calculating a proportion of total scheduled visits. The authors reported 80% of scheduled massage visits were completed by patients. The researchers also performed significance tests to determine if there were any differences between groups on patient adherence, finding no significant difference. These details tell us that 80% patient adherence to a once or twice per week 60-minute massage therapy treatment protocol is sufficient to achieve clinically important benefits. We also know that the once or twice per week 30-minute protocol was not sufficient to achieve the same benefits.[6]

Cost

When we discuss cost, we are referring to the amount charged to patients and insurance companies for the care provided, as opposed to the cost for healthcare organizations to provide treatments. Cost of treatment is a significantly influential barrier that should be addressed in treatment publications. Cost is an essential consideration, because it often influences access to care for many patients, in fact perhaps the majority. Treatment publications should address the issue of cost and compare the different treatment options in terms of cost. However, it can be difficult for researchers to ascertain valid cost information, other than for the treatments administered through their own studies. Furthermore, even though researchers most likely could report cost information on the treatments administered in their studies, this information is usually not reported. In some publications, researchers will report whether patients were charged for the research treatment. Research treatments often are provided for free. In that case, treatment cost would be essentially meaningless information. Also, even if researchers reported the cost of treatment, the amounts would likely not apply elsewhere. Cost is an investigational area in which significant improvements are needed. Generally, it will be up to you to locate cost information separate from the treatment publications that you read, although you might be able to glean certain cost information from treatment publications.

For example, in the massage therapy treatment article[6] the once-per-week 60-minute protocol was effective. This indicates that a lower-cost option (once-per-week 60-minute protocol) is as effective as a higher-cost option (twice-per-week 60-minute protocol). If a patient was considering massage therapy as a treatment for knee OA, you would have reason to inform him or her that 60 minutes of Swedish massage therapy once per week could be beneficial based on results of the 2012 clinical trial. However, the authors in the study provided no data on the usual care protocol, so you have no information on the cost of massage therapy compared to the cost of usual care. It would be

necessary for you to gather cost information on other care options or for the patient to do so, if cost was a deciding factor for the patient.

With that in mind, we performed a search in PubMed for "cost of massage therapy" (with quotes) and no publications were returned. We also conducted a more general search through an Internet search engine for "cost of Swedish massage therapy" (without the quotes), which returned over 22 million hits. The third hit on the page was a webpage called "Massage Cost—What Does A Massage Cost?" It was an article written by Anitra Brown for About.com (no publication date was provided). The author claimed that massage costs start at $75 per hour in small cities and $90 per hour in larger cities. Of course, these claims were unreferenced.[25]

We then performed a search of massage therapy providers in our community and found a range of prices. The price was $20 per hour at the local university massage therapy clinic[26] and $50 per hour at several of the other businesses in town. Thus, if a patient in our community was considering massage therapy as a treatment for OA of the knee, then the cost for 8 weeks of treatment (based on the dosage reported in the clinical trial) would range from $160 to $400.

It might seem like we went to a lot of trouble to gather cost information about massage therapy. However, the above searches only took about 2 minutes and gleaned the information we would need to answer a question about the cost of massage therapy for a patient in our community. You might not always have those 2 minutes to spare, but it can be helpful in guiding patients on selection of treatment modalities. Patients might not themselves have the time, resources, or skills to quickly locate and evaluate this kind of information, and your efforts in this area could help them overcome a barrier that is often quite significant: cost.

Access

As with cost, access is a topic that is often not addressed in treatment research but would be beneficial to have information about. Cost is a factor that determines access; other factors include availability of treatments, availability of qualified providers, availability of required equipment or other resources, transportation to get to the treatment facility or to pick up a prescription, and language consonance between providers and patients. Access varies significantly by geographic location, by socioeconomic status, and by education level.

Healthcare disparities is a field of study that focuses on access to health care. In fact, "healthcare disparities" is a MeSH for studies in this field. A significant amount of study focuses on disparities. However, the topic is usually studied separately from treatment research, rather than incorporated into treatment studies. As with information on cost, it is often necessary to perform a separate search for information on access when considering treatment options. Even so, questions of access to care are often commonsense concerns that can be addressed by asking a patient directly about them. Published information on access to a specific type of treatment, although informative, might not help in determining if an individual patient has access to the treatment. Access to treatment is more of a public health topic than an individual health topic.

In treatment publications, it is important for researchers to address issues of access and describe barriers. This information will help healthcare organizations make decisions about how to best expend resources. Many organizations and communities have limited financial resources to invest in healthcare services. Strategic decisions are made every day regarding which types of treatments to provide in a given practice or organization based on the needs of the population and patients' ability to pay for the services. Organizations and practices also have to take into account the necessary qualifications and experience required for a given treatment to be provided. The more complex and risky a given treatment, typically the more credentials and licenses required to perform it.

Consider cancer therapies. Cancer treatment is often multimodal and interprofessional, involving surgery, pharmaceuticals, radiation, oral health care, pain management, management of medication interactions, rehabilitation, mental health

support, and interventions to support patient caregivers. It might be necessary to have the personnel and other resources in all of these areas in order to provide adequate cancer treatment (depending on the type and severity of cancer to be treated). Each area of specialization might require a separate practitioner or team of practitioners. Suffice it to say that access to care of this kind is limited due to its cost and complexity.

Time

The final treatment selection factor to consider is time: the amount of time to perform the treatment, the amount of time needed for the treatment to reach efficacy, the amount of time for a patient to travel or be transported to the treatment facility, and the amount of time needed to recover from the treatment. Publications related to a specific treatment modality should explain relevant temporal issues. In the massage therapy study,[6] the researchers undertook the questions of how much time each treatment needed to last and how many weeks of treatment were needed in order to achieve a minimal clinically important difference. The article did not address the question of time for patients to transport themselves to massage therapy treatments, but this would likely be an issue you would consider together with a patient if massage therapy was being considered.

In treatment studies, researchers should compare temporal issues across different treatment options as well as different doses. It might be too complex to compare every combination in a single study. You might need to look for several publications related to a given treatment and try to determine if there are temporal differences between treatment/dose combinations.

TREATMENT ALGORITHMS AND EXPERT GUIDELINES

Treatment algorithms and expert guidelines are common forms for presenting treatment information. They are typically produced by special interest organizations, such as the American Heart Association, or by government organizations, such as the Agency for Healthcare Research and Quality (AHRQ). Many point-of-care information sources (e.g., DynaMed, PIER, and MD Consult) provide access to treatment algorithms and expert guidelines.

A *treatment algorithm* is often presented as a decision chart that provides an outline of the treatment process. An *expert guideline*, also referred to as a *practice guideline* or a *best practice*, details the recommended care associated with a given condition. Treatment algorithms and expert guidelines can represent opinion, or they can represent high-level research. A well-designed treatment algorithm or practice guideline will include references as well as designations regarding the strength and type of evidence supporting the recommendations they present. **Figure 9–2** is an example of an algorithm associated with managing osteoarthritic knee pain. This hypothetical algorithm was derived from a publication by the American Osteopathic Association (AOA).[27] The algorithm incorporates the information in the article with the concept of patient-centered care. It also includes the option of massage therapy, which was not mentioned in the AOA article. The AOA article includes a treatment algorithm of its own. If you have access to the article (see entry 27 in the references for this chapter), we encourage you to retrieve it and examine how the algorithm is presented in light of following discussion about treatment algorithms and evidence.

Treatment algorithms should be evaluated by the same criteria as other healthcare information sources. It can be challenging, however, to determine the evidence that supports a specific treatment algorithm. In some cases, researchers will conduct a study to evaluate the outcomes associated with utilization of a treatment algorithm. In most cases, the algorithm is presented without any discussion of associated outcome research. More often than not, treatment algorithms represent basic information and belong near the bottom of the evidence pyramid. They can be quite useful, but you will require additional information before following them.

Whereas algorithms tend to present abbreviated recommendations for quick reference, practice guidelines tend to be more detailed and grounded

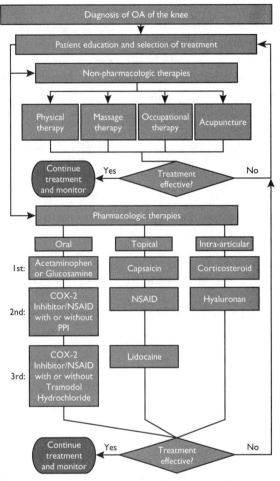

Figure 9–2 Algorithm for Managing Osteoarthritic Knee Pain

in supporting research. For example, the American Academy of Orthopaedic Surgeons (AAOS) produced a practice guideline for nonarthroplasty treatment of OA of the knee.[28] The types of interventions addressed in the guideline include patient education, lifestyle modification, complementary and alternative therapy, mechanical interventions, analgesic medications, intra-articular corticosteroid injections, needle lavage, and surgical interventions. The recommendations were developed by a workgroup that referenced existing systematic reviews completed by the AHRQ as well as the Osteoarthritis Research Society International (OARSI). The group also performed its own systematic reviews for any treatments not addressed by the other two bodies of research.

The practice guideline describes the methods for identifying and including studies, including which databases were used to locate the publications. The working group initially identified 278 systematic reviews, of which 48 were sufficiently on topic to be retrieved and evaluated. Among them, seven systematic reviews met the inclusion criteria. The authors presented a table that outlined the ranking criteria used to rate the levels of evidence. We present an excerpt from the table (**Table 9–2**) focused on the treatment studies.[28]

The authors additionally graded each recommendation in the guideline according to the following scheme:[28]

- **A:** Good evidence (Level I studies with consistent findings) for or against recommending the intervention.
- **B:** Fair evidence (Level II or III studies with consistent findings) for or against recommending the intervention.
- **C:** Poor quality evidence (Level IV or V) for or against recommending the intervention.
- **I:** Insufficient or conflicting evidence does not allow a recommendation for or against the intervention.

The working group presented 22 recommendations with associated evidence levels and grades, grouping the recommendations according to treatment categories. We present the full list of recommendations of the study to exemplify the various disciplines that are involved in treating this health condition. Note that the guideline does not address all possible treatments. As the authors explain:

> This guideline should not be construed as including all proper methods of care or excluding methods of care reasonably directed to obtaining the same results. The ultimate judgment regarding any specific procedure or treatment must be made in light of all circumstances presented by the patient and the needs and resources particular to the locality or institution.[28]

Patient Education and Lifestyle Modification

Recommendation 1: The authors suggest patients with symptomatic osteoarthritis (OA) of the knee be encouraged to participate in self-management educational programs such as those conducted by the Arthritis

Table 9–2 Criteria for Rating of Evidence in Practice Guideline for Osteoarthritis of the Knee

Level of Evidence	Therapeutic Studies Investigating the Results of Treatment
Level I	• High-quality RCT with statistically significant difference but narrow confidence intervals • Systematic review of Level I RCTs (and study results were homogenous)
Level II	• Lesser-quality RCT (e.g., < 80% follow-up, no blinding, or improper randomization) • Prospective comparative study • Systematic review of Level II or Level I studies with inconsistent results
Level III	• Case-control study • Retrospective comparative study • Systematic review of Level III studies
Level IV	• Case series
Level V	• Expert opinion

Source: American Academy of Orthopaedic Surgeons. *Treatment of osteoarthritis of the knee (nonarthroplasty).* December 6, 2008. [Online database: National Guideline Clearinghouse]. Available at: http://guideline.gov. Accessed July 23, 2012.

Foundation, and incorporate activity modifications (e.g., walking instead of running; alternative activities) into their lifestyle. (Grade B, Level II)

Recommendation 2: Regular contact to promote self-care is an option for patients with symptomatic OA of the knee. (Grade C, Level IV)

Recommendation 3: The authors recommend patients with symptomatic OA of the knee, who are overweight (as defined by a body mass index [BMI] > 25), should be encouraged to lose weight (a minimum of 5% of body weight) and maintain their weight at a lower level with an appropriate program of dietary modification and exercise. (Grade A, Level I)

Rehabilitation

Recommendation 4: The authors recommend patients with symptomatic OA of the knee be encouraged to participate in low-impact aerobic fitness exercises. (Grade A, Level I)

Recommendation 5: Range of motion/flexibility exercises are an option for patients with symptomatic OA of the knee. (Grade C, Level V)

Recommendation 6: The authors suggest quadriceps strengthening for patients with symptomatic OA of the knee. (Grade B, Level II)

Mechanical Interventions

Recommendation 7: The authors suggest patients with symptomatic OA of the knee use patellar taping for short-term relief of pain and improvement in function. (Grade B, Level II)

Recommendation 8: The authors suggest lateral heel wedges not be prescribed for patients with symptomatic medial compartmental OA of the knee. (Grade B, Level II)

Recommendation 9: The authors are unable to recommend for or against the use of a brace with a valgus directing force for patients with medial unicompartmental OA of the knee. (Inconclusive, Level II)

Recommendation 10: The authors are unable to recommend for or against the use of a brace with a varus directing force for patients with lateral unicompartmental OA of the knee. (Inconclusive, Level V)

Complementary and Alternative Therapy

Recommendation 11: The authors are unable to recommend for or against the use of acupuncture as an adjunctive therapy for pain relief in patients with symptomatic OA of the knee. (Inconclusive, Level I)

Recommendation 12: The authors recommend glucosamine and/or chondroitin sulfate or hydrochloride not be prescribed for patients with symptomatic OA of the knee. (Grade A, Level I)

Pain Relievers

Recommendation 13: The authors suggest patients with symptomatic OA of the knee receive one of the following analgesics for pain unless there are contraindications to this treatment:

- Acetaminophen (not to exceed 4 grams per day)
- Nonsteroidal anti-inflammatory drugs (NSAIDs)

(Grade B, Level II)

Recommendation 14: The authors suggest patients with symptomatic OA of the knee and increased gastrointestinal (GI) risk (age ≥ 60 years, comorbid medical conditions, history of peptic ulcer disease, history of GI bleeding, concurrent corticosteroids, and/or concomitant use of anticoagulants) receive one of the following analgesics for pain:

- Acetaminophen (not to exceed 4 grams per day)
- Topical NSAIDs
- Nonselective oral NSAIDs plus gastro-protective agent
- Cyclooxygenase-2 inhibitors

(Grade B, Level II)

Intra-Articular Injections

Recommendation 15: The authors suggest intra-articular corticosteroids for short-term pain relief for patients with symptomatic OA of the knee. (Grade B, Level II)

Recommendation 16: The authors cannot recommend for or against the use of intra-articular hyaluronic acid for patients with mild to moderate symptomatic OA of the knee. (Inconclusive, Level I and II)

Needle Lavage

Recommendation 17: The authors suggest that needle lavage not be used for patients with symptomatic OA of the knee. (Grade B, Level I and II)

Surgical Intervention

Recommendation 18: The authors recommend against performing arthroscopy with debridement or lavage in patients with a primary diagnosis of symptomatic OA of the knee. (Grade A, Level I and II)

Recommendation 19: Arthroscopic partial meniscectomy or loose body removal is an option in patients with symptomatic OA of the knee who also have primary signs and symptoms of a torn meniscus and/or a loose body. (Grade C, Level V)

Recommendation 20: The authors cannot recommend for or against an osteotomy of the tibial tubercle for patients with isolated symptomatic patello-femoral osteoarthritis. (Inconclusive, Level V)

Recommendation 21: Realignment osteotomy is an option in active patients with symptomatic unicompartmental OA of the knee with malalignment. (Grade C, Level IV and V)

Recommendation 22: The authors suggest against using a free-floating interpositional device for patients with symptomatic unicompartmental OA of the knee. (Grade B, Level IV)

When you are considering the information presented in an algorithm or a practice guideline, you can evaluate them in the same manner as any other healthcare information resource. In some instances, the item you are evaluating will provide information on the levels of evidence, the references utilized, and the grades of the recommendations. In other instances the item you are evaluating will not provide these details and will require more careful scrutiny.

STUDIES OF HARM

Studies of harm take several forms. Harm studies can examine the natural course of a disease (that is to say harm from lack of treatment), harm caused by complications from individual diagnostic or treatment interventions, or harms caused by interactions between diagnostic interventions and/or treatments. Studies of harm raise ethical considerations. Generally, studies of harm are observational in nature, mainly in the form of case-control and cohort studies, although most randomized control studies on a given diagnostic or treatment modality also include assessment of harm. When new treatments and diagnostic procedures are studied, data are collected related to adverse events in order to determine if any unexpected harms are present. Harm information is essential to the selection of treatment and diagnostic modalities. Few if any interventions are free of harm for all patients. It is not always possible to comply with the principle of *do no harm* due to adverse responses to interventions.

In studies of harm, we look for data on increase in absolute risk, the number needed to harm

(NNH), odds ratios, and explanations of the balance between benefit and harm in the study population. As a rule, the strongest evidence for questions related to harm comes from systematic reviews and meta-analyses. In the absence of such studies, large, randomized control trials are the next best evidence, although this type of research is not often performed with questions of harm due to ethical considerations. These higher levels of evidence might be difficult to find for a given question related to harm. However, harm information is often included in treatment studies that examine safety and efficacy.

In order to locate studies that include information on harm, we recommend the following search terms:

- Interactions
- Complications
- Side effects (or side-effects)
- Adverse events
- Harm
- Safety
- Tolerability
- Adherence

Example: Evidence of Harm Question

We recommend replicating the following example to practice EBP search strategies. The topic selected was based on availability of multiple high-level publications. Note that we have not included screenshots for this search because the websites change so often that the images would likely be inaccurate by the time you read this.

We were interested in the harms associated with medications used to treat rheumatoid arthritis. In order to locate the best available evidence on the topic, we started with PubMed and used the MeSH search feature to identify the MeSH in which articles related to rheumatoid arthritis are categorized. The MeSH was "Arthritis, Rheumatoid." After clicking on this MeSH link, PubMed brought up a list

of subheadings with checkboxes. From this list, we selected "drug therapy" and then added these options to the Search Builder. We then ran the search and used the filters to limit results to "Meta-analysis and Systematic Review." This brought up 620 publications on the topic. We then added several of the harm-related terms from the list presented earlier to our search. The resulting search string was as follows:

"Arthritis, Rheumatoid/drug therapy"[Mesh] AND (safety OR tolerability OR "side effects" OR "adverse events" OR interactions OR complications)

This strategy reduced the list to 245 results. Next we limited our search to the last 5 years in order to get the most current information. This brought the results list down to 135 items. This list was short enough that we were willing to glance through it to see if a highly relevant outcome was showing. Another effective strategy for performing this search would be to use the Clinical Queries feature in PubMed. We also performed this search using the same search string and received the same results in the Clinical Queries area.

In the list was a comparative effectiveness study performed by AHRQ entitled, "Summary of AHRQ's Comparative Effectiveness Review of Drug Therapy for Rheumatoid Arthritis (RA) in Adults—An Update."[29] This publication was available for free as a full-text online publication. It was published in January–February of 2012. The list also had a publication from 2011 entitled, "Comparative Effectiveness Research (CER): A Summary of AHRQ's CER on Therapies for Rheumatoid Arthritis."[30] These two articles met our criteria of being high-level evidence, being recent, and being focused on our clinical question.

The first article included a table listing the harms of various medications in comparison to one another as well as the strength of evidence for each study. The harms reported in the studies included discontinuation, cardiovascular events, cerebrovascular events, hepatic events, and infection.

Note that you can familiarize yourself with harms associated with specific interventions by searching for general information about the intervention itself. For instance, with medications numerous databases and other resources can be searched that provide details on harms. Medications usually also have information provided with them in the package insert that lists known harms. It would not be prudent to rely entirely on such resources, but they are helpful in beginning to educate yourself about the treatment. Alas, not all types of interventions have such readily accessible general sources of harm information.

STUDIES OF PREVENTION

The term **prevention** is defined as, "actions aimed at eradicating, eliminating, or minimizing the impact of disease and disability, or if none of these is feasible, retarding the progress of disease and disability."[11] Generally, prevention focuses on illnesses that can be acquired, as opposed to illnesses that are inherited. However, an emerging and rapidly growing area of research is that related to the prevention of genetic mutations that cause numerous illnesses, especially with regard to cancer. The goal of preventive health care, according to the American Board of Preventive Medicine, is "to protect, promote, and maintain health and well-being and to prevent disease, disability, and death."[31]

Originally, preventive medicine as a field focused on communicable diseases, identifying the causes of diseases, finding their sources, and determining the mode of transmission. One of the great breakthroughs in medical science was also a seminal moment for the field of disease prevention. In the 1850s, Louis Pasteur performed experiments whose results supported the germ theory of disease, "which holds that germs attack the body from outside."[32] At that point in European history, many authorities believed that tiny organisms such as germs "could not possibly kill larger ones such as humans."[32]

However, in 1864 the French Academy of Sciences accepted his results. Later Pasteur extended his theory to explain the causes of many diseases, including anthrax, cholera, tuberculosis, and smallpox.[32] He also identified methods for their prevention by vaccination. Pasteur is perhaps best known for his development of vaccines for rabies and for a process for removal of bacteria from certain liquids (wine, beer, and milk) through boiling and cooling, a process that came to be known as *pasteurization*. Another famous and foundational prevention example was the discovery in the 1850s by John Snow that the water provided by Southwark and Vauxhall Water Company in London was the source of a cholera outbreak.[33] Closing the wells used by the company halted the outbreak.

Types of Prevention

Today, prevention research has a number of broad areas of focus, such as the prevention of occupational injury, the prevention of lifestyle-caused illnesses, the prevention of disease progression, the prevention of psychiatric illness, and so on. Preventive health care has come to be divided into four types, as follows:

1. **Primary prevention**, *which aims to reduce the incidence of disease by personal and communal efforts, such as decreasing environmental risks, enhancing nutritional status, immunizing against communicable diseases, or improving water supplies. It is a core task of public health.*

2. **Secondary prevention**, *which aims to reduce the prevalence of disease by shortening its durations. If the disease has no cure, it may increase survival and quality of life; it will also increase the prevalence of the disease. It seldom prevents disease occurrence; it does so only when early detection of a precursor lesion leads to complete removal of all such lesions. It is a set of measures available to individuals and communities for the early detection and prompt intervention to control disease and minimize disability, e.g., by the use of screening programs. It is a core task of preventive medicine. Both early clinical detection and population-based screening usually aim at achieving secondary prevention. In certain diseases these activities may also contribute to tertiary prevention.*

3. **Tertiary prevention**, *which consists of measures aimed at softening the impact of long-term disease and disability by eliminating or reducing*

impairment, disability, and handicap; reducing suffering; and maximizing potential years of useful life. It is mainly a task of rehabilitation.

4. **Quaternary prevention**, *which consists of actions that identify patients at risk of overdiagnosis or overmedication and that protect them from excessive medical intervention. Actions that prevent iatrogenesis (adverse effects of preventive, diagnostic, therapeutic, surgical and other medical, sanitary, and health procedures, interventions or programs).[11]*

Thus, studies of prevention focus on the above four types of prevention, although the researchers themselves often do not categorize studies according to the type of prevention.

Prevention Resources

Perhaps the most well-known sources for information on prevention are the CDC and the USPSTF. Both organizations fund research in prevention and provide guidelines for healthcare practitioners as well as the public based on current research. Prevention information can also be found through other healthcare information sources, such as special-interest organizations, PubMed, the World Health Organization, and others.

The USPSTF is an especially effective resource for guidance on prevention activities because of its mission:

The U.S. Preventive Services Task Force (USPSTF or Task Force) is an independent group of national experts in prevention and evidence-based medicine that works to improve the health of all Americans by making evidence-based recommendations about clinical preventive services such as screenings, counseling services, or preventive medications.[34]

The guidelines produced by the USPSTF include specifics on levels of evidence, grades of recommendations, and references to original sources. The way that the USPSTF guidelines are presented makes it easier for readers to rate the strength of the evidence and to determine if the information provided is trustworthy. As of the writing of this chapter, the website address for the USPSTF is www.uspreventiveservicestaskforce.org.

While we are on the subject of the USPSTF, in November of 2011 the USPSTF submitted a report to Congress entitled *High-Priority Evidence Gaps for Clinical Preventive Services* (located at www.uspreventiveservicestaskforce.org/annlrpt/index.html as of the writing of this chapter). The intent behind the report was explained as follows:

. . . by identifying these evidence gaps and prioritizing these areas for research, it will inspire public and private researchers to collaborate and target their efforts to generate new knowledge and fill current evidence gaps so that in the near future, the USPSTF will be able to develop definitive recommendations on these important topics.[34]

The gaps were grouped into three categories and reported as follows:[35]

Screening tests that deserve further research:
1. Screening for Coronary Heart Disease with New and Old Technologies
2. Screening for Colorectal Cancer with New Modalities
3. Screening for Hepatitis C
4. Screening for Hip Dysplasia in Newborns

Behavioral intervention research topics that deserve further research:
1. Moderate- to Low-Intensity Counseling for Obesity
2. Interventions in Primary Care to Prevent Child Abuse and Neglect
3. Screening for Illicit Drug Use in Primary Care

Evidence gaps relating to specific populations and age groups that deserve further research:
1. Screening for Osteoporosis in Men
2. Screening and Treatment for Depression in Children
3. Screening and Counseling for Alcohol Misuse in Adolescents
4. Aspirin Use to Prevent Heart Attacks and Strokes in Adults Ages 80 Years and Older

Recommendations from the USPSTF are structured similarly to the practice guideline we discussed earlier under the topic of treatment algorithms and practice guidelines.

BIOSTATISTICS IN TREATMENT, HARM, AND PREVENTION

Resources on treatment, harm, and prevention will include many different types of biostatistics. Although biostatistics is a central topic in this chapter, there is too much information to address every concept. As such, we will discuss several of the more common biostatistics found in resources on treatment, harm, and prevention, especially those found in research publications.

Relative Risk

Relative risk is "the ratio of the risk of an event among the exposed to the risk among the unexposed."[11] Or, put another way, it is the event rate in one group divided by the event rate in the other group. Relative risk is also referred to as the risk ratio (RR):

$$RR = \frac{EER}{CER}$$

The rule for interpreting the RR is as follows:

- RR > 1.0: The risk of the outcome of interest is increased for one group.
- RR < 1.0: The risk of the outcome of interest is decreased for one group.
- RR = 1.0: The risk of the outcome of interest is equal between groups.

Relative risk should only be calculated when using a cohort research design. Keep in mind that a score close to 1.0 is likely to indicate no difference. You will need to look at the accompanying p-value and confidence interval to determine if a specific RR value represents a statistically significant difference.

Consider the following hypothetical example. A comparison between two groups receiving treatment A versus usual care produces a relative risk of 2.3 with a 95% confidence interval of 0.7–3.9 and a p-value of 0.23. The confidence interval for the RR number crosses 1.0, meaning that

the true relative risk could be decreased, rather than increased, as the 2.3 RR value indicates. Furthermore, the p-value is high enough that we can conclude that it is not less than alpha, because we would likely never see an alpha value higher than 0.23. Typical values for alpha are 0.001, 0.01, and 0.05. Rarely, we might see 0.10. Even if we are most generous and use 0.10 for alpha, the p-value is not less than 0.10 and the RR value is not statistically significant.

Relative risk is based on probabilities of an event, rather than odds of an event. The event rate for each group is a proportion of those with the outcome divided by the total number of individuals in the group (e.g., in a contingency table the formulas are $\frac{a}{a+b}$ for the probability in the exposed group or $\frac{c}{c+d}$ for the probability in the unexposed group). This differs from calculating odds, which is the number with the outcome divided by the number without the outcome (e.g., $\frac{a}{b}$ for the odds in the exposed group or $\frac{c}{d}$ for the odds in the nonexposed group).

There is no rule for how far an RR score needs to be beyond 1.0 in order to be significant. In some situations an RR of 1.5 might be statistically significant and in other situations an RR of 10.0 might not be statistically significant. As we have said, you will need to read the associated p-value and confidence interval in order to determine if an RR value is statistically significant.

This usage of relative risk is especially applicable to studies of harm and prevention, although it can be used in treatment studies as well.

Example: Relative Risk

Consider the following example of relative risk from a recent study. A 2012 randomized control trial by Wijesinghe et al.[36] examined the effectiveness of high-concentration oxygen (experimental group) compared to titrated oxygen to achieve O_2 saturation between 93–95% (usual care group) in the treatment of community-acquired pneumonia (CAP). The researchers included data from 150 emergency department patients with suspected CAP.

The main outcome measure was the proportion of patients with a rise in $PtCO_2$ of 4 mm Hg or greater at 60 minutes. $PtCO_2$ is the transcutaneous partial pressure of carbon dioxide.[37] $PtCO_2$ was used to estimate arterial $PaCO_2$. $PaCO_2$ is partial pressure of carbon dioxide in the arterial blood.[37] The proportion of patients in the high-concentration oxygen group that achieved the target $PtCO_2$ level (36/72) was higher than that of the usual care group (11/75).

> How would you categorize this study, as a study of treatment, harm, or prevention?

The RR was 3.4 (95% CI: 1.9–6.2). This means that the group receiving high-concentration oxygen had a 3.4 times greater probability of achieving the desired level of $PtCO_2$ than the titrated oxygen group. Note that in this case the risk of interest is a good outcome, achieving $PtCO_2$ 4 mm Hg or greater at 60 minutes. The confidence interval also tells us that the difference was statistically significant because it does not cross 1.0.

Relative Risk Reduction and Relative Risk Increase

Like relative risk, **relative risk reduction** (**RRR**) and **relative risk increase** (**RRI**) can be reported in various kinds of studies. RRR and RRI are another way of expressing relative risk. Relative risk reduction is "the difference in event rates between two groups expressed as a proportion of the event rate in the untreated group."[11] The difference between RRR and RRI is that one represents a reduction in risk (RRR) and the other represents an increase in risk (RRI). They are calculated in essentially the same way:

$$RRR = \frac{CER - EER}{CER}$$

That is to say that RRR is the control event rate minus the experiment event rate divided by the control event rate.

Example: Relative Risk Reduction

The following is an example of a study that utilized RRR and RRI. A systematic review of literature was performed in 2012 by Pietrosimone et al.[38] to "determine the relative risk reduction associated with prophylactic knee braces in the prevention of knee injuries in collegiate football players." In instances when the RRR value was negative, then the value was reported as RRI, which was simply the absolute value of the RRR statistics. The primary outcome measure was incidence of ligamentous knee injuries.

The researchers identified seven studies that met their inclusion criteria. Three of the studies reported a RRR and the other four studies reported a RRI, as follows:

RRR
- RRR = 58 (95%CI: 25 to 76)
- RRR = 10 (95%CI: –26 to 36)
- RRR = 56 (95%CI: 13 to 77)

RRI
- RRI = 17 (95%CI: –71 to 19)
- RRI = 114 (95%CI: –492 to 23)
- RRI = 49 (95%CI: –69 to –31)
- RRI = 42 (95%CI: –70 to –18)

The first RRR value is 58. This means that in that particular study athletes who used the brace had 58 times lesser probability of experiencing a ligamentous knee injury. The confidence interval tells us that the population RRR value is most likely somewhere between 25 and 76 (according to that particular study). The RRR for the second study listed was 10, meaning that athletes who used the brace had a 10 times lesser probability of experiencing a ligamentous knee injury. However, the confidence interval for that statistic ranged from –26 to 36. A negative RRR is actually a RRI. Based on the confidence interval, it is possible that the brace could result in an increase in probability of injury. Note that in the four studies showing an increase in relative risk three of the four RRI confidence intervals also crossed zero.

The authors summarized their results as follows: "Confidence intervals for the RRR in three of the studies [sic] were very large and crossed zero, suggesting that a true prophylactic effect was unlikely."[38] They concluded by saying:

> *Therefore, due to the inconsistent findings within the literature, we deem the current evidence regarding the efficacy of prophylactic knee bracing in reducing knee injuries inconclusive . . . Better-quality randomized controlled trials will allow us to accurately determine whether prophylactic knee bracing in collegiate football players is efficacious or harmful.*[38]

Odds Ratio

The *odds ratio* (OR) is the ratio of the odds of an event occurring in one group to the odds of an event occurring in another group. The OR is a measure of association that is calculated in retrospective studies. To calculate an odds ratio, researchers begin by calculating the odds of an event in each group (the exposed group and the unexposed group; i.e., the control group). An odds ratio is most commonly used in epidemiological studies and studies of harm.

An odds ratio makes little sense in treatment research, because treatment research is more likely to be prospective rather than retrospective. A retrospective treatment study would involve identifying a treatment of interest that is suspected of causing a given outcome, dividing a random selection of charts into cases and controls, and then determining if the patient records support a significant association between the treatment and the outcome. In most cases, such a study would be a study of harm because the outcome of interest would be some type of undesirable outcome. That is not to say that a case-control treatment study could not be performed; it is just uncommon. The main point here is that when you come across an odds ratio you should check to see if the study is retrospective. If it is prospective, an odds ratio is likely not the correct statistic, and the underlying design of the study might be flawed.

Prevention studies also are often prospective in nature, but retrospective prevention studies are performed, in which case an odds ratio would be an appropriate statistic.

Example: Odds Ratio

A case-control study was performed to estimate vaccine effectiveness (VE) for prevention of hospitalization due to pandemic influenza (H1N1). The cases were patients aged 18 to 65 with a 10-day history of acute respiratory infection (ARI) who had tested positive for H1N1.[39] Controls were patients in the same age range who had an ARI but were negative for H1N1. The researchers then compared those who had received a flu vaccination and those who had not in each of the groups to determine if breakthrough infections were more likely among the vaccinated or unvaccinated group.

> While we are on the subject of flu vaccinations, what type of prevention is a vaccine?

The researchers compared several types of vaccinations, including 2009/2010 pandemic flu vaccination, 2009/2010 seasonal flu vaccination, 2008/2009 seasonal flu vaccination, 2007/2008 seasonal flu vaccination, pneumococcal vaccination, and pandemic vaccination offered by an employer.[39] We will look at just one of the comparison results—those receiving the 2009/2010 pandemic flu vaccination among nonhospitalized patients.

With an odds ratio:

- OR > 1.0: The odds are increased.
- OR < 1.0: The odds are decreased.
- OR = 1.0: The odds are equal.

The odds ratio for the 2009/2010 pandemic flu vaccination was 0.5 (95% CI: 0.0–4.8).[39] An OR of 0.5 means that those who had the pandemic flu vaccination had 0.5 (lesser) odds of developing H1N1 compared to those who did not have the vaccination. Note, however, the confidence interval of 0.0–4.8. This indicates that among those vaccinated with the 2009/2010 pandemic flu vaccine, the true odds of developing H1N1 were most likely somewhere between 0.0 and 4.8.

The 2009/2010 pandemic flu–vaccinated patients could have had greater odds of developing H1N1 (4.8) or zero odds (0.0) of developing H1N1. When the confidence interval for an odds ratio crosses 1.0, it means that there was no significant difference. In this example, this fact is supported by the *p*-value associated with the odds ratio of 0.62.[39] The *p*-value is not less than alpha (even though we have not stated what alpha was for this study, the lowest level of alpha used would be 0.10 and the *p*-value of 0.62 is clearly no less than that). Thus, the odds of developing H1N1 with the 2009/2010 pandemic flu vaccination were no different than the odds of developing H1N1 without the 2009/2010 pandemic flu vaccination among nonhospitalized patients.

We will not go through the steps of calculating odds ratios here. The formula for the odds ratio is $\frac{ad}{bc}$. In the example we just discussed, the odds ratios presented were adjusted for time period and age. Furthermore, the study was underpowered for detecting differences among nonhospitalized patients. The reason for low statistical power was a low proportion of H1N1 cases and the small numbers of vaccinated patients. There were only 24 vaccinated patients and 117 nonvaccinated patients in the pandemic flu vaccination comparison. In fact, none of the 24 vaccinated patients in this group developed H1N1.[39]

Hazard Ratio

A **hazard ratio** (**HR**) is a measure of how often a particular adverse event occurs in one group compared to another group over time. The element of time is the primary distinguishing characteristic of a hazard ratio. It is essentially a relative risk calculation weighted according to time across a survival curve during the course of a study. The hazard is the slope of the survival curve, and the hazard ratio compares the slope between two groups.[40] Generally, hazard studies look at serious adverse events and/or death. You can use the following rule to interpret hazard ratios:

- HR > 1.0: Means greater hazard
- HR < 1.0: Means lesser hazard
- HR = 1.0: Means equal hazard

Example: Hazard Ratio

A study was performed to determine the difference in risk for not being screened for colorectal cancer among patients who received no automated outreach and patients who received automated outreach.[41] Automated outreach involved an interactive voice response (IVR) call followed by a mailed fecal immunochemical test. The adjusted HR was 3.75 (95% CI: 3.6–3.91). This means that those who did not receive automated outreach messages had a 3.75 times greater hazard (of not being screened for colorectal cancer) over time.

Absolute Risk, Absolute Risk Reduction, Absolute Risk Increase

Absolute risk (AR) is another way of stating the event rate or incidence rate of a group. Absolute risk is helpful for determining the clinical importance of an event. When relative risk, relative risk reduction, and relative risk increases are reported, they can be misleading because they are proportions. Absolute risk is calculated for each group, and then the AR for the experimental group is subtracted from the AR for the control group to determine absolute risk reduction.

Absolute risk reduction (ARR) is merely the mathematical difference (subtraction) between the event rate in the control group and the event rate in the treatment group:

$$ARR = EER - CER$$

Unfortunately, AR, ARR, and ARI (absolute risk increase) are not often reported. A number of critiques of the literature have suggested that the AR and ARR or ARI always be reported along with RR, RRR, and RRI. The main question with AR, ARR, and ARI is whether the risk difference is clinically meaningful.

Example: Absolute Risk and Absolute Risk Reduction

Consider the following example. In a 2012 publication of a cohort study on patients with acute lung injury, researchers examined the effect of mechanical ventilation on 2-year mortality.[42] The experimental intervention was to limit volume and pressure of the mechanical ventilation treatment, which is a treatment referred to as *lung-protective mechanical ventilation*. The researchers found an ARR of 4% for those patients who had received at least 50% adherence to lung-protective ventilation and an ARR of 7.8% for those who received 100% adherent treatment. The baseline mortality level among this patient population was 49.7%.

This means that the 2-year mortality rate among the 50% adherence group was approximately 45.7% and the 2-year mortality rate among the 100% adherence group was 41.9%.[42] In total, adherence was achieved for 41% of 485 patients. The researchers did not specify how many patients received 50% adherence and how many received 100% adherence. They did, however, define adherence as a minimum of 50%. Thus, we can estimate that 199 patients received at least 50% adherent treatment.

With a mortality rate of 45.7%, the number of deaths among this group would have been 91.[42] If this group had not received the treatment, based on the numbers reported in the study, we would estimate the number of expected deaths to have been 99 (i.e., 199 × 49.7%). This produces a difference of 8 deaths, meaning that 8 additional patients are estimated to have survived longer than 2-years as a result of lung-protective mechanical ventilation. This is a very concrete number that likely has relevance to clinicians and to both patients and their families.

Number Needed to Treat, Number Needed to Harm, and Number Needed to Screen

Three additional statistics that simplify the results of treatment, harm, and prevention studies are the **number needed to treat** (NNT), the **number needed to harm** (NNH), and the **number needed to screen** (NNS). These three statistics are similar in their definitions:

- *NNT:* "The number of persons needed to be treated, on average, to prevent one more event."[11] The formula for NNT is 1/ARR.

- *NNH:* "The number of persons needed to be treated, on average, to produce one more adverse event."[11] The formula for NNH is 1/ARI. ARI is used because the risk of adverse events is increased, rather than reduced.

- *NNS:* "The average number of persons who must undergo a screening test and the ensuing diagnostic and therapeutic procedures in order to prevent one case of the disease of interest."[11] The formula for NNS is the same as for NNT: 1/ARR.

Example: NNT and NNH

A meta-analysis was performed to determine efficacy and safety of three medications used to treat rheumatoid arthritis (infliximab, etanercept, and adalimumab).[43] These medications are classified as anti-tumor necrosis factor alpha (anti-TNFα) drugs. The researchers calculated the NNT and NNH for each medication. The primary outcome measure was the American College of Rheumatology (ACR) efficacy response criteria. An ACR score of 20 was deemed a clinically important response. The three medications proved to be similar in terms of treatment efficacy, with an NNT of 4 (with a range of 3 to 6). This means that treating four patients with any one of the studied medications would produce one additional clinically important improvement in symptoms. The range reported with the NNT is similar to a confidence interval. It tells us that the true NNT is most likely somewhere between 3 and 6.

With regard to NNH, a variety of adverse events were evaluated. Overall, the combined NNH for side effects was 27. This means that treating 27 patients with one of these medications produces one more patient who experiences side effects (such as infection, injection site reaction, and infusion reactions). This tells us that side effects from these medications are fairly common. In fact, that is just what the authors said: "Side effects were more common among patients receiving anti-TNFα drugs than controls."[43]

CHAPTER SUMMARY

Treatment, harm, and prevention studies are important areas of information in health care.

Studies of treatment are perhaps the most common type of biomedical research. Prevention studies are becoming increasingly important, and significant resources are focused in this area. Harm studies are less common, but questions of harm are frequently included in treatment research. Treatment, harm, and prevention research can be helpful in facilitating the selection of treatment modalities in collaborative decisions made with patients and their families.

Issues to investigate when engaging in EBP associated with selection of treatment include efficacy, indications/contraindications, side effects, complications, administration and dosage, adherence, cost, access, and time. In some cases, studies will address all of these issues. More often, however, it will be necessary for you to search for multiple sources of information in order to find evidence or information related to all of these considerations. Your ability to synthesize and communicate about the research and general information with patients will greatly impact the efficacy of the care you provide.

You will gain the greatest benefit from approaching these topics of treatment, prevention, and harm from the three approaches to EBP: prospective, concurrent, and retrospective. Furthermore, with experience and time you will become increasingly informed on the body of knowledge related to treatment, harm, and prevention in your field of practice. As such, the amount of time needed to locate and evaluate information will be reduced. Furthermore, with time and experience EBP will become habit and feel like an incorporated part of the care process.

Treatment studies explore many types of questions related to an array of issues, such as efficacy of treatment, interactions between treatments, factors that influence treatment adherence or treatment discontinuation, cost of treatment, patient preferences, and access to treatment.

Harm studies examine the natural course of a disease (i.e., harm from lack of treatment), harm caused by complications from individual diagnostic or treatment interventions, or harms caused by interactions between diagnostic and/or treatment modalities. Generally, studies of harm are observational in nature, mainly in the form of case-control and cohort studies.

Prevention studies examine outcomes from interventions that focus on eradicating, eliminating, or minimizing the impact of disease and disability. If this is not feasible, the studies should seek to retard the progress of the disease and resulting disability.

The use of certain search terms for each type of study can help improve your success in locating information in each specific area. We provided lists of search terms specific to prevention and harm studies in this chapter. The search terms for treatment studies are more varied and the list much longer. Hence, we did not provide a list for those types of studies. However, the treatment selection topics discussed in this chapter do offer a reasonable set of treatment-related search terms.

We discussed several biostatistics that are commonly reported in treatment, harm, and prevention publications, including the relative risk (RR), the relative risk reduction (RRR), the odds ratio (OR), the hazard ratio (HR), the absolute risk (AR), the absolute risk reduction (ARR), the number needed to treat (NNT), the number needed to screen (NNS), and the number needed to harm (NNH). We looked at examples of publications that reported these statistics and explored their meaning. It is well worth your time to practice calculating the statistics that can be calculated using a contingency table. The only statistic discussed in this chapter that cannot be calculated using a contingency table is the hazard ratio.

We also recommend as a study strategy that you locate an article that uses each type of statistic discussed in this chapter and see if you can construct a contingency table based on the information provided in the article. You should also evaluate the article in terms of the level of evidence, risks of bias in the design (if it is a research article), and the comprehensiveness of the article (in terms of the topics addressed in this chapter). Additionally, it is well worth your time to browse through the topics listed by the U.S. Preventive Services Task Force and the Centers for Disease Control and Prevention. We encourage you to become familiar with sources that provide practice guidelines and treatment algorithms in your field.

EXERCISES

Matching

Match the vocabulary term to its definition.

Vocabulary Terms

1. Indications

2. Adverse Event of Special Interest

3. Method of Administration

4. Relative Risk

5. Iatrogenesis

6. Primary Outcome Measures

7. Secondary Prevention

8. Primary Prevention

9. Tertiary Prevention

10. Dose

11. NNT

12. Efficacy

13. NNS

14. Relative Risk Reduction

15. Interaction

16. Quaternary Prevention

17. Hazard Ratio

Definitions

a. the average number of persons who must undergo a screening test and the ensuing diagnostic and therapeutic procedures in order to prevent one case of the disease of interest

b. the technique for performing a treatment (e.g., holding an instrument at a specific angle)

c. the circumstances in which a given treatment *should* be used

d. adverse effects of preventive, diagnostic, therapeutic, surgical, and other medical, sanitary, and health procedures, interventions or programs

e. the circumstances in which a given treatment *should not* be used

f. undesirable experiences associated with the use of a medical product in a patient that results in death, hospitalization, disability or permanent change, congenital anomaly/birth defect, or requires intervention to prevent permanent impairment or damage

g. frequency of administration and quantity of treatment

h. actions that identify patients at risk of over-diagnosis or over-medication and that protect them from excessive medical intervention (e.g., actions that prevent iatrogenesis)

i. the number of persons needed to be treated, on average, to produce one more adverse event

j. an action or set of actions that aims to reduce the incidence of disease by personal and communal efforts

k. the ability of an intervention to produce the desired beneficial effect

l. the difference in event rates between two groups expressed as a proportion of the event rate in the untreated group

m. how a treatment reaches its target location

n. additional end points that are evaluated but are not the specific focus of the intervention

o. an action or set of actions that aim to reduce the prevalence of disease by shortening its duration

p. the proportion of how often a particular adverse event occurs in one group compared to another group over time; the element of time is the primary distinguishing characteristic of this measure

q. the degree to which patients are able to sustain a treatment regimen according to how it was prescribed

18. Absolute Risk

19. Contraindications

20. NNH

21. Minimal Clinically Important Differences

22. Mode of Administration

23. Treatment Algorithm

24. Odds Ratio

25. Secondary Outcome Measures

26. Adherence

r. mutual or reciprocal action or influence

s. the number of persons needed to be treated, on average, to prevent one more event

t. a decision chart that provides an outline of the treatment process

u. the smallest difference in score in an outcome of interest to patients that is perceived as beneficial and would mandate a change in treatment

v. end points that are intended to be directly impacted by the intervention and measured in a clinical trial

w. another way of stating the event rate or incidence rate of a group

x. the ratio of the risk of an event among the exposed (or treatment group) to the risk among the unexposed (or control group)

y. an action or set of actions aimed at softening the impact of long-term disease and disability by eliminating or reducing impairment, disability, and handicap; reducing suffering; and maximizing potential years of useful life

z. the ratio of the odds of an event occurring in one group to the odds of an event occurring in another group

Application Questions

Review the following hypothetical example and answer the following questions. You might find it helpful to review the construction of a contingency table before proceeding with the problem set.

Researchers were interested in determining adverse events of special interest (AESI) associated with the use or nonuse of prescribed stimulant medication among children and adolescents. Stimulants often are prescribed for the treatment of attention-deficit/hyperactivity disorder (ADHD). In this hypothetical example, researchers accessed de-identified Medicaid records. Patients were divided into two groups: those who were currently using a stimulant medication and those who were not using a stimulant medication. (Note that for the sake of simplicity we are not accounting for the fact that there would be patients who were formerly prescribed stimulant medications. In a real study performed on this topic, past stimulant use would be an important consideration.)

The researchers looked retrospectively (going back 10 years) in the records of patients aged 4 to 18 years for incidents of stroke, acute myocardial infarction, or sudden cardiac death. The total patient years evaluated was 2,321,311. There were 132 AESI, 51 of which were among the current stimulant–use cohort. There were a total of 1,165,951 patient years among the current stimulant–use cohort, and 1,155,360 patient years among the nonuse cohort.

1. What type of study is represented by the above description?
   a. RCT
   b. Cohort study
   c. Case-control study
   d. Systematic review
   e. Case study

2. This study is an example of which of the following kinds of research?
   a. Diagnosis research
   b. Prevention research

c. Treatment research

d. Harm research

e. Epidemiological research

3. Based on the type of research, which of the following biostatistics would make the most sense to quantify the difference between current stimulant use and nonuse in terms of risk of AESI?

a. NNT

b. PPV

c. Sensitivity

d. NNS

e. OR

4. What were the AESI in the study?

5. What is the probability of an AESI among the exposed group? Among the nonexposed group?

6. Complete the following contingency table based on the information provided in the description (we have filled in the total patient years for you).

	AESI	No AESI	Patient Years
Current stimulant use	a	b	
Nonuse	c	d	
			2,321,311

7. Calculate the OR based on the data in the table.

8. Explain what the OR means.

9. Which biostatistic could be reported if the researchers graphed the AESI over time for each treatment and used the slope of the resulting survival curves to compare the two treatments?

a. HR

b. NNH

c. RR

d. AR

e. NPV

10. Considering all of the issues of treatment selection, which issues do the study provide information on to assist in making a decision about whether to treat a child or adolescent with stimulant medication?

REFERENCES

1. U.S. National Library of Medicine. Medical subject heading database. Available at: www.ncbi.nlm.nih.gov.libpublic3.library.isu.edu/mesh?term = treatment. Accessed July 10, 2012.

2. Dorland's medical dictionary for health consumers. [Online database]. Search provider: Farlex Free Medical Dictionary. 2007. Available at: http://medical-dictionary.thefreedictionary.com/efficacy. Accessed July 10, 2012.

3. Centers for Disease Control and Prevention. *Vaccines and preventable diseases: Varicella vaccine effectiveness and duration of protection.* Information for health care providers. Available at: www.cdc.gov/vaccines/vpd-vac/varicella/hcp-effective-duration.htm. Accessed July 10, 2012.

4. Hajiro T, Nishimura K. Minimal clinically significant difference in health status: The thorny path of health status measures. *Eur Respir J.* 2002;19:390–391.

5. American College of Rheumatology. Western Ontario and McMaster Universities osteoarthritis index (WOMAC). June 2012. Available at: www.rheumatology.org/practice/clinical/clinicianresearchers/outcomes-instrumentation/WOMAC.asp. Accessed July 11, 2012.

6. Perlman AI, Ali A, Njike VY, Hom D, Davidi A, Gould-Fogerite S, et al. Massage therapy for osteoarthritis of the knee: A randomized dose-finding trial. *PLoS One.* 2012;7(2):e30248.

7. Perlman AI, Sabina A, Williams AL, Njike VY, Katz DL. Massage therapy for osteoarthritis of the knee: A randomized controlled trial. *Arch Intern Med.* 2006;166(22):2533–2538.

8. Angst F, Aeschlimann A, Michel BA, Stucki G. Minimal clinically important rehabilitation effects in patients with osteoarthritis of the lower extremities. *J Rheumatol.* 2002;29:131–138.

9. Escobar A, Quintana JM, Bilbao A, Arostegui I, Lafuente I, et al. Responsiveness and clinically important differences for the WOMAC and SF-36 after total knee replacement. *Osteoarthritis Cartilage.* 2007;15:273–280.

10. Medscape Reference. *Drugs, diseases, and procedures: Varicella virus vaccine live.* ND. Available at: http://reference.medscape.com/drug/varilrix-varivax-varicella-virus-vaccine-live-343177. Accessed July 12, 2012.

11. Porta M. *A dictionary of epidemiology*, 5th ed. Oxford, UK: Oxford University Press; 2008.

12. U.S. Food and Drug Administration. *Safety: What is a serious adverse event?* Updated June 23, 2011. Available at: www.fda.gov/safety/medwatch /howtoreport/ucm053087.htm. Accessed July 12, 2012.

13. ClinicalTrials.gov. *A multicentre, single-arm, open-label safety study of lenalidomide plus dexamethasone in previously treated subjects with multiple myeloma*. Updated May 15, 2012. Available at: www.clinicaltrials.gov. Accessed July 12, 2012.

14. U.S. National Library of Medicine. PubMed Health. A.D.A.M. medical encyclopedia: *Multiple myeloma*. Reviewed March 4, 2012. Available at: www.ncbi.nlm .nih.gov/pubmedhealth/PMH0001609/. Accessed July 12, 2012.

15. U.S. Food and Drug Administration. *Frequently asked questions about therapeutic biological products*. Updated December 24, 2009. Available at: www.fda.gov/Drugs/DevelopmentApprovalProcess /HowDrugsareDevelopedandApproved/Approval Applications/TherapeuticBiologicApplications /ucm113522.htm. Accessed July 12, 2012.

16. Centers for Disease Control and Prevention. *Vaccinations and immunizations: Varicella vaccine safety and monitoring*. Reviewed April 5, 2012. Available at: www.cdc.gov/vaccines/vpd-vac /varicella/hcp-vacc-safety-monitor.htm. Accessed July 12, 2012.

17. MedlinePlus. Merriam-Webster. Medical dictionary. 2012. Available at: www.merriam-webster.com /medlineplus/interaction. Accessed July 12, 2012.

18. MD Consult. *Ascorbic acid, vitamin C: Interactions*. ND. Available at: www.mdconsult.com. Accessed July 12, 2012

19. The Joint Commission. *Medication reconciliation*. Sentinel event alert, Issue 35. 2006. Available at: www.jointcommission.org/SentinelEvents /SentinelEventAlert/sea_35.htm. Accessed July 12, 2012.

20. Cassel CK (ed.). *Geriatric medicine: An evidence-based approach*. 4th ed. New York: Spring-Verlag; 2006.

21. *Collins English dictionary: Complete and unabridged*. 10th ed. 2009. Available at: http://dictionary.reference .com/browse/adherence. Accessed July 22, 2012.

22. *Collins English dictionary: Complete and unabridged*. 10th ed. 2009. Available at: http://dictionary .reference.com/browse/compliance. Accessed July 22, 2012.

23. *American heritage medical dictionary*. Boston: Houghton Mifflin; 2007.

24. Seltzer DL. *Language tips: Compliance, adherence, or concordance & more on furthermore and moreover*. November 11, 2009. Available at: http:// languagetips.wordpress.com/2009/11/11/language -tips-compliance-adherence-or-concordance-more -on-furthermore-and-moreover/. Accessed July 22, 2012.

25. Brown A. About.com: *What does a massage cost?* ND. Available at http://spas.about.com/od/massa2 /a/massagecost.htm. Accessed July 23, 2012.

26. College of Technology. Massage therapy program. ND. Available at: www.isu.edu/ctech/massagetherapy /schedule.shtml. Accessed July 23, 2012.

27. Barron MC, Rubin BR. Managing osteoarthritic knee pain. *J Am Osteopath Assoc*. 2007;107(suppl 6): ES21–ES27.

28. American Academy of Orthopaedic Surgeons. *Treatment of osteoarthritis of the knee (nonarthroplasty)*. December 6, 2008. [Online database: National Guideline Clearinghouse]. Available at: http://guideline.gov. Accessed July 23, 2012.

29. Singh JA, Cameron DR. Summary of AHRQ's comparative effectiveness review of drug therapy for rheumatoid arthritis (RA) in adults—an update. *J Manag Care Pharm*. 2012;18(4 Suppl C):S1–18.

30. Oderda GM, Balfe LM. Comparative effectiveness research (CER): A summary of AHRQ's CER on therapies for rheumatoid arthritis. *J Manag Care Pharm*. 2011;17(9 Suppl B):S19–24.

31. American Board of Preventive Medicine. *What is preventive medicine?* [Webpage]. 2011. Available at: http://www.abprevmed.org/aboutus.cfm. Accessed July 23, 2012.

32. BBC. *History: Louis Pasteur (1822–1895)*. ND. Available at www.bbc.co.uk/history/historic_figures /pasteur_louis.shtml. Accessed July 23, 2012.

33. Snow J. *On the mode of communication of cholera*. London: John Churchill; 1860.

34. Agency for Healthcare Research and Quality. U.S. Preventive Services Task Force. ND. Available at: www.ahrq.gov/clinic/uspstfix.htm. Accessed July 23, 2012.

35. U.S. Preventive Services Task Force. *First annual report to congress on high-priority evidence gaps for clinical preventive services*. November 2011. Available at: www.uspreventiveservicestaskforce. org/annlrpt/index.html. Accessed July 23, 2012.

36. Wijesinghe M, Perrin K, Healy B, Weatherall M, Beasley R. Randomized controlled trial of high concentration oxygen in suspected community-acquired pneumonia. *J R Soc Med*. 2012;105(5):208–216.

37. *Dorland's medical dictionary for health consumers*. [Online database]. Search provider: Farlex Free Medical Dictionary. 2007. Available at http:// medical-dictionary.thefreedictionary.com/PaCO2. Accessed July 23, 2012.

38. Pietrosimone BG, Grindstaff TL, Linens SW, Uczekaj E, Hertel J. A systematic review of prophylactic braces in the prevention of knee ligament injuries in collegiate football players. *J Athl Train.* 2008;43(4):409–415.

39. Hellenbrand W, Jorgensen P, Schweiger B, Falkenhorst G, Nachtnebel M, Greutélaers B, et al. Prospective hospital-based case-control study to assess the effectiveness of pandemic influenza A(H1N1)pdm09 vaccination and risk factors for hospitalization in 2009–2010 using matched hospital and test-negative controls. *BMC Inf Dis.* 2012:12;127.

40. LoBiondo-Wood G, Haber J. *Nursing research.* 6th ed. St. Louis, MO: Mosby; 2006.

41. Kempe KL, Shetterly SM, France EK, Levin TR. Automated phone and mail population outreach to promote colorectal cancer screening. *Am J Manag Care.* 2012;18(7):370–378.

42. Needham DM, Colantuoni E, Mendez-Tellez PA, Dinglas VD, Sevransky JE, Dennison Himmelfarb CR, et al. Lung protective mechanical ventilation and two-year survival in patients with acute lung injury: prospective cohort study. *BMJ.* 2012;344:e2124. doi: 10.1136/bmj.e2124.

43. Alonso-Ruiz A, Pijoan JI, Ansuategui E, Urkaregi A, Calabozo M, Quintana A. Tumor necrosis factor alpha drugs in rheumatoid arthritis: systematic review and metaanalysis of efficacy and safety. *BMC Musculoskelet Disord.* 2008;9:52.

ANSWERS TO EXERCISES

Matching

1. C
2. F
3. B
4. X
5. D
6. V
7. O
8. J
9. Y
10. G
11. S
12. K
13. A
14. L
15. R
16. H
17. P
18. W
19. E
20. I
21. U
22. M
23. T
24. Z
25. N
26. Q

Applications Questions

1. Answer: c. Explanation: The study is retrospective, and the two groups are divided into cohorts based on a specific exposure.

2. Answer: d. Explanation: The study focuses on harm caused by complications from a treatment intervention.

3. Answer: e. Explanation: Of the listed biostatistics, odds ratio is the best choice. An odds ratio is utilized with retrospective research designs for comparing groups with regard to an outcome of interest.

4. The three AESIs in this study were stroke, acute MI, and sudden cardiac death.

5. The probability of AESIs among the exposed group was 0.0044%; that is, 51 incidents divided by 1,165,951 patient years: $\frac{51}{1,165,951}$. The probability among the nonexposed group was 0.0070%; that is 81 incidents divided by 1,115,360 patient years: $\frac{81}{1,115,360}$.

6. Contingency Table:

	AESI	No AESI	Totals
Current Stimulant Use	51	1,165,900	1,165,951
Nonuse	81	1,155,279	1,155,350
Totals	132	2,321,179	2,321,311

7. Odds ratio (OR) = 0.62
8. The OR means that the odds of a child or adolescent experiencing a stroke, acute MI, or sudden cardiac death while on stimulant medication treatment are less than the odds of having one of these events while not on a stimulant medication. (Note that this does not mean the stimulant medication has a protective effect!)
9. Answer: a. Explanation: A hazard ratio compares the slope of the survival curve for multiple treatments.
10. The above study would provide information primarily about complications. It would not be informative about side effects, efficacy, indications/contraindications, interactions, administration and dosage, adherence, cost, access, or time. It would be necessary to access other sources to facilitate a well-informed treatment selection decision.

CHAPTER 10

Evidence-Based Practice and Pharmaceutical Information

Teresa Shelton, MPAS, PA-C and
Bernadette Howlett, PhD

INTRODUCTION

One of the most frequent encounters healthcare providers have with medical evidence is through the pharmaceutical or medical device sales pitch. This pitch can come in the form of direct marketing to patients or visits from sales representatives. The majority of patients are on some type of medication, which can have implications for nearly all types of health encounters (e.g., interactions with other treatments or side effects that inhibit the patient's ability to adhere with other treatments). This chapter focuses on interacting with the pharmaceutical industry and its representatives, although the information we provide in this chapter can apply to other healthcare related sales, such as medical devices. The information in this chapter is relevant to clinicians, therapists, pharmacists, and allied healthcare professionals. It does not matter whether or not you prescribe medications; any healthcare professional who provides treatments or counsels patients regarding medications should have knowledge about pharmaceuticals. Everyone from the prescribing clinician, the nurse who counsels on how to use the medication, the

pharmacist and the tech who dispense and discuss the treatment risks and benefits, the physical therapist, and even a phlebotomist require knowledge about pharmaceuticals.

For example, consider a patient using medication that inhibits blood clotting. The patient should be made aware of any additional treatment that could increase bruising or cause uncontrolled bleeding. This could be something as seemingly benign as continuous use of ibuprofen or baby aspirin. If a patient is receiving both a blood thinner and ibuprofen, then certain physical therapy treatments might need to be adjusted or avoided.

Let's consider the pharmaceutical issues related to a hypothetical shoulder-repair patient prescribed physical therapy after a surgical procedure. The patient experienced postoperative complications from a pulmonary embolus, which led to the prescription of a potent daily blood thinner. With physical therapy, patients are often advised to take an anti-inflammatory medication, such as ibuprofen or naproxen, to relieve pain. However, these over-the-counter medications can increase risk of bleeding. Additionally, vascular injury risk is higher with exercise and physical therapy. It is important for the therapist to be able to advise the patient on limiting the use of nonsteroidal anti-inflammatory drugs (NSAIDs), such as ibuprofen and naproxen. (Some NSAIDs are prescribed and others are available without a prescription.) Physical therapy might need to be delayed for a patient in this situation, which could also delay the patient's return to function or lead to other complications. If you were the therapist, you should expect questions regarding patient expectations and evaluate the interactions, risks, and benefits of all treatment options. Your ability to assess the research related to medications is paramount when making clinical decisions, whether you are the prescribing provider or the provider who administers medications.

A key objective of this chapter is to give you information about how the pharmaceutical industry approaches sales and how to use evidence-based practice (EBP) to inform decisions made in the treatment plan about the proper use of pharmaceuticals. Even if you are not a prescribing clinician or pharmacist, you are likely to encounter the impact of marketing aimed to influence your patients, and you should be aware of its particular influence on the patients themselves.

This chapter includes information on pharmaceutical sales representatives (**PSRs**), including their qualifications, training, and sales techniques, such as providing gifts and samples. The chapter also discusses the productive utilization of your PSR. Information on pharmaceutical costs and other considerations for clinicians are also provided, as well as efficient tools for researching new treatments and obtaining continuing education credits, which some fields of practice require for licensure. A review of direct-to-consumer advertising pros and cons is offered, along with drug package insert data. An end-of-chapter exercise is provided for you to "tease out" the content of a sample sales brochure that relates to the dialogue you are about to read. You are presented with this information from both the perspective of a former PSR and a certified physician assistant currently practicing medicine as a family practitioner.

Controversy exists with regard to the motives of pharmaceutical companies. The following set of quotes represents an array of views from varying sources regarding the pharmaceutical industry and its impact on patients and their caregivers:

- "The pharmaceutical industry, at its root, has honorable and noble motives, which are to: extend life, improve the quality of life, and provide cost-effective treatments."[1]
- "Physicians prescribe pharmaceuticals throughout their professional lives, but because new drugs are being approved and marketed so quickly, it is likely that most current medical students will ultimately prescribe a great many medicines about which they had received no training in medical school or residency . . . in the year 2000 alone, the FDA approved 89 new drug products."[2]
- "Industry, physicians, and patients have benefited from physicians' interactions with drug and device representatives for decades . . . and at least some harm has been done."[3]
- "Perhaps Congress or state legislatures should consider increasing regulation to make drugs more accessible to patients, rather than be concerned about the profit margins of (the pharmaceutical industry). Pharmaceutical sales teams are a force to be reckoned with, comparable to an army prepared to enter a battle, equipped with powerful tools to take down anyone who stands in their way."[4]

These quotes represent a dichotomy between those who support the pharmaceutical industry and those who do not. Some view the pharmaceutical industry as being driven purely by profit motives, whereas others view it as being driven to improve health outcomes and quality of life. If not for pharmaceutical companies, who will take the considerable financial and ethical risks of research and development? Conversely, who protects patients and advocates for cost-effective and sustainable use of treatments? These are likely universal ethical considerations and not a true dichotomy. You cannot stand on one side and take into account all of the issues you need to consider as a healthcare professional. As such, this chapter does not advocate for either position, but rather attempts to present a balance between both views.

Let's start the discussion on pharmaceutical sales with a sales call involving hypothetical statin drugs. The following sales script represents a typical conversation between a PSR and a prescribing clinician named Teresa:

PSR: "Teresa, the last time we visited we spoke about the relative efficacies of Bogustatin and SuperStatin for your patients with high cholesterol levels. You mentioned Bogustatin is the cholesterol medication you use first line for your patients. May I ask why?"

Teresa: "It is the gold standard medication with the most scientific evidence for safety and efficacy. I mainly use the drug because I don't get as many patients calling me about side effects when I send them home with it."

PSR: "So if I am hearing you correctly, Teresa, a key reason you choose one statin over another for your patients that need to reduce their cholesterol levels is their side effect profile?"

Teresa: "For choosing statin medications, it is a definite consideration, but not the only one. I keep efficacy in mind along with safety."

PSR: "I have some recent postmarketing surveillance conducted with over 6,000 family practice and internal medicine patients with over 10,000 patients referenced in the U.S. The data show patient discontinuation rates and the reasons why those patients stopped taking their statin medication. Would you be interested in seeing what was determined about Bogustatin?"

Teresa: "If you can give me a quick summary. I have patients waiting."

PSR: "Of course. Thank you for your time today. This graph (see **Figure 10–1**) illustrates that the main reason patients discontinued Bogustatin was due to intolerance of side effects, predominantly headache and back pain. The research states that the number of patients who discontinued the drug due to pain in extremities was less than half of those who stopped taking Bogustatin. In fact, the highest reported adverse event that occurred in only 6% of patients taking SuperStatin was a headache, which patients reported as mild and transient. How commonly do these events result in noncompliance with Bogustatin in your patients?"

Teresa: "More than I'd like, but not that often."

PSR: "You may find this interesting, then, Teresa. The other concerning fact determined by this surveillance is that up to 40% of these patients who discontinued the medication chose not to consult with their provider prior to stopping the drug, and they told their provider up to several months later, at their next scheduled appointment. This was a factor in a lack of improvement in their lipid levels. If this is happening among patients nationally, is it possible your patients might not be telling you that they aren't as satisfied as you may think?"

Teresa: "I guess you have a point, but what information do you have that says SuperStatin is better?"

PSR: "I'm glad you asked. In these charts (**Figure 10–2**), you can see that efficacy rates among patients using Bogustatin and SuperStatin are statistically similar. Based on what you've seen today, do you have enough information to consider trying SuperStatin in patients that need to lower their cholesterol levels?"

Teresa: "I'll look over these studies and consider it."

PSR: "Thank you for giving your patients an opportunity for equal efficacy and fewer major side effects with SuperStatin and for allowing me to show you how SuperStatin reigns superior over other medications in its class. I look forward to meeting you next time and hearing what you and your patients think."

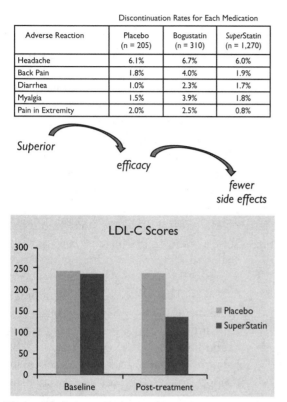

Discontinuation Rates for Each Medication

Adverse Reaction	Placebo (n = 205)	Bogustatin (n = 310)	SuperStatin (n = 1,270)
Headache	6.1%	6.7%	6.0%
Back Pain	1.8%	4.0%	1.9%
Diarrhea	1.0%	2.3%	1.7%
Myalgia	1.5%	3.9%	1.8%
Pain in Extremity	2.0%	2.5%	0.8%

Superior

efficacy

fewer side effects

Figure 10–1 SuperStatin Brochure Page

The sales call is a conversation in which the PSR aims to seek objections or concerns expressed by the healthcare provider related to the use of the product. The goal of the visit is to provide FDA- and corporate-approved messages that identify solutions for the provider's patients. The above interaction is typical of a 5-minute conversation a clinician might have with a PSR. Drug representatives aim to make a compelling argument by using statistics to compare medications to one another and a placebo via the reiteration of clinical trial facts. The PSR's intention is not to convince you to do something that is not based on evidence, but rather to get your commitment to try the product with your patients.[2] PSRs expect you to conduct your own trial of their medication. (In clinical practice, when a medication is prescribed for the first time with a patient, it is often referred to as "trialing" the drug. This usage does not imply performing a clinical trial, but rather trying the drug out with a patient for the first time. You could think of this as an *N of 1 trial*.)

Now that the PSR has reviewed the scientific data that demonstrate that your patients will

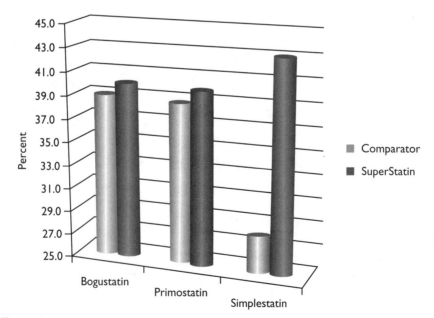

Figure 10–2 Efficacy Comparison Between SuperStatin and Other Statins

tolerate the medication, the PSR assumes that you can count on it to perform well for your patients. What *you* need to decide is whether the information that you deemed worth your time to obtain from your PSR meets the criteria you are required to consider before prescribing a medication and, if so, whether or not the drug merits an initial trial with a few patients.

In March 2006, Roberto Cardarelli et al. from the Department of Family Medicine/Center for Evidence-Based Medicine published a meta-analysis entitled, "A Cross-Sectional Evidence-Based Review of Pharmaceutical Promotional Marketing Brochures and Their Underlying Studies: Is What They Tell Us Important and True?" [5] Based on their review of 20 studies, they found the following: "75% of the studies were found to be valid, 80% were funded by the pharmaceutical company, 60% of the studies and the corresponding brochures presented patient-oriented outcomes, and 40% were compared to another treatment regimen." What does this tell us? Three-quarters of the studies were well done, the majority of them were funded by pharmaceutical companies, over half of the studies and brochures spoke only about patient-centered results (outcomes that matter), and less than half of the studies aimed to make a direct comparison to other branded drugs, presumably in their class.

You can, therefore, expect that the studies brought to you by the PSR will show his or her new medication in a positive light while comparing it to placebo and/or an older, generically available drug that is not used as frequently due to higher side effects than a newer-generation medication. It is important for you to know that there will be a deficit in head-to-head medication comparisons presented to you by a PSR. Head-to-head trials are somewhat rare in drugs new to the U.S. pharmaceutical marketplace. (Note that the FDA requirements for Phase III human trials and approval to market do not require head-to-head direct medication comparisons. The medication is compared only to placebo.) This chapter will compare gold standards in statin medications from hypothetical head-to-head trials against one another and discuss what comparisons are presented to you by a PSR when direct comparisons between two drugs do not exist.

It is vital to determine the impact a new medication can have on you and your practice as well as your patients. Consider the likelihood that your patients will be more satisfied if they try a medication that is new to both of you. What is the risk to you and your service as a trusted provider (or to the health of your patients) if you prescribe this medication? Do you anticipate fewer phone calls from patients regarding side effects when adding a new medication to the list you have established as your practice standard? Nursing staff and medical assistants who answer these calls will be the first to inform prescribers of whether patients are satisfied or have a problem with the medication, and an initial trial of the medication can make or break your confidence in this medication for the future. Bear in mind that the job of your PSR is to identify why you use a competitor's medication as a practice standard and show you how prescribing his or her company's medication could better benefit your practice as well as your patients' health. From there, the PSR and the company will let the product speak for itself through your patients' comments and compliance.

THE PHARMACEUTICAL SALES REPRESENTATIVE

This section describes the process of getting a job as a pharmaceutical representative. This information is provided to help you understand the basic credentials and training of the people who promote medications. The training is often quite rigorous and ongoing. PSRs have extensive training not only in pharmaceutical science, but also in effective communication.

Basic Professional Requirements

PSRs who work in the primary care setting must be trained in selling a product to a variety of provider types. The following are the typical minimum requirements for obtaining a position as a PSR:

- The candidate must have a bachelor's degree and a minimum cumulative GPA of 3.0 or higher from a 4-year university.
- In most cases, the candidate will have 2 years of business-to-business sales experience and documentation of proven success in increasing market share of a product for a company.
- The candidate will undergo a rigorous interview process, including several meetings, with numerous hours of discussion regarding his or her personal behaviors and decision-making skills. The candidate also must be able to prove his or her sales success.
- A detailed background check, including verification of a college degree(s), and several references are also required.
- The successful candidate will be the one person out of about 60 qualified applicants who stood out as the best person for the job.

In order to work in a specialty sales force, prior experience is an important prerequisite. Right now, many people who have experience are looking for a new position due to budget cuts, generic production of branded medications, or poor sales of a medication they were previously representing. One major factor in the redistribution of a sales force (i.e., layoffs) is the merging of companies or corporate buyouts, which will happen frequently in a PSR's career. In only 4 years in the industry, I applied to only two companies but ultimately worked for four by the time I retired due to mergers, acquisitions, and restructuring of sales forces. (Note: the first-person perspective shared in this chapter comes from the lead author of this chapter.)

In our current economic climate, you might be asking why anyone would continue to work in an industry that undergoes frequent restructuring. PSRs are expected to evolve along with these changes. One of the main reasons for becoming a PSR is that the benefits are good and that there are many opportunities for upward movement with new and exciting challenges. My personal opinion, and why I stayed in the industry through so many changes, was that the lifestyle of a PSR is good compared to other business management and sales positions that I had been in. Target bonuses are awarded each quarter on top of a competitive base salary, and someone who likes autonomy in their job, travel opportunities, and exposure to the medical environment would be attracted to this type of sales position. Getting into the industry is highly competitive, and to stand out takes commitment and a long history of good sales performance. You can see why PSRs take their jobs seriously (and also why they dress so nicely).

Pharmaceutical Representative Training

The following elaboration is relevant to you as a healthcare provider because you should be aware of the knowledge base as well as the corresponding limitations of pharmaceutical sales training. A PSR's job is not to provide care; it is to influence your prescribing habits.[6] The first year of training of a new PSR involves three phases. In my personal experience, the first phase consisted of 4 weeks of sequestration in a hotel room near my home sales territory where I reviewed several manuals and CDs to learn about the basics of life science and biology. Each day my individual trainer (an experienced PSR working in the field for my new company) would meet with me in the morning and afternoon to answer questions regarding key points in the material. He would administer tests on anatomy, physiology, and pharmacology (including pharmacodynamics and pharmacokinetics) as well as on the drug marketplace. I was expected to know the data on the void to be filled by the new medication I would be selling. An overview of managed care organizations and detailed data on how certain healthcare systems pay their healthcare providers were also provided. I was tested on my comprehension of this information. After passing these exams with a minimum of a 90% grade, I was then qualified to enter phase 2 and attend the national sales skills development seminar for 2 weeks at the home office. This training focused on the use of scientific data and how to sell the product using EBP.

A large part of honing our sales skills was to incorporate key phrases that were approved by the corporate office into each sales interaction. These messages also had to be formally approved by the FDA before they could be printed on our sales brochures or presented to clinicians. The following is a hypothetical example of a non-FDA-approved statement:

> *The rate of pain in the extremities on Bogustatin is significantly higher than with SuperStatin, as reported by patients during phase III clinical trials.*

A more accurate, and FDA-approved, way to state comparative data would be:

> *In relative clinical trials for FDA approval, Bogustatin's rate of pain in extremities was 2.5%, and in the clinical trials of SuperStatin only 0.8% of patients reported this adverse event.*

Although such a message would be approved by the FDA, oftentimes it is not clear how many total patients were in each trial and what methods the two studies had in common. It is not possible to validate either message as a true comparison.

Ongoing training occurred quarterly, with periodic sales messages or new market data released for online and at-home study. For the launch of each new medication brought to market, a regional sales meeting would be held, which would include role-play practice in front of peers in a district or region. On the last day of the training conference, I met personally with a working healthcare practitioner and targeted prescriber with whom I was to carry out the new sales message in a "conversational sales" interaction. The conversational sales strategy includes identifying the personality of the sales target (the clinician). One such technique is called the personality palette.

The Personality Palette

Pharmaceutical representatives are trained to identify their own strengths and weaknesses, including self-behavior patterns, and those of others that influence decision making. Having this skill allows the PSR to select the individualized sales strategy that will be more likely to influence a successful outcome—a prescription written for their

medication. One example of this individualization skill is Dr. Taylor Hartman's "color code,"[7] which groups personalities into four colors:

- *Reds:* Authoritative, "the power wielders"
- *Blues:* Compassionate, "the do-gooders"
- *Whites:* "The peacekeepers"
- *Yellows:* Amiable, "the fun lovers"

Variability in local communities taken into account, you will generally find that Reds comprise 25% of the population, Blues 35%, Yellows 20%, and Whites 20%. I was taught a variation on Hartman's system. The four divisions I learned in my sales career were Reds, Yellows, Blues, and Greens (**Figure 10-3**):

- *Reds:* Authoritative
- *Blues:* Amiable
- *Yellows:* Compassionate
- *Greens:* Process-oriented and scientific

Many of us have a color or identifying trait that dominates our personality. Once the PSR identifies your dominant personality, he or she can tailor messages to your decision-making style to ensure that your time is not wasted and that productive conversations happen during each meeting with you.[4] According to Teven et al., "A successful PSR effectively manages the impressions he or she makes with healthcare professionals. Given the goal-directed nature of influencing physicians . . . individual difference variables have the potential to impact the success or failure of sales transactions."[6]

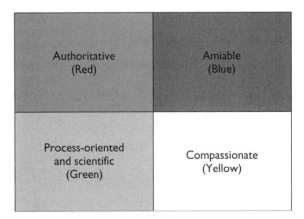

Figure 10-3 Personality Palette

Sales call scripts are written to include statements targeting the four main personalities and their corresponding colors. The calls can change between sales industry sources, but the overall theme is the same among most references:

- **Red/authoritative:** The provider makes quick decisions based on business-related data from peers.

  Sales approach: The PSR offers one 30-second tidbit on how patients will be more satisfied with the drug, which means less work for the doctor once the samples are given out. Doctors' reports of higher patient satisfaction with their choice of treatment and health care are provided.

  Sales technique: The PSR shows clinical results with solid p-values. Anecdotal references generally work well if the expert referred to is a respected leader of that clinician's peer group.

- **Yellow/compassionate:** The provider makes decisions slowly based on patient outcomes and feelings.

  Sales approach: The PSR will use a graph to illustrate how the side-effect profile for this new drug is more favorable than the competitor's medication or to the current generically available gold standard. He or she describes how this treatment option will benefit patients over the other medication available.

  Sales technique: The PSR presents a glossy chart showing the gold standard's percentage of common side effects and the new medication's lower percentage of those same side effects, all due to less frequent dosing and ease of use.

- **Blue/amiable:** The provider makes quick decisions based on the relationship between the new product and ease of use.

  Sales approach: The PSR uses patient statements and positive images to "paint the picture" of the diseased patient before and after the use of the new medication.

  Sales technique: The PSR will discuss the before and after results to show better quality of life for patients using the product and offer

viable statistics. The PSR will likely use patient photos and glossy charts to tie in patient satisfaction and positive outcomes for improved quality of life.

- **Green/process-oriented and scientific:** The provider makes decisions based on hard facts and requires a significant amount of statistics to slowly come to a decision. The provider will usually agree to look over the journal data.

  Sales approach: The PSR will discuss the science. Greens want details on how the drug binds to its corresponding receptor better than the competition's drug. The PSR will show how the p-values and confidence intervals were evaluated among the same types of patients in the placebo and treatment groups. The longer the drug has been on the market, the more information is available to the provider. Many of these types of providers say they will not trial a product with their patients until it has been on the market for at least 2 years with extensive postmarketing data available on safety and efficacy.

  Sales technique: The PSR will bring out the official article reprint and show the p-values and concluding statements favoring the new product over another or placebo.

Performance Evaluation of a PSR

The PSR is charged with creating a business plan and a routing plan for which providers in their territory they should be interacting with the most and which sales messages and approaches are most successful in influencing clinicians to initiate a trial of the product with their patients. The company has a means of tracking prescriptions, and through the distribution of samples the PSR can determine which providers are offering the medication to patients. PSR performance is evaluated in terms of sales in his or her territory.

Connors, citing the *Albany Law Review*, explains the use of data mining to improve success of pharmaceutical sales strategies: "In addition to sales reps' personal knowledge of doctors' prescribing patterns, clinicians' prescribing habits are tracked by data mining companies who sell data, allowing companies to determine which sales tactics are most effective."[4]

THE COST OF PHARMACEUTICALS: CAN WE BE BRIBED?

Pharmaceutical salespeople have recommended drugs to clinicians for over 100 years. In an article published in the *Annals of Thoracic Surgery* in 2007, Dr. K. Iverson stated: "In 2002, the big Pharmaceutical Research and Manufacturers of America (PhRMA) companies spent about $22 billion marketing to physicians and only about $26 billion on research . . . they also spent about $3.3 billion marketing directly to consumers."[3]

This creates the potential for an ethical dilemma, because such marketing might influence physician-prescribing behavior without necessarily benefiting the patient.[4] Fugh-Berman et al. reported that, "Many studies have shown that pharmaceutical marketing affects prescribing choices."[8] Wilkes et al. concurred, stating, "The manner in which doctors obtain information about new and changing pharmaceuticals obviously has the potential to have a profound impact on healthcare costs, pharmaceutical companies' profits, and the quality of health care. Patterns learned in medical school undoubtedly influence physicians' future behaviors."[2] Additionally, "promotions targeting physicians account for the majority of drug industry spending on marketing and promotion."[4] A statistic from 2007 states that there exists one PSR for every five physicians.[2]

Recent economic reports show that in 2010 U.S. pharmaceutical companies spent $68 billion for research and development of pharmaceutical products. However, this was a 3% decrease from the previous year, which some believe reflects "a growing disillusionment with poor returns on pharmaceutical R&D [research and development]."[9]

To offer some perspective, in 2010 the National Institutes of Health (NIH) invested more than $30.9 billion in medical research.[10]

In the United States, a formidable amount of money is spent on pharmaceuticals. Nine percent of the annual total cost of health care in the United States is attributed to the use of pharmaceuticals.[2] Pharmaceutical companies are extremely profitable. A look at the *Fortune* 500 list of the most profitable companies in 2010 shows that after WalMart and Exxon Mobil, numbers one and two, respectively, Pharmaceutical Research and Manufacturers of America (PhRMA) companies were ranked 4th ($13.4 billion), 7th ($12.9 billion), and 10th ($12.2 billion) in highest profits for the year.[11]

Pharmaceutical companies need to recoup their investments. Some of the more secure investments can be multicenter drug trials. In a meta-analysis entitled, "Quantitative Analysis of Sponsorship Bias in Economic Studies of Antidepressants," Baker et al. determined that sponsored drug trials resulted in clearly more favorable patient and study outcomes for that particular company's drug versus the comparator medication.[12]

Gifts

In an essay, Connors states that there are generally three kinds of gifts that physicians receive from PhRMA companies: "reminder items, moderately priced items, and expensive items."[4] Reminder items include ink pens, sticky notes, patient surveys on a particular illness, and patient education materials. In the past, coffee mugs and the aforementioned gifts were permitted in most clinics. Due to revisions in PhRMA guidelines, pharmaceutical companies no longer offer noneducational materials to physicians.[4] In addition, a number of academic and medical institutions have adopted policies that prohibit the receipt of these types of tchotchkes (small, free gifts).

Rules vary per clinic with regard to the receipt of lunches and educational presentations for new products or for new FDA-approved indications for older products. These are considered a moderately priced item, costing approximately $20 to $100 per event.

One product that has been used as a reference tool for many years by medical students is *The Merck Manual*. As a gift, *The Merck Manual* would be considered a moderately priced item, costing approximately $65 at retail price. The online description of *The Merck Manual* is as follows:

> *The 18th Edition of The* Merck Manual *is packed with essential information on diagnosing and treating medical disorders to help health care professionals and medical students deliver the best care. The world's most widely used medical reference now features expanded clinical focus on each disorder, as well as more specific guidance on patient examinations.*[13]

The text is also available for purchase online.

Expensive gifts include research grants and honoraria for speaking engagements in which physicians educate their peers on the latest research that highlights a specific company's new medication. Patient surveys and questionnaires substantiate the impression that gifts to physicians increase the individual cost of medications and also influence the type of medication prescribed to patients.[4]

At this time, much of what PhRMA has distributed to office-based clinicians is in the form of journal article reprints and other educationally purposed items, such as patient education brochures detailing instructions for product use and expected adverse drug reactions (ADRs). In addition to samples, coupons for discounted copays at the pharmacy and patient assistance application forms (for highly discounted medications offered by the manufacturer) might be kept as resources in medical clinics. Many of us have heard about the "good old days" of physician indulgence with exotic vacations or night club sprees given in exchange for prescriptions, but those types of "gifts" no longer exist per new PhRMA guidelines.[4]

Wilkes and Hoffman performed a study to evaluate the responses of medical students to a pharmaceutical representative presentation about a drug.[2] The study involved a mock presentation conducted by pharmacy students, one of whom was a former pharmaceutical representative. The general idea was to educate students about the tactics of pharmaceutical marketing and some of the misinformation and omitted data that can be communicated by PSRs and to get students to think critically about the information they receive. Information was also presented to the students regarding the impact that gifts have on some clinicians' prescribing habits. Once it was revealed to the students that this was a mock presentation, the students indicated that they felt less confident about the validity of the information given to them during the presentation. The authors stated that, "About one-third of our students felt that voluntary guidelines would be an effective method of assuring that drug company promotional and educational activities are accurate and fairly balanced. More than three-fourths felt that the FDA should aggressively punish drug companies that violate established rules regarding balance and accuracy."[2]

In the effort to clarify or distinguish between education and promotion, a number of governmental guidelines and industry-initiated guidelines have been put in place. In April 2003, federal guidelines to regulate the relationship and interactions between the pharmaceutical industry and clinicians were amended by the Office of the Inspector General (OIG) for the U.S. Department of Health and Human Services that suggest a "buyer beware" type of warning. Even small gifts, as well as educational projects, are likely to result in prescriptions or purchases of medical devices or treatments used for patients.[3]

As of the most recent laws passed by the Food and Drug Administration (FDA) and created by PhRMA in 2002, promotional materials or gifts given to clinicians by the pharmaceutical companies are now limited. Gifts worth more than $100 are prohibited. The Advanced Medical Technology Association (AdvaMed) developed a similar code in 2003. The Council on Ethical and Judicial Affairs for the American Medical Association (AMA) also has drafted guidelines on accepting gifts from medical device manufacturers and pharmaceutical companies. Izserson et al. explain that AMA guidelines mirror those of PhRMA, stating that gifts should, "primarily entail a benefit to patients and should not be of substantial value" (i.e., less than $100).[3]

Samples and the Benefits of PhRMA Companies

It has been stated that more patients have benefited from this partnership between the pharmaceutical industry and clinicians than have the pockets of doctors or members of the PhRMA industry. Patients benefit from the wide distribution capabilities of PhRMA companies. For example, when insulin was discovered in May of 1921 and mass production was required to deliver the needed hormone to diabetics worldwide, a large pharmaceutical manufacturer ramped up its production and helped millions of patients obtain the medication within 6 months.[5] Vaccinations for outbreaks such as the swine flu have been available in a timely manner thanks to a PhRMA company. Furthermore, many medical schools are able to provide new treatments to patients through the research funded by pharmaceutical companies.

Additionally, free samples can dramatically enhance patient care.[14] Samples and patient-assistance coupons are redeemable for reasonable copays, and some companies have programs that provide free or discounted prescriptions to needy patients. When clinicians determine that patients need access to novel therapies that insurance will not cover, and patients cannot afford, clinicians provide not only their services as diagnosticians and educators, but also a free trial of a medication. For patients on fixed incomes, this can make or break their compliance to treatment.

Let's evaluate the economics of this situation. According to Iverson et al., "samples prod physicians to prescribe . . . more expensive drugs much faster (instead of generics), and the cost of samples is $2 to $3 billion annually to the company."[3] When that amount is translated into total retail costs, the company loses approximately $13 to $15 billion plus the cost of the PSR to deliver those sample medications and speak with the clinicians who hand the samples out to their patients.

Another way of looking at this is to consider the fact that the cost of health care is increasing in proportion to the increasing expenditures for prescription medications. In 2004, seniors paid an average of $2,322 for their medications.[3] Annual prescription usage in the United States and Medicare preventive healthcare benefits are increasing,[14] which may account for more clinic visits and more consistent medication management and prescriptions.

A link on the Medicare website connects patients to a pharmaceutical assistance program sponsored by drug manufacturers (RxAssist). This program helps patients who have less favorable outcomes from generic medications afford the brand-name medication. Through these programs the price of the brand-name medication is usually based on income and medical need . . . The end result is that the patient gets the needed medication for free for up to a year.[12] Individual members of PhRMA have their own links on the RxAssist website for patients and healthcare providers with frequently asked questions (FAQs) on free medications and discount cards.[15] Low-income patients can also seek care at government-funded community health centers, many of which have pharmacies. They receive free or low-cost branded and generic products.

In an article by Dubois evaluating the effects of pharmaceutical promotions, he stated that for the practice of medicine, "the basis of continuous quality improvement efforts whose goal is that similar patients should generally receive similar interventions . . . patients should receive interventions that have proven clinical benefit and represent a cost-effective option."[16] As demonstrated in the discussion above, we, as clinicians, can offer new therapies to patients via cost-effective options.

TIPS ON HOW TO USE YOUR PSR WISELY

In an *Albany Law Review* article, Connors discussed the higher purpose of PSRs, stating that their "[I]nteractions should be focused on informing healthcare professionals about products, providing scientific and educational information, and supporting medical [research and] education."[4]

The following tips can help to ensure that your time spent with PSRs is productive and efficient:

- Request any head-to-head drug or treatment comparisons their company or independent schools of medicine have performed using their drug.
- If they only have articles illustrating placebo-controlled trials, request to see those that are randomized and double-blinded (where applicable).
- Ask for the confidence intervals and p-values of statistics that the PSR has interpreted for you. If they are not valid, let the PSR know that you need more information from a peer-reviewed journal article prior to a trial of the drug.
- Ask the PSR to locate and present any unpublished trials for newer indications being sought or to back up anecdotal reports on the use of the new medication over the gold standard.
- Here are statements you can use when you decline a marketing approach from a PSR: "I don't initiate my own trial of any new medications until there are at least 2 years of postmarketing surveillance available" or "Show me data regarding ADRs and morbidity and mortality from Phase IV trials."

SOME THINGS TO WATCH FOR

Picking apart a competitor's package insert is a popular PSR strategy. The solution is for you to look for adverse drug reactions and sample sizes and anything that would not apply to the affected (illness-ailment being treated) patient population versus their product's methods, data, and p-values. Comparison of package inserts does not provide an apples-to-apples comparison, yet it might be presented as such by the PSR.

The PSR might use results of animal studies to establish side-effect profiles. For example, tolterodine is a medication used to treat overactive bladder. One of the most common side effects of medications in this class is dry mouth. This happens because the medication is selective for receptors in the mouth as well as the bladder. Tolterodine has been reported in animal studies as selecting receptors in the bladder rather than receptors in other locations. CenterWatch describes the selectivity of the drug as follows:

> Tolterodine is a competitive muscarinic receptor antagonist. Both urinary bladder contraction and salivation are mediated via cholinergic muscarinic receptors. In the anesthetized cat, tolterodine shows a selectivity for the urinary bladder over salivary glands; however, the clinical relevance of this finding has not been established.[17]

Note this information means that the clinical finding has not been confirmed in humans.

As a PSR, I had numerous conversations with clinicians who asked if the medication I was promoting (which was an alternative to tolterodine) was as selective for the bladder as tolterodine, implying that they had been informed of tolterodine's superior bladder selectivity. I was unable to offer a valid comparison because the adverse event data I had for the medication I was promoting were from human trials, not animal trials. The lesson here is that clinicians need to consider the type of research performed.

In some instances, the PSR might fail to offer information on adverse effects[2] unless requested to do so by the clinician. It is important that you ask for this information and also look for it through other sources.

Sometimes PSRs will refer to the drugs they sell by their trade names while referring to competitor drugs by their generic names. This practice is used because the trade names are usually more appealing and memorable than the generic names.[2]

PERFORMING TIMELY RESEARCH

You should research how the medical community ranks the medication or treatment offered by a PSR. One way to keep current is to join a journal club. A journal club is a group of clinicians who work together to keep up with the most recent FDA-approved medications. Presenters will select important articles and provide a detailed critique of the studies, their clinical importance, and their generalizability.[18] Another resource is *The Medical Letter on Drugs and Therapeutics*. This newsletter offers objective, peer-reviewed evaluations of new FDA-approved drugs and new information on previously approved drugs.

The following are some other ways of staying on top of new drugs and treatments:

- Attend Continuing Medical Education (CME) conferences or complete CME courses online. You can sign up for emails of CME credit updates (MedScape) in treatment and research for a quick and easy means of staying up-to-date.
- If you work in a hospital setting, use the hospital's computer research system.
- Establish reliable ways of looking up common facts (e.g., Google Scholar, your profession's national website, AAFP, UpToDate, Epocrates, MedScape).
- Identify a set of ways to look up obscure facts.
- Browse at least one general journal regularly. Invest time to discover new sources of useful information (e.g., peer-reviewed journals, respected colleagues).
- Develop critical-appraisal skills.

If a PSR refers to a particular study, read the actual study to verify any claims that were made. Statistically significant data might not be beneficial or applicable to all of your patients. In an analysis of pharmaceutical advertisements presented in 10 of the leading medical journals, distortions (that are prohibited by the FDA) were found in 36% of the graphs in the advertisements.[19] Keep this in mind when deciding to trial a new drug.

DIRECT-TO-CONSUMER MARKETING

As you are well aware, consumers are increasingly being targeted directly by the pharmaceutical industry through advertisements in the media and the Internet, which are often difficult to counter.[3] Advertisements are found on television, radio, the Internet, and in magazines. Which medications come to mind when you think of direct-to-consumer advertising of pharmaceuticals? Two of the most common today are erectile dysfunction and a cholesterol medication. Patients often ask providers if they need a medication after seeing an ad on television where a "friend" (usually the erectile dysfunction ad) or they themselves had a personal medical complaint (I think my cholesterol is high). Per FDA regulations with regard to the content of direct-to-consumer (DTC) advertisements, if the name and indicated use of the product is mentioned in the ad, then the full list of side effects must be stated during the commercial or within the print or online advertisement.

One of the benefits of DTC advertisements is that it might get the general public to seek preventive care, which gives us an opportunity to head-off heart disease and strokes in the early stages of the disease process, as in the case of hypercholesterolemia. Pharmaceutical companies would claim that they enable us to make a difference before the patient is symptomatic. As a means of bringing new patients into your office, DTC advertisements promote preventive care. The idea is to initiate the treatment of conditions prior to getting severe enough that they are life-threatening.[4]

The World Health Organization (WHO) offers strong support for preventive health care to reduce the number of chronic health conditions: "Not only are chronic conditions projected to be the leading cause of disability throughout the world by the year 2020; if not successfully prevented and managed, they will become the most expensive problems faced by our healthcare systems."[20] According to the WHO, people with diabetes "generate healthcare costs that are two to three times those without the condition" and that "costs of lost production due to diabetes are estimated to be five times the direct healthcare costs."[20] When screening and prevention services are utilized, as in the Kaiser Permanente model of integrated health care, improvements can be seen across a variety of conditions, including heart disease, asthma, and diabetes, and hospital admission rates.[21] Our point here is this: If DTC ads help bring patients to the door and we can clarify their medical needs and give them factual answers, perhaps the money spent on advertising is more useful to us and our patients than previously thought.

Figure 10–4 offers an example of one of the few types of direct marketing currently permitted in clinician offices. This example is for our hypothetical medication, SuperStatin, and it is designed to motivate consumers to seek the medication. Note the wide array of indications listed. Many patients, perhaps the majority, would be able to check at least one of the options. I encourage you to look for other examples of this type of promotional material.

Another DTC marketing strategy is television advertising. In the past, pharmaceutical companies were not allowed to advertise on television. This changed in 1997 when the FDA completed a study examining the relationship between product promotion and medication usage. The FDA concluded that the evidence showed that product promotion did not result in excessive use.[16] In light of these findings, the FDA removed the ban on television advertising of pharmaceuticals.[4] During the next 2 years, the DTC advertising of pharmaceuticals,

and statins in particular, increased dramatically. During the same period, the number of patients using these drugs increased by 60%. Some say that DTC advertising results in greater use of various therapies by more "marginal" candidates, and that in the case of statins the typical users would be those at lower risk.[16]

PACKAGE INSERTS

Package inserts (PIs) include information you can use as a guideline for proper use and prescribing of medications. The following is a breakdown of each section within the package insert. We have noted the areas of importance that merit special attention:

1. **DESCRIPTION**
   - Chemical composition and all ingredients, including active medications; inactive coatings, such as starches; enteric coatings; or specific drug delivery-system for extended release.
2. **CLINICAL PHARMACOLOGY**
   - Class of medication.
   - Pharmacodynamics (how the drug works on the body).
   - Pharmacokinetics (how the body uses the drug).
     a. Absorption.
        ○ Includes the effect of food, if any, in the stomach when taking the medication.
        ○ Includes the need, or lack thereof, of a specific gastric pH.
     b. Distribution.
        ○ Protein-binding percentages and free drug circulating in plasma.
     c. Metabolism.
        ○ Active and inactive metabolites, liver versus other metabolic pathways.
        ○ Common pathways in liver: CYP450, CYP3A4, CYP2A6, and CYP2D6.
     d. Excretion.
        ○ Plasma concentrations, including half-life, area under the curve (AUC), C_{max}, and T_{max}.

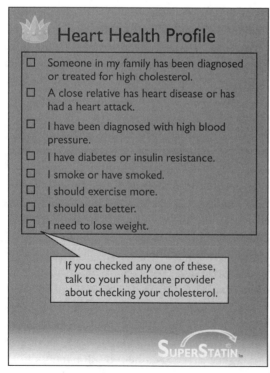

Figure 10–4 Direct-to-Consumer Survey for SuperStatin

○ Elimination of the drug in feces, urine, etc.

- Pharmacokinetics in special populations.
  a. Age.
  b. Pediatric (unless specifically created for use in children, most new medications will not have been evaluated for children).
  c. Gender (males vs. females with excretion and parent drug levels).
  d. Race.
  e. Renal insufficiency (dose adjustments).
  f. Hepatic insufficiency (dose adjustments).
- Drug–drug interactions.
  a. Not usually available unless new trials have been performed, but might note that drugs that use the same excretory or metabolic pathway have the potential to interact.
  b. Electrophysiology (will be included if CNS [central nervous system] side effects are part of that class of medications).

3. **CLINICAL STUDIES**
- Study methods are summarized and a table of results based on set trial outcomes and end points is presented.
- This is the critical analysis area for clinicians, because baseline to end-of-treatment changes with *p*-values are provided in these graphs.

4. **INDICATIONS AND USAGE**
- Specific diagnosis for which the drug was studied and approved for use during the FDA-approved clinical trials.

5. **CONTRAINDICATIONS**
- Black Box Warning: absolute contraindication for drug use that could lead to death in patients with specific lifestyle habits or comorbid conditions.
- Absolute contraindications, including comorbidities that predispose patients to a poor outcome or adverse event that might not be life threatening but definitely life altering.

6. **PRECAUTIONS**
- General
  a. Cautions for patients due to the effectiveness of the drug or common side effects (e.g., for an overactive bladder medication, the caution that urinary retention might result).
  b. Cases in which the medication can be used but clinicians and patients should be advised that potential benefits must outweigh potential risks of use.
- Information for patients
  a. Cases in which adverse events might be amplified.
  b. Special considerations for usage (e.g., after meals, with meals, empty stomach).
- Drug interactions
  a. Use of two medications in the same class.
  b. Issues with pharmacokinetic profiles of medications similar to this one.
  c. Any known problems that arose during clinical trials with the use of specific medications and this medication.
- Carcinogenesis, mutagenesis, impairment of fertility
  a. Results of animal trials and human trials with defects occurring at higher-than-indicated doses of the trial drug.

7. **SPECIAL CONSIDERATIONS FOR USE**
- Pregnancy
  a. TERATOGENIC EFFECTS: Any observed birth defects in pregnant animals during Phase II animal trials.
  b. PREGNANCY CATEGORY: FDA Use-in-Pregnancy Ratings. For more information on the FDA drug rating system, see the FDA website.
    ○ **Category A**: Controlled studies show no risk. Adequate, well-controlled studies in pregnant women have failed to demonstrate

a risk to the fetus in any trimester of pregnancy.

○ **Category B:** No evidence of risk in humans. Adequate, well-controlled studies in pregnant women have not shown increased risk of fetal abnormalities despite adverse findings in animals,
Or

○ In the absence of adequate human studies, animal studies show no fetal risk. The chance of fetal harm is remote, but remains a possibility.

○ **Category C:** Risk cannot be ruled out. Adequate, well-controlled human studies are lacking, and animal studies have shown a risk to the fetus or are lacking as well. There is a chance of fetal harm if the drug is administered during pregnancy, but the potential benefits might outweigh the potential risk.

○ **Category D:** Positive evidence of risk. Studies in humans, or investigational or postmarketing data, have demonstrated fetal risk. Nevertheless, potential benefits from the use of the drug might outweigh the potential risk. For example, the drug might be acceptable if needed in a life-threatening situation or serious disease for which safer drugs cannot be used or are ineffective.

○ **Category X:** Contraindicated in pregnancy. Studies in animals or humans, or investigational or postmarketing reports, have demonstrated positive evidence of fetal abnormalities or risk that clearly outweighs any possible benefit to the patient.

• Nursing mothers: Excretion of active drug or its active metabolites in breast milk, and the percent of active drug that might be passed on to the nursing infant.

• Pediatric use: Included if safety and effective dose have been studied.

• Geriatric use: Included if trial patients over the age of 65 or 75 have experienced similar or enhanced adverse events, with dose reduction recommendations based on trial patients.

8. **ADVERSE REACTIONS**
• **CHART PRESENTED TO YOU BY THE PSR:** The adverse events data are illustrated in this section. Look for a table that lists all of the ADRs, the most common ADRs and percentages, with trial medication (listed with dose-specific increases in ADRs or not) and placebo comparisons.
• **POSTMARKETING SURVEILLANCE:** Phase IV trials, serious or spontaneous ADRs that occurred just after the medication was used, which might be linked to medication use. All of these ADRs must be reported.
• **OVERDOSAGE MANAGEMENT:** Any overdose experience since the drug has been placed on the market, including foreign trials or postmarketing surveillance ADRs reported in humans, and how the overdose or misuse of the drug was treated, with the outcome for the patient stated.

9. **DOSAGE AND ADMINISTRATION**
• Very relevant data, because this is the most effective dose for the specific patients studied, with the fewest side effects at that dose.
• Dose modifications are listed here for special populations, as well as titration guidelines for minimizing adverse events early in the medication's use.

10. **HOW SUPPLIED**
• A description of what the tablets, capsules, patches, liquids, or injections look like in their packaging and the quantities per unit/bottle/syringe.
• This is important information for you to know and be able to reference, because many patients go abroad to get cheaper versions of branded drugs.
• Many medications (especially in a pediatric practice) are only indicated for adults, because that is the patient population that was studied in FDA-approved clinical trials.

One final issue to consider with regard to pharmaceutical and medical devices is off-label use of medications. A colleague(s) might have anecdotal data regarding some promising result from the use of a medication garnered from a recent conference or from personal experience that has not yet been published in a peer-reviewed journal. Ask your colleague for the evidence about the suggested off-label use. The FDA allows off-label uses with the expectation that clinicians base this usage upon sound medical evidence. FDA guidance for off-label usage is as follows:

> If physicians use a product for an indication not in the approved labeling, they have the responsibility to be well informed about the product, to base its use on firm scientific rationale and on sound medical evidence, and to maintain records of the product's use and effects. Use of a marketed product in this manner when the intent is the "practice of medicine" does not require the submission of an Investigational New Drug Application (IND), Investigational Device Exemption (IDE), or review by an Institutional Review Board (IRB). However, the institution at which the product will be used may, under its own authority, require IRB review or other institutional oversight.[22]

CHAPTER SUMMARY

"Pharmaceutical manufacturers often appear to forget their moral purpose . . . if that means providing false or misleading data to physicians and consumers, then so be it."[16] This quote is a rather harsh means of implying that there is a lack of ethics that is somehow unique to pharmaceutical companies. All companies exist to make a profit and, as consumers, many of us hope to gain from the products we buy. That being said, unless the PSR provides you with a head-to-head clinical trial comparing the two medications you are discussing, you should keep in mind that their statements could be a loose interpretation of each product's package insert, with different patients and trial protocols. Again, this is not a malevolent attempt to coerce prescribers into writing a prescription that is inappropriate for their patients, although some providers do believe that pharmaceutical companies and their representatives have no place in a healthcare setting. Gaining knowledge about new pharmaceutical treatment options requires a significant time investment. PSRs are one source of this information. Engaging in effective EBP will enable you to take the most benefit from interactions with PSRs while avoiding the pitfalls of pharmaceutical or other types of marketing. As Fletcher et al. stated, "The information found must be concentrated, because clinicians in the midst of patient care cannot afford the inefficiency of sorting through unwanted information to find what is relevant. Finally, it must be accurate, because the stakes are high both for patients' lives and for society's resources."[18]

With regard to data that pertain to your patients and specific treatment goals for those patients, your PSR can be an excellent person to rely on for updates on costs, insurance coverage, and recently published trials. The PSR is also a great resource for free or discounted medications directly from the manufacturer through patient assistance programs. Additionally, where else can you find someone willing to debate the merits of each medication in their class? PSRs are well trained in the pros and cons of their medication as well as all others used to treat the same disease. Small nuances might differentiate medications within an entire class of drugs that might seem identical to us as providers. PSRs are anxious to share their knowledge to help healthcare providers identify a solution, and they hope you choose their product as the solution to your patients' problems. Clinicians are highly motivated to offer a solution for patients who have failed to achieve therapeutic goals or were not able to tolerate the side effects they had when using the gold standard. Of course, the PSR would prefer that you use his or her medication first. However, it is more likely that you will choose the new medication for the next patient for whom that specific type of medication is indicated.

If you prefer to receive information via nonpharmaceutical–sponsored sources, seek CMEs and hospital-sponsored lectures instead of inviting PSRs to your office. If you are not in a private practice, try to seek employment with an organization that supports your ethics and practice preferences.

Depending on your profession, if you are a prescriber you might earn required CME credits for each licensing interval and be provided with recent data with which to make educated prescribing decisions. Many healthcare professionals look to these resources for the majority of their updates and will attend at least one conference per year to augment their knowledge of new research and treatment options.

EXERCISE

In this exercise, you will review pertinent information regarding Bogustatin and SuperStatin, the fictitious cholesterol-lowering drugs described in this chapter. You will use the figures in this chapter and the fictitious SuperStatin brochure presented in the chapter appendix.

1. Refer to the package insert for SuperStatin (chapter appendix) and the ad that was shown to the clinician during the sales call in the clinic (Figure 10–1). Pay special attention to the "n" for each drug. What relevance does this have on the outcome of the adverse drug reaction percentages and overall impression of side effects reported for each drug tested?

2. Refer to Figure 10–2 and the sales statements associated with the claims of efficacy for SuperStatin versus Bogustatin. Are they statistically similar? What information do you have to verify this? (Hint: Try the package insert for SuperStatin.)

3. Refer to Figure 10–1. What visual cues are there to suggest that SuperStatin is more favorable than its comparators, Bogustatin and placebo?

4. Refer to Figure 10–4, which is the "Heart Health Profile." In this direct-to-consumer survey, which could appear in any magazine targeting homemakers or middle-aged men, consumers are asked a number of questions regarding their health and are prompted to consult with their doctor about their cholesterol if they meet any of the criteria. What

response is expected from patients with regard to their next visit to their healthcare provider?

REFERENCES

1. *Fundamentals of pharmaceutical sales*. 4th ed. Walpole, MA: Informa Training Partners; 2003.
2. Wilkes MS, Hoffman JR. An innovative approach to educating medical students about pharmaceutical promotion. *Acad Med*. 2001;76(12):1271–1277.
3. Iserson KV, Cerfolio RJ, Sade RM. Politely refuse the pen and note pad: Gifts from industry to physicians harm patients. *Ann Thorac Surg*. 2007;84:1077–1084.
4. Connors AL. Big bad pharma: An ethical analysis of physician–directed and consumer-directed marketing tactics. *Albany Law Review*. 2009;73(1): 243–282.
5. Cardarelli R, Licciardone JC, Taylor LG. A cross-sectional evidence-based review of pharmaceutical promotional marketing brochures and their underlying studies: Is what they tell us important and true? *BMC Fam Pract*. 2006;7:13.
6. Teven JJ, Winters JL. Pharmaceutical representatives' social influence behaviors and communication orientations: relationships with adaptive selling and sales performance. *Human Communication*. 2006;10(4):465–486.
7. Hartman T. *The Hartman personality profile: Also known as the color code*. Available at: www.colorcode.com. Accessed August 4, 2012.
8. Fugh-Berman AJ, Scialli AR, Bell AM. Why lunch matters: Assessing physicians' perceptions about industry relationships. *J Contin Educ Health Prof*. 2010;30(3):197–204.
9. Hirschler B. *Drug R&D spending fell in 2010, and heading lower*. Reuters. June 27, 2011. Available at: www.reuters.com/article/2011/06/26/pharmaceuticals-rd-idUSL6E7HO1BL20110626. Accessed August 2, 2012.
10. National Institutes of Health. NIH budget: Research for the people. Reviewed March 1, 2012. Available at: www.nih.gov/about/budget.htm. Accessed August 2, 2012.
11. CNN Money. *Top companies: Most profitable*. 2010. Available at: http://money.cnn.com/magazines/fortune/fortune500/2010/performers/companies/profits/. Accessed August 2, 2012.
12. Baker CB, Johnsrud MT, Chrismon ML, Rosenheck RA, Woods SW. Quantitative analysis of sponsorship bias in economic studies of antidepressants. *Br J Psychiatry*. 2003;183:498–506.

13. Porter R. (ed.). *The Merck Manual of Diagnosis and Therapy.* 19th ed. West Point, PA: Merck Sharp & Dohme Corp; 2011.

14. Cooper RJ, Schriger DL, Wallace RC, Mikulich VJ, Wilkes MS. The quantity and quality of scientific graphs in pharmaceutical advertisements. *J Gen Intern Med.* 2003;18(4):294–297.

15. RXAssist.org. Patient assistant program center: Frequently asked questions about patient assistance programs. ND. Available at: http://rxassist.org/faqs /default.cfm. Accessed August 4, 2012.

16. Dubois RW. Pharmaceutical promotion: Don't throw the baby out with the bathwater. *Health Aff.* February 2003; published ahead of print February 26, 2003, doi:10.1377/hlthaff.w3.96.

17. CenterWatch. *Drug information: Detrol LA (tolterodine tartrate).* Available at: www.centerwatch .com/drug-information/fda-approvals/drug-details .aspx?DrugID = 658. Accessed June 30, 2012.

18. Fletcher RH, Fletcher SW. Evidence-based approach to the medical literature. *J Gen Intern Med.* 1997;12:5–14.

19. Cooper RJ, Schriger DL, Wallace RC, Mikulich VJ, Wilkes MS. The quantity and quality of scientific graphs in pharmaceutical advertisements. *J Gen Intern Med.* 2003;18(4):294–297.

20. World Health Organization. Integrating prevention into health care. *Indian J Med Sci.* 2002;56(12): 619–621.

21. Feachem GA, Sekhri NK, White KL. Getting more for their dollar: A comparison of the NHS with California's Kaiser Permanente. *BMJ.* 2002;324:135–143.

22. United States Food and Drug Administration. *Regulatory information: "Off-Label" investigational use of marketed drugs, biologics, and medical devices* – information sheet. [Webpage]. Updated August 10, 2011. Available at: http://www.fda.gov /RegulatoryInformation/Guidances/ucm126486 .htm. Accessed October 9, 2012.

ANSWERS TO EXERCISE

1. SuperStatin had more patients in its trials than did Bogustatin. This reduced the percent of reported side effects in comparison to the other drugs tested with a smaller number of patients. The comparisons may not be accurate in regard to expectations for patient side-effect outcomes, and SuperStatin may be more similar among the comparator drug than demonstrated by the percentages shown:

   - SuperStatin: 6% of 1,270 = 76.2 patients had headaches.
   - Bogustatin: 6.7% of 310 = 20.77 patients had headaches.

   This is approximately four times fewer patients tested than SuperStatin. If we multiply 20.77 by 4, we find this is approximately 80 patients versus 76. Thus, they are essentially the same.

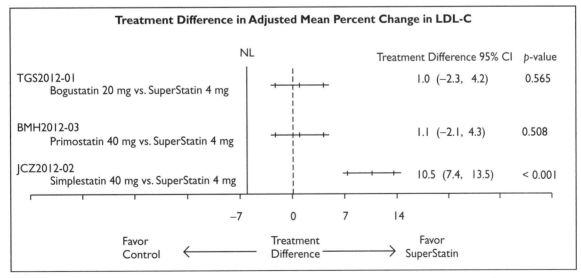

Figure 10–5 Forest Plot Comparing Hypothetical Medications Bogustatin, Primostatin, and Simplestatin

302 | **Part** II | APPLICATIONS OF EVIDENCE-BASED PRACTICE

Let's compare the other side effect that is reported much less with SuperStatin versus Bogustatin—pain in extremities:

- SuperStatin: 0.8% × 1,270 = 10.16 patients had pain in extremities.
- Bogustatin: 2.5% × 310 = 7.75 patients had pain in extremities.

If we multiply this by 4, we might assume that nearly 30 patients would have this side effect when Bogustatin is tested in a similar number of patients as SuperStatin and a reasonable assumption would be that less patients would discontinue SuperStatin over Bogustatin because of pain in the extremities. SuperStatin has an advantage here.

2. Yes, they are statistically similar, because the p-value for the efficacy of SuperStatin compared to Bogustatin is greater than 0.5. (Look at the forest plot [refer to Figure 10–5] from the package insert.) The chart displays three head-to-head comparisons of different medications against SuperStatin. SuperStatin and Bogustatin performed similarly in terms of LDL-C, while SuperStatin greatly outperformed Simplestatin.

3. Three things are readily apparent:
   - In the adverse events reporting section, the font is larger for SuperStatin.
   - Whenever Super is used, it is italicized and larger to make it stand out.
   - The eye is led via arrows toward the positive outcomes of the trial, indicating that SuperStatin solves a problem.

4. Patients may be prompted to ask their physicians questions such as the following:
   - "Do my genetics play a role in my health? Am I at risk for a heart attack because my father had one?"
   - "What lifestyle changes affect my heart? Should I make a change?"
   - "Is my blood pressure high? Should I start checking it?"
   - "What does cholesterol have to do with my heart? What is my level?"
   - And, most important, the goal question of the survey: "Should I be taking SuperStatin?"

SuperStatin Package Insert*

PRESCRIBING INFORMATION

Description

SuperStatin (suporvastatin) is an inhibitor of the enzyme HMG-CoA reductase. It is a synthetic lipid-lowering agent for oral administration.

The chemical name for suporvastatin is tricalcium spiro bis(3,2,1)-octane-8.1′-cycloquinofluorodihydroxy-4-hectenoate). The structural formula is:

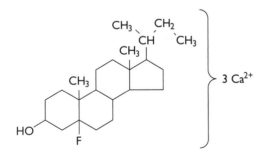

The empirical formula for suporvastatin is C38H23 3CaF6N3O10 and the molecular weight is 790.13. Each SuperStatin round ivory film-coated tablet is

* Brett E. Shelton contributed to the graphics and layout for Appendix A.

debossed with a crown on one side and a "4" on the opposite side. Each tablet contains 4 mg of suporvastatin and is to be given orally. Suporvastatin is a pale ivory odorless powder. Each tablet also contains the following inactive ingredients: sucrose, cellulose, talc, calcium carbonate, stearic acid, ferric oxide, white wax, and carnauba wax.

CLINICAL PHARMACOLOGY

Mechanism of Action

Suporvastatin competitively inhibits HMG-CoA reductase, which is an enzyme involved in the biosynthesis of cholesterol. The agent competes with this substrate to inhibit cholesterol synthesis in the liver. The uptake of LDL from the blood-stream to the liver is changed to decrease the total cholesterol in the plasma and cholesterol receptors in the liver respond by decreasing very low density lipoprotein synthesis.

Pharmacodynamics

In a randomized, double blind, placebo-controlled, double-dummy, 3-way parallel, active-comparator study with flippyfloxacin in 201 healthy participants, SuperStatin was not associated with clinically meaningful QTc interval prolonquation or increased heart rate at daily doses of up to 12 mg (3 times the recommended daily maximum dose).

Pharmacokinetics

Absorption: One hour after oral administration, less than 60% of suporvastatin is absorbed. Peak plasma concentrations (C_{max}) and area under the curve (AUC) occur between 5–6 hours postdose. Effect of Food: Administration with a high-fat meal resulted in decreased bioavailability and reduced absorption but did not significantly reduce suporvastatin AUC. Suporvastatin was noted to have a moderately higher percent change from baseline for LDL-C following morning dosing. The drug is mostly absorbed in the duodenum of the small intestine but not in the distal GI tract.

Distribution: Suporvastatin is more than 97% bound to albumin in human plasma, and its mean volume of distribution is approximately 120 L. Suporvastatin and its metabolites are inert to blood cell interaction.

Metabolism: Suporvastatin is minimally metabolized by CYP2D6. The major metabolite in the plasma is vandalone, which is formed by a phenyl-type conjugate and is inactive.

Excretion: The mean plasma half life is approximately 16 hours. Radioactivity tests on orally administered suporvastatin 4 mg dose demonstrated a 25% mean excretion rate in urine and a mean of 73% excretion rate in feces within 5 days.

Pharmacokinetics in Special Populations

Geriatric: In a pharmacokinetic study which compared healthy elderly (> 65 years old) and young volunteers, suporvastatin C_{max} and AUC were 24% and 8% higher in the elderly, respectively. This showed no effect on efficacy or safety in elderly subjects from clinical studies.

Race: In pharmacokinetic studies, suporvastatin C_{max} and AUC were 18% and 3% lower, respectively, in

African American or Black healthy volunteers compared with the C_{max} and AUC of Caucasian and Hispanic healthy volunteers.

Gender: In a pharmacokinetic study which compared healthy female and male volunteers, suporvastatin C_{max} and AUC were 40% and 30% higher, respectively in females, but this had no effect on the efficacy or safety of SuperStatin in women in clinical studies.

Hepatic Impairment: The ratio of suporvastatin C_{max} and AUC between patients with mild hepatic imparment and healthy volunteers was 1.2. The ratio of suporvastatin C_{max} and AUC between patients with moderate hepatic impairment and healthy volunteers was 3.3. Mean half-life for moderate hepatic impairment, mild hepatic impairment, and healthy volunteers were 22, 18, and 16 hours, respectively.

Renal Impairment: Patients with moderate renal impairment (glomerular filtration rate of 30 to < 60 ml/min/1.73 m^2) and those with end-stage renal disease receiving hemodialysis demonstrated suporvastatin AUC levels at 80% and 82% higher than those of healthy volunteers, respectively. The suporvastatin C_{max} is 50% and 35% higher, in these same patients, respectively. The effect of suporvastatin in patients of mild and severe renal impairment levels is unknown.

Drug-Drug Interactions: The route of metabolism of suporvastatin is via the CYP2D6 pathway with the formation of the inactive metabolite of vandalone.

Warfarin: In healthy patients using warfarin, the steady-state pharmacodynamics for INR and PT levels and pharmacokinetics were unaffected by the use of SuperStatin 4 mg daily. Patients should continue to monitor INR and PT levels while using SuperStatin with warfarin.

CLINICAL STUDIES

Study 1 = Placebo controlled study; A multicenter, randomized, double-blind, double-dummy, placebo controlled study was performed to evaluate the efficacy of SuperStatin (suporvastatin) compared with placebo in 412 patients with primary hyperlipidemia. SuperStatin (suporvastatin) was given as a

Table 1: Mean Change in LDL-C from Baseline to Posttreatment at 12 Weeks and Percent Change in LDL-C at 12 Weeks

	Placebo (N = 205)	SuperStatin (N = 207)
Baseline	244	240
Posttreatment	240	137
Percent change	–3%	–43%

single 4 mg daily dose for 12 weeks and significantly reduced plasma LDL-C compared to placebo.

Study 2 — Active-controlled Study with Bogustatin (TGS2012-01)

SuperStatin was compared to the HMG-CoA reductase inhibitor Bogustatin in a multicenter, randomized, double-blind, double-dummy, active-controlled Phase III study of 525 patients with primary hyperlipidemia. Patients began a 10-week washout period of only diet and exercise and were then randomized to a 12-week treatment with either SuperStatin or Bogustatin (Figure 1). Results of lipid reduction are shown in Figure 1. The study outcome demonstrated that for the mean percent change in LDL-C from baseline to 12-weeks, SuperStatin 4 mg daily was comparable in efficacy to 20 mg daily of Bagustatin. Mean treatment difference (95% CI) was 1%.

Active–controlled study with Primostatin (BMH2012-03): SuperStatin was compared to the HMG-CoA reductase inhibitor Primostatin in a multicenter, randomized, double-blind, double-dummy, active–controlled Phase III study of 473 patients with primary hyperlipidema. Patients began a 10-week washout period of only diet and exercise and were then randomized to a 12-week treatment with either SuperStatin or primostatin (Figure 1). Results of lipid reduction are shown in Figure 1. The study outcome demonstrated that for the mean percent change in LDL-C from baseline to 12 weeks, SuperStatin 4 mg daily was comparable in efficacy to 40 mg daily of primostatin. Mean treatment difference (95% CI) was –1.1%.

Active–controlled study with Simplestatin (JCZ2012-02): SuperStatin was compared to the HMG-CoA reductase inhibitor Simplestatin in a multicenter, randomized, double-blind, double-dummy, active-controlled Phase III study of 650 patients with primary hyperlipidemia. Patients began a 10-week washout period of only diet and exercise and were then randomized to a 12-week treatment with either SuperStatin or Simplestatin (Figure 1). Results of lipid reduction are shown in Figure 1. The study outcome demonstrated that for the mean percent change in LDL-C from baseline to 12-weeks, SuperStatin 4 mg daily was superior in efficacy to 40 mg daily of Simplestatin. Mean treatment difference (95% CI) was –0.5%.

INDICATIONS AND USAGE

SuperStatin (suporvastatin) is a HMG-CoA reductase inhibitor indicated for patients with primary hyperlipidemia and mixed dyslipidemia as an adjunctive therapy to diet and exercise to reduce elevated levels of total cholesterol (TC) and low-density lipoprotein cholesterol (LDL-C).

CONTRAINDICATIONS

SuperStatin is contraindicated in patients with the following conditions:

- Known hypersensitivity to the drug or its ingredients, as demonstrated by rash, pruritus, and urticaria, which were reported during SuperStatin clinical trials.

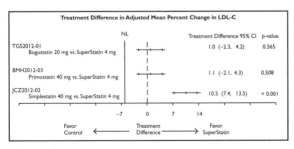

Figure 1: The treatment differences in efficacy in LDL-C change from baseline between SuperStatin and active controls in the Phase III studies

- Those with active liver disease as demonstrated by elevated liver function tests, including elevations in transaminases.
- Women who may become pregnant or are currently pregnant. Due to the mechanism of decreasing cholesterol and therefore possible biologically active substances and hormones derived from cholesterol, there is potential harm to the developing fetus. No clinical trials have been performed on pregnant women to determine safety or efficacy in this patient population.
- Nursing mothers. SuperStatin, like all other HMG-CoA reductase inhibitors in its class, is contraindicated in pregnant or nursing mothers. In animal studies, SuperStatin was shown to pass into breast milk. This class of medications has the potential to cause serious adverse reactions in nursing infants.

PRECAUTIONS

Skeletal Muscle Effects

Cases of myopathy and rhabdomyolysis with acute renal failure secondary to myoglobulinuria have been reported with HMG-CoA reductase inhibitors, including SuperStatin. For this reason, SuperStatin should be prescribed with caution in patients with predisposing factors for myopathy. These factors include increased age (> 65 years old), hepatic impairment, renal impairment, and uncontrolled hypothyroidism. In patients using fibrates and niacin to lower lipid levels with SuperStatin, the risk of myopathy increases.

Lipid controlling medications should not be used in cases of dehydration, acute renal failure, sepsis, or hypotension until equilibrium has been attained and blood tests verify normal return to function. Advise all patients to report tenderness, weakness, unexplained muscle aches, and fever.

Liver Enzyme Monitoring and Conditions Commonly Associated with Abnormalities in Liver Function Tests

Increases in liver function tests (AST/ALT, for example) have been reported with the use of

HMG-CoA reductase inhibitors. In clinical trials, SuperStatin showed transient elevations in these transaminases. It is recommended that liver function tests be performed prior to SuperStatin therapy at 12 weeks of therapy as well as periodically at 6 months thereafter. Should an increase of 3x the upper limits of normal persist, a reduction in dose or discontinuation of the drug is recommended.

SuperStatin should be used with caution in patients who consume substantial quantities of alcohol.

Information for Patients

Dosing Time

SuperStatin may be taken at any time of day, with or without food.

Muscle Pain

Patients should notify their healthcare provider of any medications they use, including over-the-counter drugs. They should also report any muscle aches, pains, or weakness in a timely manner.

DRUG INTERACTIONS

The concomitant use of SuperStatin with some other medications may enhance suporvastatin exposure, including fibrates, niacin, and some antibiotics, including tetracyclines and penicillin.

Warfarin (see pharmacokinetics section)

In healthy patients using warfarin, the steady-state pharmacodynamics for INR and PT levels and pharmacokinetics were unaffected by the use of SuperStatin 4 mg daily. Patients should continue to monitor INR and PT levels while using SuperStatin with warfarin.

Carcinogenesis, Mutagenesis, Impairment of Fertility

There was an absence of drug-related tumors in a 90-week carcinogenity study in mice given suporvastatin, with systemic maximum exposures (AUC)

at 20 times the clinical maximum exposure of 4 mg per day. In another 90-week carcinogenicity study in rats given suporvastatin there was an increase in the incidence of pituitary gland tumors. These tumors occurred at doses of 25 mg/kg/day, which is over 200 times the daily human systemic exposures at the 4mg per day dose.

Suporvastatin was not mutagenic in viral and bacterial tests, including mononucleosis and Escherichia coli.

Suporvastatin exhibited no effects on male and female rat fertility; however, when 1 mg/kg/day was administered to male and female rabbits, mortality from gastric toxicity was suspected as a cause of mortality. Decreased viability of fetuses was not observed.

USE IN SPECIFIC POPULATIONS

Pregnancy: Teratogenic Effects (see Contraindications); Pregnancy: Category X; Nursing Mothers (see Contraindications)

As studies in pregnant and nursing mothers have not been conducted, it is not known whether suporvastatin is secreted in human breast milk. However, trial data in animals has demonstrated secretion in animal breast milk and it is therefore thought to have adverse effects on the nursing infant. Women who require treatment with an HMG Co-A reductase inhibitor such as suporvastatin should be advised not to nurse their infants or to discontinue the use of the drug prior to nursing an infant.

Pediatric Use

Use of SuperStatin in pediatric patients, including patients under the age of 18 years old has not been established and therefore safety and efficacy in this patient population is unknown.

Geriatric Use

Of the 1,270 patients randomized to use SuperStatin in clinical studies, 572 (45%) were 65 years and older. Efficacy and safety between elderly and younger patients were not significantly different,

yet greater sensitivity to the drug in some older patients should not be ruled out entirely.

Hepatic Impairment

SuperStatin is contraindicated in patients with active liver disease, as may be demonstrated by persistent elevations in liver function blood tests such as elevated transaminases.

Renal Impairment

Patients with moderate renal impairment (glomerular filtration rate of 30 to < 60 mL/min/1.73 m^2) and those with end-stage renal disease receiving hemodialysis should take SuperStatin at a starting dose of 4 mg every other day for the first 3 months of use and have renal function tests performed at baseline and at 12 weeks of use.

ADVERSE REACTIONS

The following adverse reactions were discussed in the Precautions section of the label: Rhabdomyolysis and Liver Enzyme Monitoring.

Clinical Studies Experience

The frequency of adverse events and reactions varies among study populations and as such may not mimic or reflect the frequency of adverse reactions observed in clinical practice. Patients ranged in age from 18–87 years, with 51% females and 49% males. Approximately 87% of the patients were Caucasian, with the remaining races in descending order: Asian, Indian, African American, and Hispanic, or other.

Note: Other adverse reactions also reported from clinical studies but of lesser frequency included nasopharyngitis, influenza, ingrown toenails, and acne.

The following blood analysis laboratory test abnormalities were also reported: elevated AST, ALT, ALK PHOS, albumin, and glucose.

OVERDOSAGE

No specific treatment is recommended for overdosage of suporvastatin. Patients should be

Table 2: Adverse Reactions Reported by > 1% of Patients Treated with SuperStatin and Placebo in 12-Week Controlled Studies

Adverse event occurring in <1% of patients	Placebo (N = 205)	SuperStatin 4 mg QD (N = 207)
Headache	6.1%	5.8%
Fatigue	10.0%	7.0%
Diarrhea	1.0%	1.6%
Back pain	1.8%	2.2%
Myalgia	1.5%	2.3%
Pain in extremity	2.0%	1.3%

administered supportive care for symptoms and renal and hepatic functions monitored.

DOSAGE AND ADMINISTRATION

General Dosing Information

The starting and maintenance doses of SuperStatin in most populations is 4 mg/day. In patients with hepatic or renal impairment, the dosing frequency is lowered to 4 mg every other day. After 12 weeks of use, lipid levels should be analyzed and dosage adjusted accordingly.

Limitations of Use

Doses of SuperStatin greater than 4 mg per day were associated with an increase in adverse events, such as headache and pain in extremities.

Antibiotics

If patients are in need of antibiotics such as tetracy-clines and penicillins, SuperStatin should be discontinued for the duration of the antibiotic therapy.

HOW SUPPLIED

SuperStatin tablets 4 mg (round ivory film-coated tablet is debossed with a crown on one side and a "4" printed on the opposite side) are supplied as follows:

30 count HDPE bottle—NDC 98765-432-01

7 count blister (PVC/Paper backed foil)—NDC 98765-432-02

Store at room temperature 20 degrees C to 25 degrees C (68 to 77 degrees F)

Rx only

Manufactured by: BennieGabby Pharmaceuticals, Inc. Pharmatown, OR 01234 USA.

Address Medical Inquiries to:
www.SUPERSTATIN.com

Implementation and Evaluation in Evidence-Based Practice

Ellen J. Rogo, PhD

INTRODUCTION

Practitioners should appraise the trustworthiness of the evidence, assess the relevance of the evidence to the context expressed in a PPAARE (problem, patient/population, action, alternative, results, and evidence) question, select an action and implement it, and then evaluate the results. After this process has been completed, the practitioner should reflect on the experience and learn from it.

Before a decision can be made about what action to take, the evidence found by searching various databases has to be read several times to critically analyze its trustworthiness. Yes, I said that the evidence will have to be read multiple times before a judgment can be made with regard to its quality. Based on my experience as an educator, students who are new to evidence-based practice (EBP) commonly have the expectation of reading a scientific study or systematic review one time and then being able to critically analyze its components. This notion generally leads to frustration, whereas students who commit to reading the document at least three times have a much better success rate in determining its trustworthiness.

My advice to students and practitioners new to EBP is to print a hard copy of the evidence whenever possible. However, beware of the number of pages in a document. For example, some Cochrane Systematic Reviews in the full-article version are sometimes hundreds of pages. Another useful strategy to use when reading the evidence multiple times is to have the document in hand and interact with the content by underlining important aspects or writing questions or comments about the content in the margins. For instance, I always underline the purpose of the study or systematic review. Why? The purpose (or intent or aim) sets the stage for determining the alignment of the content with the subsequent methods, results, discussion, and conclusions sections. Second, use the margins to write any questions you might have that might require you to go to another resource, such as a textbook or statistics dictionary, to look up information. I frequently use this strategy when I am trying to determine whether the statistical analysis was appropriate for the data collected. I also write comments in the margins related to the strengths and limitations of the evidence.

The first time you read the evidence start with the abstract. The abstract includes a summary of the content and provides the reader with the "big picture" before reading the details in the rest of the document. The intent of the first reading of the entire publication, then, is to understand the content by underlining important aspects of the study and writing questions in the margins. Seek the answers to your questions before continuing to a second reading of the document.

With the second reading of the document, you should focus on analyzing the components of the evidence based on criteria for determining its trustworthiness. A series of questions is presented later in the chapter to assist you with the analysis of quantitative and qualitative studies.

During the third reading, comments about the strengths and limitations of the evidence can be written in the margins to help make a final appraisal of the trustworthiness of the content and to assess its relevance and usefulness to the context of the PPAARE situation.

The process of critical analysis of scientific literature is a skill that takes practice to develop. As the old adage goes, "practice makes perfect." Having someone to mentor you in this process is advisable. Educators and colleagues who are experienced can be mentors and help you learn this process.

APPRAISE THE TRUSTWORTHINESS OF QUANTITATIVE EVIDENCE

The trustworthiness of the evidence is appraised to determine if it is worthy of being used in making a decision about a healthcare action. Critical appraisal is necessary to establish the strengths and limitations of the evidence. When appraising the quality of a research study or other source of healthcare information, remember that there is no perfect study. Therefore, it is important to identify the study's limitations and to make a judgment as to whether the strengths of the study outweigh the weaknesses.

Trustworthiness of quantitative research is based on an appraisal of internal validity, external validity, reliability, and objectivity.[1] Establishing **internal validity** is done by appraising the methods section of the research report to determine whether the research design, sampling procedures, research protocol, data collection instruments, and procedures actually contributed to measuring what the researchers intended to measure. For example, when measuring blood pressure during data collection the stethoscope and sphygmomanometer need to accurately measure the systolic and diastolic pressure. Steps should be taken to calibrate and recalibrate the sphygmomanometer on a regular basis to ensure the accuracy of the data collected. When researchers employ the use of an instrument to determine conditions such as depression, the validity of that instrument to actually measure the condition should be established. Validity of newly developed instruments can be established through the use of a content validity index.[2-4] The validity of new diagnostic tests can be compared to the validity of existing tests. Failure of the researchers to establish the validity of the data collection instrument reduces the trustworthiness of the evidence.

External validity focuses on the ability to generalize the findings to the population from which the sample was derived and generalize the results in a realistic context. When establishing the external validity related to the sample, a critical appraisal of how the sample was selected (e.g., randomized versus convenience) and assigned to intervention and control groups is essential (e.g., random versus nonrandom assignment). When researchers use a sample of convenience, it limits the external validity and the ability to generalize the findings to the entire population. The research protocol should be carefully appraised to determine whether the intervention procedures were realistic for implementation in a practical sense.

The term *intervention* applies to many types of re-search, including studies of diagnostic interventions, treatment interventions, prevention interventions, and screening interventions. In prospective comparative studies, the *intervention group* includes subjects who have the condition or exposure of interest. The *comparison group* includes subjects who do not have the condition or exposure of interest. The comparison group might have no intervention/exposure, might have a placebo, or might have an active intervention (such as the usual standard of care or another intervention that has already been utilized in patient care).

For instance, some interventions are provided for an extended period of time, which would not be realistic in a practice setting due to issues related to the patient's time commitment or cost.

An inverse relationship exists between internal and external validity. As internal validity increases, external validity decreases, and vice versa. In an experimental study where the research protocol is implemented in a highly controlled environment and the internal validity is high, the external validity and the ability to generalize to another setting is reduced. Likewise, to control for internal validity a researcher can use a homogeneous sample; however, the impact on the ability to generalize to a population other than that represented by the characteristics of the homogeneous sample is limited.

Internal and external validity are influenced by **extraneous variables**. Extraneous, or **intervening**, variables are undesirable variables that interfere with the intended purpose of the investigation by introducing error to the study and affecting the dependent variable or outcome.[5] When extraneous variables affect the independent variable and the internal validity of a study, they are called confounding variables. Researchers need to control for extraneous variables; otherwise, the trustworthiness of the study is decreased. Whenever these variables cannot be avoided, the researcher should clearly delineate them as limitations in the discussion section

of the research report. **Table 11–1** provides an overview of common extraneous variables related to the sampling strategy and the research methods as well as ways to control or balance their effects.

The reliability of the data is appraised by determining the consistency or reproducibility of the manner in which the data were collected. When clinical data are being collected by one researcher, **intra-rater reliability** needs to be established to show that the data collected on one participant is consistent with the data collected on the other participants. When multiple researchers are collecting data, the first step is to establish intra-rater reliability to ensure consistency within each data collector. The second step is to determine the consistency of data collection among all of the researchers, which is referred to as **inter-rater reliability**. Researchers generally discuss the procedures used to establish intra-rater and inter-rater reliability. These procedures can include collecting data on a small number of participants one day and then collecting the data points on the same subjects 1 week later. The consistency of the measurements is generally reported by **Cohen's kappa**; a coefficient of 0.8 or higher is considered a trustworthy level. Cohen's kappa is a correlation statistic telling us how well the first data point predicts the second data point. The correlation needs to be strong in order for the researchers to have inter-rater reliability.

The researchers must also discuss the reliability of the data collection instrument, such as a survey to measure knowledge level or a tool to measure quality of life. One common procedure for establishing the reliability of a data collection instrument is the **test–retest method**, whereby the survey or tool is administered to a small group of participants at one time and then the same instrument is administered 1 week later to the same subjects. The level of agreement between the test scores and retest scores are compared using a correlation coefficient. There are several types of correlation tests used for this purpose, depending on the scale of the data. A Pearson product-moment coefficient (r) is reported for interval or ratio data, a Spearman rank order

Table 11-1 Extraneous Variables and Strategies to Control or Balance the Effects

Category of Variables	Description	Control or Balance Strategy
Sample	• Characteristics of the sample are not representative of the intended population. • Sample size is too small for the effect size. • Sample groups are formed based on extreme scores at the low or high scores (statistical regression). • Changes in the participants due to time (e.g., physiological and cognitive development). • Discontinuance rate (attrition or mortality).	• Use a random sampling method for selection and random assignment. • Conduct a sample size calculation before the study begins. • Match participants with high scores to those with low scores in the sample groups. • Use a research design with a control group or use a cross-sectional versus a longitudinal design. • A 20% discontinuance rate is acceptable with a comparable number from the intervention and control or comparison group. • Study completion needs to be based on attaining the sample size determined by a preliminary sample size calculation, which must account for the expected discontinuance rate.
	• Participants change their knowledge, values, or behavior because they are aware they are being studied (Hawthorne effect). • Participants experience a change in their disease or condition because they believe they have been given the intervention (placebo effect).	• Use a research design with a control group. • Use a research design with a control group.
Methods	• Repeated measurements using the same data collection instrument can sensitize participants' knowledge, values, or actions. • An occurrence outside of the study sensitizes the participants' knowledge, values, or actions. • Bias of the data collector. • Data collection instruments do not accurately measure the data. • Experimenter's characteristics (e.g., enthusiasm, age, gender) affect how the participant responds to the intervention.	• Use a research design with a control group or a posttest-only design. • Use a research design with a control group. • Use data collectors who are "blind" as to the assignment of participants in the intervention and control/comparison groups or use two data collectors. • Use calibrated equipment and a standard protocol to collect clinical data; validity is established for the data collection instrument. • Standardize the manner in which the intervention is provided using a script or an audio or visual (e.g., CD or DVD) presentation.

coefficient for ordinal data, and a Kuder-Richardson coefficient for dichotomous data.

Objectivity requires the researcher to remain unbiased, honest, and precise. The researcher must strive to avoid making unconscious choices when planning, conducting, and reporting the results of the study. Conducting research with a collaborative team is one way to control for objectivity, because a system of checks and balances can be employed among members of the team or multiple data collectors can be used to confirm each other's data. Another strategy is to use data collectors and researchers analyzing the data who are "**blind**" as to which group (the intervention or the comparison group) the participants are assigned.

Another aspect of objectivity is related to conflict of interest. A conflict of interest might occur if the author of a publication or his or her family members receive compensation with regard to the study. Many publishers require authors to disclose a conflict of interest related to the study. A declaration that there is no conflict of interest helps establish the trustworthiness of the evidence.

Table 11–2 lists the fours aspects of determining the trustworthiness of a quantitative study and general questions to ask as you are reading a research report. In addition, we provide you with a series of questions to assist you in your quest to determine the trustworthiness of a quantitative study (see **Table 11–3**).

CRITICAL APPRAISAL OF A QUANTITATIVE STUDY

Research reports describing quantitative studies are published in a variety of media, including print and online formats. Open access journals and sites allow free access to research reports. Some journals require a subscription for access, and practitioners who do not have access to the journals can pay a fee to view the report. Regardless of the journal or site in which a report appears, practitioners must understand three things about the publication process when appraising a study.

First, an article published in a **peer-reviewed** source is reviewed by experts in the discipline and judged worthy of publication. However, some health sciences disciplines make a distinction between peer-reviewed and **refereed publications**. A refereed publication is also reviewed by experts, but generally the publication is geared towards reporting primary research studies, systematic reviews, and meta-analyses. However, some peer-reviewed sources publish articles to inform professionals of information related to practice that are not high-level evidence. If your discipline makes this distinction, Ulrichsweb contains a list of refereed journals (note that a subscription is required to access information at http://ulrichsweb .serialssolutions.com).

Second, publishers have guidelines that authors adhere to when writing their manuscript. For instance, the CONSORT (CONsolidated Standards Of Reporting Trials) guidelines provide criteria for authors to use to report randomized controlled trials (RCTs). Furthermore, some guidelines specify a word limit such as 4,000 words. This limit poses a challenge to authors who want to publish very detailed reports of their study.

Third is the issue of publication bias, whereby those studies not reporting significant differences are not published at all or not in a timely fashion.

Table 11–2 Four Aspects of Determining the Trustworthiness of a Quantitative Study

Aspect of the Study	Question to Ask
Internal validity	Did the study accurately measure what it intended to measure?
External validity	Can the results be generalized to a population or to a real-life context?
Reliability	Were the data measured consistently?
Objectivity	Was the conduct of the study unbiased?

Table 11–3 Questions to Establish Trustworthiness of a Quantitative Study

Publication Section	Content	Questions	Appraisal (check one box)
Located on the first and/or last page of the publication	Authors' names, credentials, affiliations, and conflict of interest	• Are the authors' credentials and educational background appropriate to conduct this type of study? • Are the authors affiliated with an educational program, health institution, or practice setting? • Do the authors report a conflict of interest?	☐ Strength ☐ Limitation ☐ Not evident ☐ Not applicable
Presented on the first or last page of the publication	Funding source	• Does the funding source have a vested interest in a beneficial outcome of the study?	☐ Strength ☐ Limitation ☐ Not evident ☐ Not applicable
Introduction	Purpose	• Is the intent of the study clearly stated? • Are the variables being investigated identifiable? • Are the outcomes of the study identifiable? • Is the population under study identifiable?	☐ Strength ☐ Limitation ☐ Not evident ☐ Not applicable
Introduction	Hypotheses and research questions	• Are the hypotheses in alignment with the intended purpose? • Are the variables under study identifiable in the hypotheses (e.g., independent and dependent variables)? • Is one hypothesis written for each dependent variable under study? • Are the research questions in alignment with the intended purpose? • Are the variables under study identifiable in the research questions? • Is one question written for each variable under study?	☐ Strength ☐ Limitation ☐ Not evident ☐ Not applicable
Methods	Research design	• Is the design selected in alignment with the purpose? • Is the design appropriate to reach the stated outcome? • Is a control or comparison group used when its use strengthens the validity of the outcome? • Are the researchers blind to the assignment of participants (when it makes sense)? • Are the participants blind to their assignment (when it makes sense)? • Does the design limit the number of extraneous variables?	☐ Strength ☐ Limitation ☐ Not evident ☐ Not applicable

Table 11–3 (*continued*)

Publication Section	Content	Questions	Appraisal (check one box)
Methods	Sample	• Did the authors describe the population that the sample is intended to represent? • Was the sampling frame used appropriate for the purpose of the study? • Was the inclusion and exclusion criteria clearly described, and was it appropriate for the intended outcome? • Was the assignment of participants to treatment and control/comparison groups random or nonrandom, and was the method appropriate? • Was the sample size sufficient to include all applicable variability? • Was a sampling calculation discussed?	☐ Strength ☐ Limitation ☐ Not evident ☐ Not applicable
Methods	Research protocol	• Was the protocol for conducting the study described thoroughly and in enough detail? • Was the protocol followed appropriate for the purpose? • Did the study continue long enough to have valid outcomes? • Was the protocol consistently administered to the participants in each group? • Did the researchers take steps to control for extraneous variables? • Was the protocol ethical and approved by an Institutional Review Board (IRB)?	☐ Strength ☐ Limitation ☐ Not evident ☐ Not applicable
Methods	Data collection	• Were the data collection methods appropriate for the intended purpose of the study? • Were the data collection procedures consistently applied to the participants? • Was the validity and reliability of the data collection instrument established at a high enough level? • Was the reliability of the data collectors established at a high enough level?	☐ Strength ☐ Limitation ☐ Not evident ☐ Not applicable
Results	Sample	• Were important demographics of the intervention and control/comparison group similar and, if not, did it impact the results? • Were treatment and control groups similar at the baseline measurement of the outcome variables and, if not, did this difference impact the results? • How were eligible participants accounted for throughout the study?	☐ Strength ☐ Limitation ☐ Not evident ☐ Not applicable

(*continues*)

Table 11–3 (*continued*)

Publication Section	Content	Questions	Appraisal (check one box)
		• Was the discontinuance rate comparable between the treatment and control or comparison group?	
Results	Data analysis	• What did the power analysis indicate? • Were data analyzed using an on-protocol or intention-to-treat analysis, or both? • If intention-to-treat analysis was used, what method was used to input missing data? • Were the statistical analyses appropriate for the level of data (i.e., nominal, ordinal, interval or ratio)? • Were the statistical analyses appropriate to test the hypotheses and answer the research questions?	☐ Strength ☐ Limitation ☐ Not evident ☐ Not applicable
Results	Findings	• Are findings presented relative to each hypothesis and research question? • Are findings reported as statistically significant or not significant? • When confidence levels are reported, are the upper and lower limits acceptable to implement a change to your practice? • Do the findings have practical or clinical significance?	☐ Strength ☐ Limitation ☐ Not evident ☐ Not applicable
Discussion		• Did the researchers thoroughly explain their interpretation of the findings? • Were the explanations logical? • Did the researchers compare their findings to the findings of previous studies and provide a rationale on why they differ? • Did the researchers thoroughly identify and discuss the limitations? • What are the implications for practice? • What future research recommendations are made?	☐ Strength ☐ Limitation ☐ Not evident ☐ Not applicable
Conclusions		• Are the conclusions in alignment with the intended purpose of the study? • Do the conclusions logically follow from the findings and interpretation?	☐ Strength ☐ Limitation ☐ Not evident ☐ Not applicable

This situation leaves the professional without valuable scientific literature that should be used to make decisions within their healthcare setting. However, publication bias is not evident in every professional journal or open access site.

STRUCTURE OF A QUANTITATIVE RESEARCH REPORT

Most research reports follow a similar format for publication of quantitative investigations. One way to critically appraise the trustworthiness of a publication is to evaluate the structure of the publication. The first page of the report contains the title of the report and the authors' names, credentials, and affiliations. An abstract of the research follows and provides an overview of the purpose, methods, results, and conclusions. The first section of the report contains an introduction to the scientific literature related to the topic studied. This information establishes the need for this investigation based on knowledge gained from previous studies and the rationale for conducting the current study. By the end of the introduction, the purpose of the study should be readily identifiable.

The next section of the research report, the methods section, describes the methods used to conduct the study. The methods relate to the research design, sampling strategy, research protocol, data collection instruments, and procedures. The authors also address steps taken to establish validity and reliability. In addition, the methods describe the statistical analysis applied to the data. The findings of the statistical analysis are presented in the results section of the research report, along with a description of the participants completing the study and those who discontinued participation.

The discussion section is where the researchers provide an explanation of their interpretation of the findings. Also within this section, the results of the current study are compared to the results of previous studies to provide the reader with similarities and differences for comparison. The limitations are discussed in light of the methods used to conduct the study. Next, the implications for practice are described with regard to the findings and interpretation. Suggestions for future research are contained in this section or in the conclusions section. A conclusion is a judgment made by the researchers related to the purpose of the study based on the findings and interpretation. References used in the report are provided after the conclusions. At the beginning or end of the report, the acknowledgments, the authors' disclosure of a conflict of interest, and the source of funding, if any, can be found.

Now that you have an overview of the content of a research report, it is time to begin developing your critical-analysis skills to determine the trustworthiness of the quantitative study.

Critical Analysis

The first consideration for assessing the trustworthiness of the research report is the information about the authors. The authors' credentials and educational background should be appraised to determine whether they are appropriate for conducting the study. Furthermore, their affiliations with educational institutions, health institutions, or practice settings are considered, as well as their declaration of a conflict of interest. The second consideration is the source of funding for the study. The funding source is less trustworthy when the agency has a vested interest in the outcomes of the study. Consider the following example.[6]

Psychological Family Intervention for Poorly Controlled Type 2 Diabetes

Karen M. Keogh, PhD; Susan M. Smith, MD; Patricia White, PhD; Sinead McGilloway, PhD; Alan Kelly, PhD; James Gibney, MD; and Tom O'Dowd, MD.

Author Affiliations: From the Department of Public Health and Primary Care (KMK, SMS, PW, AK, TO), Trinity College, Dublin, Ireland; Department of Psychology (SM), National University of Ireland, Maynooth, Ireland; and Department of Endocrinology (JG), Trinity College, Dublin, Ireland.

Author Disclosures: The authors (KMK, SMS, PW, SM, AK, JG, TO) report no relationship or financial interest with any entity that would pose a conflict of interest with the subject matter of this article.

Funding Source: This study was funded by the Irish Health Research Board, project grant RP/2005/178.

All of the authors in this example have the educational background required to conduct the study. The strength of this research team is that it consists of interprofessional affiliations from a variety of disciplines, including public health, psychology, and endocrinology from an educational institution. None of the authors reported a conflict of interest. The funding source was a governmental agency that does not have a financial interest in the outcome. In comparison, let's say you are reading a study determining the effectiveness of two drugs manufactured by different drug companies. One of the drug companies funded the study, and the researcher who conducted the study disclosed that he was employed as a part-time consultant to the drug company providing the financial support. This information should send up a "red flag" to critically appraise the trustworthiness of the study very carefully.

As you read through the introduction to the research report, look for the purpose of the research. The intent of the study should be clearly stated, and the variables, outcomes, and population should be identifiable. Sometimes researchers include hypotheses or research questions. Hypotheses are usually presented in the null form; that is, that there is no statistically significant difference between the dependent variable in the experimental group and the control/comparison group. These hypotheses are found in studies that use parametric or nonparametric data analysis, such as experimental, quasi-experimental or **correlation studies**. Research questions are posed for studies analyzing data using descriptive statistics. Hypotheses and research questions need to be in alignment with the intent of the study. One hypothesis is written for each dependent variable under study. Likewise, one research question is written for each variable

being investigated. The following is an example from a study entitled "Web-Based Collaborative Care for Type 1 Diabetes: A Pilot Randomized Trial."[7]

The present trial sought to test the LWD [Living with Diabetes] program with a sample of moderately poorly controlled type 1 diabetes patients in an academic diabetes clinic. We hypothesized that intervention arm patients would experience larger reductions in A1C after 12 months of internet-based collaborative care compared to those receiving usual care. We also hypothesized a priori that intervention patients would report larger positive changes in diabetes-specific self-efficacy than patients receiving usual care.

The first sentence of the example contains the **purpose statement**, the Living with Diabetes intervention program and the poorly controlled type 1 diabetic population attending a university clinic. The second sentence presents the hypothesized outcome of the study related to A1C, and the third sentence states the hypothesized outcome for self-efficacy. This passage also indicates that the intervention group received usual diabetic care in conjunction with Internet-based collaborative care and the control group received usual care. Already the reader can be thinking about the next consideration for critical appraisal, the research design.

The research design should naturally follow from the intended purpose and outcome of the study. A stronger design is one that employs the use of a control or comparison group, which is double-blinded when it is possible, and that limits the number of extraneous variables affecting the validity of the outcome. Consider the following example from the previous study.[7]

The study was designed as a 12-month open-label, randomized, pretest–posttest pilot trial comparing usual care alone to usual care plus a Web-based collaborative care program.

The strength of this example is that it used a randomized approach to assigning the participants to the intervention and control group, the measurement of the two dependent variables at baseline (pretest) and at 12 months (posttest), and the use of a control group. An **open-label design** means that both the researchers and participants know to which group they were assigned. In this study, it would be impossible to employ the use of a double-blind study, because both the participants and the diabetes educator providing the intervention were aware of the Internet-based aspect of the study. To balance the effects of the open-label design, the participants in this study were randomly assigned to the intervention and control groups and allocation concealment was utilized with everyone except the study coordinator.[7]

> The allocation sequence was developed by the study statistician and programmed into an electronic database to conceal allocation from other study staff during recruitment . . . this assignment was not disclosed to participants until written informed consent had been given and all baseline data collection had been completed.

The method for selecting the sample is the next consideration when appraising scientific research. The population that the sample represents should be described, and the sampling frame should be appropriate for the intended outcome. The **inclusion criteria** are important to consider for determining whether the participants had the characteristics, diseases, or conditions to be studied. Likewise, the **exclusion criteria** eliminate potential participants with characteristics that would invalidate the research by introducing extraneous variables or exposing subjects to a contraindicated intervention. The following excerpt describes these criteria in detail.[8]

> Potential study participants were identified in the Diabetes Care clinic's electronic medical record. Patients between the ages of 21–49 years were eligible for inclusion in the study if they carried a diagnosis of type 1 diabetes, had two or more clinical encounters at the clinic and at least one AIC test result in the previous 12 months, had a most recent AIC value of 7%. . . . Potential participants were deemed ineligible during record review if they did not receive multiple daily injection therapy with insulin glargine, were currently receiving continuous subcutaneous insulin infusion (or were transitioning to pump therapy), were terminally ill, had documentation of significant mental illness or substance abuse in their charts, or did not speak and read English.

The assignment of participants to the intervention and control group should be completed using some method of **randomization**. The sample size should be sufficient to include variability of the participants' characteristics. The following description is the sampling procedure for a pilot study using a table of random numbers to assign blocks of patients to the experimental and control groups until a moderate size sample of 122 patients was obtained.[9]

> After consent and baseline data have been collected from the first 40 patients, they will be randomized into intervention and control groups by using computer generated random number tables. The main investigators will not be involved in the randomisation procedure, which will be carried out by an independent expert. The use of block randomisation means that the intervention can be delivered in a staggered manner, with some participants beginning the intervention while further recruitment continues. When the next 40 patients are recruited, they will then be randomly allocated to intervention or control groups, and so on, until 122 patients are included in the trial.

Another example of randomization is addressed in the statement, ". . . patients entering phase 2 of the study were randomized within each practice by flip of a coin to either the integrated care intervention or usual care."[8]

In the pilot study, the sample size calculation was discussed and the rationale for selecting 122 participants was provided.[9]

Taking HbA1c and Diabetes Well-being as primary outcomes, a total sample size of 76 and 86 respectively, were calculated. This was using 80% power to detect a significant *absolute* change of 0.9% in glycaemic control (this absolute change has been related to clinical outcomes in the UK prospective diabetes study, [3] and of 3 points in the Diabetes Well-being Scale-12. These calculations also allow for an anticipated "Hawthorne effect" relating to an improvement of 20% for those in the control group, by virtue of the fact that they are participating in the research. Taking the larger number of 86 participants (43 in intervention and 43 in control group), a final total number of 122 participants (61 in each group) is needed to ensure at least a 70% final response rate is met.

When a sample size calculation is not described, a power analysis can be calculated and presented with the results. Consider the following excerpt.[7]

Given the enrolled sample size, the trial had sufficient statistical power (80%) to detect a difference in A1C change of 0.65% between study groups and 99% power to detect a treatment difference of 1.0%, similar to that seen in an earlier trial of the intervention in patients with type 2 diabetes.

As the critical appraisal of the research report continues, the research protocol is evaluated to determine whether the procedures for conducting the study were described thoroughly and in enough detail for the study to be replicated in the future. The following example provides the research protocol in some detail and also refers the reader to more detail published in an intervention manual. Other criteria to consider are whether the protocol was appropriate for the intended purpose of the study, whether the study continued long enough to have valid outcomes, and whether the protocol was consistently administered to the participants in each group. Read the following example to get an idea of a research protocol.[6]

Purpose: To assess the effectiveness of a psychological family-based intervention for patients with poorly controlled type 2 diabetes.
Research Protocol: The intervention consisted of 3 weekly sessions delivered by a health psychologist (KMK) who had received 16 hours of training in motivational interviewing. The first 2 sessions lasted 45 minutes each and took place in the patient's home with their family member. The third session involved a 10–15-minute follow-up telephone call. Intervention sessions were individually tailored to participants' needs and attempted to (1) challenge and clarify any inaccurate and/or negative perceptions about diabetes, (2) examine how these perceptions influenced self-management, and (3) develop written personalized action plans to improve self-management and mobilize family support. The intervention used techniques from health psychology[18] and motivational interviewing[19] such as exchanging information, eliciting change talk, reducing resistance, building self-efficacy, problem solving, and goal setting/action planning. Details are published in the intervention manual.[17] Both the intervention and control groups continued to receive their usual diabetes care.

An assessment of the steps the researcher implemented to control for extraneous variables includes training the individual or individuals who were providing the intervention, as the previous example describes, or by showing how the person has expertise with the intervention, as depicted in the following statement: "The nurse case manager for this study (G.L.) is an advanced registered nurse practitioner with 25 years of experience as a certified diabetes educator and 10 years of experience as a primary care practitioner in diabetes."[7]

Another consideration for the research protocol is whether it is ethical and has been approved by an **Institutional Review Board** (**IRB**) or ethics committee. Any institution receiving federal money must have a formal body responsible for ensuring the protection of human rights and the conduct of ethical research according to federal codes and HIPAA (Health Insurance Portability and Accountability Act) guidelines. The following statements inform the reader that the research protocol was reviewed and approved by an appropriate body, in these cases an Institutional Review Board[8] and an ethics committee.[10]

> The protocol was approved by the University of Pennsylvania Institutional Review Board.
>
> This study was approved by the Huntingdon local research ethics committee and was carried out in accordance with the principles of the 1996 Helsinki declaration.

The data collection methods are the next component of the research report to be critically appraised. The criteria include the appropriateness of the methods with regard to the intended purpose of the study, whether the methods were consistently applied to the participants, and whether the data collection instruments were valid and reliable. In the following example, data collection methods were in alignment with the purpose of the study. Also, data were collected according to a monitoring system in the cap of the medication bottle to determine drug adherence. Guidelines were used to assess glycemic control, and the validity and reliability of the point-of-care device to record HbA1c levels was determined. However, the authors did not present the validity and reliability of the Patient Health Questionnaire.[8]

> ***Purpose:*** The objective of this study was to examine whether a simple, brief integrated approach to depression and type 2 diabetes mellitus (type 2 diabetes) treatment improved adherence to oral hypoglycemic agents and antidepressant medications, glycemic control, and depression among primary care patients.
>
> ***Data Collection:*** Adherence to antidepressants and oral hypoglycemic agents was measured at 6 and 12 weeks using electronic-monitoring data obtained from Medication Event Monitoring System (MEMS) cap on the drug container. At baseline and 12 weeks blood glycemic control was assessed in accordance with American Diabetes Association Guidelines.[35] HbA1c assays were performed using the in2it A1C Analyzer (Bio-Rad Laboratories,

> Hercules, California). Point-of-care testing using this device has acceptable precision and agreement in comparison with laboratory services.[36] Depressive symptoms were measured using the 9-item Patient Health Questionnaire (PHQ-9) at baseline, 6, and 12 weeks.

Another criterion for data collection is that the data collectors were reliable. In the previous example, more detail about the manner in which the HbA1c device was consistently used to collect data from participants would have strengthened this component of the study.

The results section of the research report is the next section to be critically analyzed based on reporting the sample characteristics, data analysis, and findings. The sample is appraised to determine the demographics of the intervention and control groups at baseline and whether the two groups were similar related to the variables being measured. The demographic information is usually presented in a table with the mean and standard deviation for age, along with the percentage of male/female participants, ethnic background, and educational level for the intervention and control groups. Other sample data can be included in the same table to establish that both groups were similar at the start of the study. For instance, in the study presented in the previous example baseline measures were reported on each of the dependent variables, including HbA1c level, depression score on the Patient Health Questionnaire, the number of medications, and functional and cognitive status scores.[8] Readers are able to view the information on the table to determine for themselves the validity of the researchers' statement: "Baseline characteristics of patients in the integrated care intervention did not differ significantly from those of patients in the usual care group."[8]

Next, the researchers need to clearly establish how the eligible participants were accounted for during and at the end of the study. The best method for presenting this information is in a figure. As an example, **Figure 11–1** presents a diagram that clearly tracks the participant flow

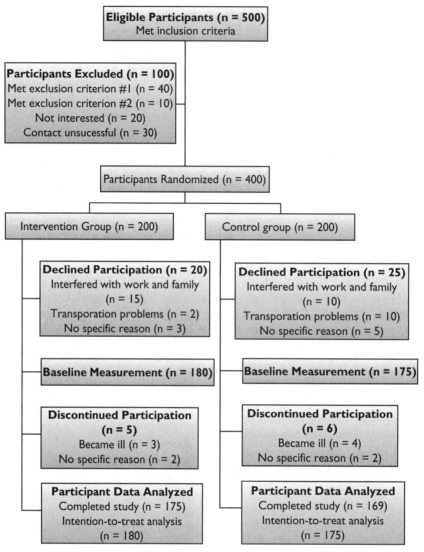

Figure 11–1 Participant Flow Diagram

throughout the entire study. From the information on the diagram, the reader can discern the number of individuals who discontinued participation from the intervention and control groups, determine the reasons, and ascertain if the rate was similar for both groups. When the rate is not comparable, the researchers should address the reasons for more dropouts from the intervention or the control group.

The last box in the diagram in Figure 11–1 presents the analyzed participant data and reports the number of participants who completed the study

and the intention-to-treat number. These two numbers represent two ways to analyze data by employing an on-protocol analysis or an intention-to-treat analysis. An **on-protocol** (also referred to as **per-protocol**) analysis uses data from participants who completed the study, whereas an **intention-to-treat analysis** uses methods to input missing data from participants who dropped out of the study. A criticism of the on-protocol analysis is that it introduces bias to the results in a better outcome for the intervention group because those participants who respond to the intervention are more likely to complete the study.[5] In contrast, the intention-to-treat analysis might bias the outcome of the intervention group because the method used to input the missing data can underestimate the intervention effects.[5] One method used to input missing continuous data is to carry forward the last measurement of the variable to the end of the study.[5] For example, if the participant's HbA1c level was measured at the 6-month interval and then the participant withdrew from the study, the 6-month measurement would be used in the 12-month data analysis. Another method to input missing data is to do a follow-up with participants who withdrew and measure the outcome even though they did not complete the intervention and include it in the data analysis. This method is deemed to represent the real-life situation that occurs in practice when patients do not adhere to treatment.[5]

The most conservative approach to data analysis is to use both the on-protocol and intention-to-treat analytic methods on the same data. When results of both analyses are consistent, the reader has more confidence in the findings. This tells us that the dropouts did not affect the outcome. When the analyses produce different findings, the researchers need to discuss the reasons for the differences.[5]

Another aspect of data analysis is appraising the appropriateness of the statistical analysis based on the level of data collected and whether the assumptions of the statistical test were met. For instance, when a *t*-test or ANOVA is used, the data have to be at the interval/ratio level and the assumption of normal distribution of the data must be met; otherwise, a nonparametric statistical analysis needs to be applied to the data. In addition, the statistical analysis must be appropriate to test the hypotheses or answer the research question(s). Hypotheses that express a cause-and-effect relationship are analyzed using statistical tests that compare outcomes of the intervention and control group or that compare the pretest measurements with the posttest measurements. Hypotheses that determine relationships are tested with correlation statistical analyses.

The results of the study are presented relative to each hypothesis and research question. Findings based on statistical analyses should be reported as significant or not significant. When confidence levels are reported, the upper and lower limits must be acceptable to implement the intervention. Another consideration is to determine whether the results, even though they might be statistically significant, are clinically significant enough to implement the intervention.

The results are usually presented in a table or other visual means to provide detailed information about the outcomes and support the findings written in the body of the research report. These representations need to have clear titles and identification of the information they portray.

The discussion section of the research report describes the researchers' interpretation of the results. The interpretation should be a logical explanation of *why* the outcomes of the study were achieved. The results of the current study are compared to previous studies, and when they differ an explanation is provided. The following excerpt is an interpretation of the results of a 3-year investigation on a self-management education program for participants with type 2 diabetes.[10]

Statistical analyses for this study were undertaken using intention-to-treat analysis, minimising bias in the reported findings. However, our study may have been underpowered to detect improvements in clinical outcomes and as a result some of our findings may be prone to type 2 error. Response rates of the study were higher than expected after 3 years of follow-up, with collection of biomedical data achieved by 83% of participants and questionnaire data by 70%, minimizing missing data and the effect this may have had on the interpretation of the study results. This compares positively with other self management education interventions that obtained long term follow-up data from 63% to 85% of the original participants.[33,35,36] Those who were followed up at 3 years were older, healthier, and less depressed at baseline than those who were not followed up. This selection bias should be considered when interpreting the results, although importantly there was no interaction with the intervention group. Additionally, missing data on individuals may have less impact in a cluster randomised trial than in an individually randomised trial.

The discussion should include an identification of the limitations that affected the outcome of the study. The researchers should critically analyze their study to determine the limitations and report them in sufficient detail. The limitations can provide suggestions for future research, as depicted in the following example.[6]

The study was not powered to detect whether there were any differences in outcomes depending on the family relationship [spouse or children], and this factor may be an area for future research. . . . Finally, it must be noted that the delivery of this intervention was challenging and time consuming, due in part to the difficulties in accessing participants despite repeated efforts.

The discussion also addresses the implications for practice, as the following example illustrates.[8]

Our study provides a sustainable solution that can be implemented in primary care or other settings for patients managing multiple medical conditions and varying degrees of complexity in pharmacotherapeutic regimens. . . . [I]nterventions that allow for tailoring content and providing tools to match the individualized needs of patients are needed. . . . Our results call for greater emphasis within health care systems and policy organizations on the development and promotion of clinical programs to enhance medication adherence, particularly among patients with chronic medical conditions and depression.

The last component in a research report is the conclusions. The statements made in the conclusions section should be in alignment with the purpose of the study and follow logically from the results and interpretation.

SYSTEMATIC REVIEWS AND META-ANALYSES

Access to systematic reviews and meta-analyses has increased as the number of research reports has become overwhelming for healthcare professionals to critically appraise during EBP. Systematic reviews and meta-analyses are at the top level of the evidence pyramid because multiple research studies are analyzed in these types of publications. The usefulness of a systematic review in the evidence-based process differs from that of a traditional literature review. A traditional literature review typically discusses all of the literature on a topic, a strategy that strengthens the breadth of the review; however, it does not provide an in-depth analysis to the professional who is trying to answer a PPAARE-focused question. The *traditional* review analyzes the literature in an unsystematic manner, whereas a systematic review uses established criteria for inclusion of studies and for determining the quality of the studies in the review. In addition, a systematic review has predetermined methods to identify studies and assess their quality. Studies must meet the criteria for quality to be included in the analysis. After analyzing and synthesizing the studies, the authors present their findings. These findings are considered a higher level of evidence based on the process of reviewing multiple independent studies. After a systematic review is conducted and several studies are deemed to have similar methodology, a meta-analysis can be applied to these studies. A meta-analysis is a statistical computation to combine the data analysis of multiple individual studies.

As an example, let us consider the following example (adapted from Patten[11]). We review four RCTs on a new intervention where three of four RCTs report a statistically significant difference between the experimental and control groups. In a traditional literature review, this finding would be reported as the intervention being effective in three of four studies. In a systematic review, the four studies would only be included if they met the inclusion criteria and were evaluated as meeting the criteria for quality.

To continue this discussion, let's say that all four of the studies were included in the systematic review and that each RCT used the same data collection instrument and similar methods to conduct the study. In each RCT, 100 participants were assigned to both the experimental and control groups, resulting in a total of 200 participants per study and a grand total of 800 for the four studies. If the mean difference between the experimental group and the control group (subtract the mean of the experimental group from the mean of the control group) for RCT 1 was 10, RCT 2 was 14, RCT 3 was 5, and RCT 4 was –5, the meta-analysis computation would add all of the RCTs' mean differences together (10 + 14 + 5 + –5 = 24) and then divide the total by the number of studies (24/4 = 6). The average of the four studies based on 800 participants would be reported as 6. This finding would be more precise than considering the findings of any one of the four studies.

This example illustrates the simplest procedure for statistical computation for a meta-analysis; however, some computations involve studies using different data collection instruments measuring the same variable but having different ranges of scores. For instance, consider a meta-analysis that includes two RCTs with the same number of participants in each study, with one study reporting the mean difference between the experimental group and control group as 50 (based on a range of possible scores from 0–100) and the other reporting the mean difference as 40 (based on a range of possible scores from 0–50). In order to equalize the different means and standard deviations for these two measurements, **Cohen's *d*** is computed to determine the effect size for each study. The statistical computation of the meta-analysis involves adding the *d* of each study and calculating an average *d* representing the effect size of the combined studies. The values for the effect size lie between –3 to +3. When *d* is ± 0.20 it is considered a small effect size, 0.50 means a medium effect size, 0.80 indicates a large effect size, 1.10 is considered a very large effect size, and any value above 1.40 indicates an extremely large effect size.[11] When sample sizes are different among studies,

further statistical computations must be calculated by weighting the studies according to the number of participants. Effect size also can be expressed as effect size **r** (**Pearson correlation coefficient**) or as r^2 (the coefficient of determination). A forest plot is the most common way to report the results of a meta-analysis.

For the EBP novice, further discussion of statistical computations used for meta-analyses is not warranted. As you move to a higher level of experience with this process, other resources can be consulted to learn more about meta-analysis computations. The novice needs to understand the process for conducting a systematic review as the precursor to a meta-analysis.

Process for Conducting a Systematic Review and Meta-Analysis

The process for conducting a systematic review and meta-analysis should use a predetermined protocol to:

- Establish that there is no conflict of interest between the authors and the funding source.
- Establish clear objectives to determine the purpose of the review and to identify the variables being considered.
- Establish search methods to locate relevant evidence (e.g., databases and search words).
- Establish eligibility criteria for selection of studies to be included in the review to avoid the limitations of publication bias and of publications in other languages besides English (e.g., RCTs; observational studies; qualitative studies; unpublished works, such as dissertations; and language of studies).
- Establish eligibility criteria for selection of studies related to the participants' characteristics, types of interventions, and outcome measures.
- Establish methods for determining the quality of the studies based on specified criteria (e.g., at least two independent reviewers

and a procedure to resolve differences when the reviewers do not agree).

- Establish a systematic method for extracting the data from the studies.
- Assess each study for risk of bias and report this information in the review.
- Establish methods for the synthesis of combining the findings of multiple studies.
- Analyze the effect size of multiple studies in a meta-analysis when further analysis is warranted.
- Establish methods for reporting the results of the systematic review or meta-analysis.
- Integrate the findings into the discussion to help the reader understand the current knowledge base in the context of the focused question it answers.

A rigorous protocol for creating systematic reviews and meta-analyses has been established by the Cochrane Collaboration. The working groups within the Cochrane Collaboration are dedicated to publishing high-quality, nonbiased publications; therefore, Cochrane-produced systematic reviews and meta-analyses are considered the "gold standard" for EBP. These types of evidence also are found in journals and open source sites; however, the quality of the protocol followed should be evaluated. Two instruments have been developed for this purpose. One measurement tool, AMSTAR (Assessment of Multiple Systematic Reviews), evaluates evidence using a series of 11 questions.[12,13] PRISMA (Preferred Reporting Items for Systematic Reviews and Meta-analyses) is more detailed, featuring a checklist that contains 27 items.[14] You can search PubMed to learn more about these tools, including their validity and reliability in determining the quality of the document and the application of these tools to your discipline.

COMPARISON OF QUANTITATIVE AND QUALITATIVE RESEARCH

To begin this discussion on quantitative and qualitative research, consider two sports, baseball and basketball. Both are games played with round balls.

The purpose of hitting the ball in baseball is to make a home run or to get the players on the bases home to score points. The uniforms in baseball consist of long pants to protect the players from sliding into bases and cleats to help the player maneuver in the dirt. The equipment needed to play the game is a bat, mitt, and a small, white, round ball. The strategy employed to play the game is very calculated, as the batting lineup is created to position the team to have the best possible chance of winning the game. In comparison, the purpose of playing basketball is to get the ball through the hoop to score points. The uniforms consist of shorts and sneakers to help players maneuver on the smooth-surface floor. The equipment used to play the game is a large orange ball. The strategy used to play the game is based on predetermined plays, but when the players are on the court their strategies are adapted to the moment of what is happening.

Both sports are unique based on the purpose, uniforms, equipment, and strategies for playing the game. Baseball is not better than basketball, and basketball is not better than baseball; they are different. The same analogy can be made between quantitative and qualitative research. Both types of research are unique in their purpose, research design, sampling strategies, data collection methods, and data analysis. Quantitative research is not better than qualitative research, and qualitative research is not better than quantitative research; they are different.

In fact, a recent trend in conducting healthcare research is to employ a mixed methods approach whereby the researcher uses a combination of quantitative and qualitative methods in the same study to collect data. Both methods of data collection can be employed simultaneously (i.e., concurrent mixed methods) or one after the other (i.e., sequential mixed methods).[15] The benefit of using a mixed methods approach is that the strengths of the quantitative methods and qualitative methods are combined to result in more comprehensive findings. In addition, the results of the quantitative portion of the study can verify the qualitative findings. The limitations of both methods

Table 11–4 Comparison of Methods to Establish Trustworthiness

Quantitative Research	Qualitative Research
Internal validity	Credibility
External validity	Transferability
Reliability	Dependability
Objectivity	Objectivity

can, "neutralize or cancel the biases of" the other method.[15] A mixed methods research design combines the best of both research paradigms, potentially, as well as their limitations.

Furthermore, establishing the trustworthiness of a qualitative study differs from the previous discussion on appraising the trustworthiness of a quantitative study. **Table 11–4** compares the components of trustworthiness for both research paradigms. Notice that the last component is the same. Objectivity in the qualitative paradigm is a deviation from the original presented by Lincoln and Guba,[1] who used the term *confirmability*. This decision to change the last component from the original term used by Lincoln and Guba is based on the previous discussion about the differences between baseball and basketball. Objectivity in qualitative research is different because the data collection instrument is the researcher and the data analysis is the researcher's interpretation of the participants' experiences. The qualitative researcher can take steps to examine his or her own personal biases in the collection and analysis of data. These strategies will be discussed in the next section.

APPRAISE THE TRUSTWORTHINESS OF QUALITATIVE EVIDENCE

The trustworthiness of qualitative evidence is necessary to determine if it is worthy of being used in making an evidence-based decision about a healthcare action. Critical appraisal establishes the strengths and limitations of the evidence reported

in the research report. When the strengths outweigh the limitations, the evidence is used to make decisions.

Judging the trustworthiness of a qualitative inquiry is based on credibility, transferability, dependability, and objectivity. **Credibility** establishes that data collection and interpretation are plausible.[1] Two strategies can be used to establish the credibility of the data collected. One strategy, **prolonged engagement**, is for the researcher to be in the field for an extended period of time to establish rapport and gain the trust of participants so that they feel comfortable disclosing their experiences during data collection.[1] In addition, collecting data for a longer period of time provides a broader perspective on the phenomenon being studied. The second strategy, **persistent observation**, is being immersed in data collection long enough to provide depth to the data collected on the phenomenon.[1] Researchers might use an approach to collect data until saturation occurs. **Saturation** occurs when new data are no longer emerging to contribute to the analysis and the analysis is well defined and demonstrates variation.[16]

Strategies to establish the credibility of the interpretation of the data include using **member checks**, a **peer reviewer**, **triangulation**, or a **negative case**.[1] Member checks can be the best way to establish credibility[1] because the participants are verifying that the researcher's analysis and interpretation of their experiences is accurate. For instance, the following two questions can be asked of the research participants: (1) Is the interpretation of your statements accurate? (2) Does the final analysis make sense based on your experiences? In a qualitative study, the peer reviewer's role is to ask hard questions about the researcher's data collection and analysis methods and to play devil's advocate and push the researcher to consider alternatives.[17] Triangulation as a strategy to establish credibility involves using (1) multiple and different participants to collect data, (2) multiple and different methods (e.g., using a combination of interviewing, focus groups, observations, and document review),

(3) multiple researchers to collect and analyze the data, and (4) multiple theories in the data interpretation.[18] Triangulation of data from multiple participants can be established by using a strategy called the **constant comparative method**. During the employment of this method, interview data are analyzed after each participant's interview and the data from one interview are compared to the data from the other interviews; therefore, data collection and analysis occur simultaneously.[19] Another strategy is to use **theoretical sampling** to gain more depth to the data analysis by re-interviewing participants or purposefully seeking out and interviewing participants who can provide a different perspective on the phenomenon. Some researchers seek out a negative case that represents a participant's alternative perspective to challenge data analysis.[1] This different perspective can confirm or disconfirm the data analysis and provide a means to consider other explanations.[1]

The qualitative report provides examples of quotations from participants to support the data analysis and to have the reader make decisions about the **transferability** of the findings to his or her own setting and situation. The quotations provide rich descriptions that, in turn, evoke feelings of having experienced the phenomenon under study.[17] Reading the rich descriptions from the participants' experiences is helpful for healthcare professionals to understand the phenomenon from a variety of perspectives; therefore, it is the readers of the research report who judge whether the findings are applicable to their context.[1] The researcher is responsible for providing the richly detailed descriptions that make the transferable judgments possible for the reader.[1]

Dependability is an assessment of the quality of the consistency of the data collected with the interpretation of the data during analysis procedures. The researcher can record decisions made throughout the analysis as an **audit trail**. Researchers can document their thoughts, decisions, questions, and interpretations as they are immersed in making sense of the data by writing memos to themselves or writing entries in a journal. This documentation can be useful to a peer reviewer or an external auditor who can read and understand the thought process of the researcher in arriving at the interpretation of the participants' experiences.

Objectivity is vital to data collection and interpretation because the researcher is the instrument used to collect and analyze the data. Qualitative researchers need to engage in **reflexivity,** which is a practice that requires critical self-reflection to become conscious of views and perspectives that might influence the inquiry.[20] Disclosure of this self-awareness should be transparent to help the reader of the research report to understand the researcher's perspective and the lens through which the data were collected and interpreted.[20] Objectivity in the data analysis can be established when at least two researchers or two research teams independently analyze the data and then negotiate their differences.

Table 11-5 presents general questions to appraise the trustworthiness of a qualitative study. **Table 11-6** contains detailed questions about each component of a research report to use in determining the overall trustworthiness of the inquiry.

CRITICAL ANALYSIS OF A QUALITATIVE STUDY

Qualitative research reports are found in the same media and follow the same structure

Table 11-5 Four Aspects of Determining the Trustworthiness of a Qualitative Inquiry

Aspect	Question to Ask
Credibility	Is the data collection and interpretation credible?
Transferability	Can these findings be applied beyond the context and participants of this inquiry?
Dependability	Is the interpretation of the data consistent with the actual data collected?
Objectivity	Did the researchers engage in reflexivity and make their self-disclosure transparent?

Table 11–6 Questions to Establish Trustworthiness of a Qualitative Inquiry

Publication Section	Content	Questions	Appraisal (check one box)
Located on the first page of the publication	Authors' names, credentials, affiliations, and conflict of interest	• Are the authors' credentials and educational background appropriate to conduct this type of study? • Are the authors affiliated with an educational program, health institution, or practice setting? • Do the authors report a conflict of interest?	☐ Strength ☐ Limitation ☐ Not evident ☐ Not applicable
Presented on the first or last page of the publication	Funding source	• Does the funding source have a vested interest in a beneficial outcome of the study?	☐ Strength ☐ Limitation ☐ Not evident ☐ Not applicable
Introduction	Purpose	• Is the intent of the study clearly stated? • Is the phenomenon being investigated identifiable? • Is the population identifiable?	☐ Strength ☐ Limitation ☐ Not evident ☐ Not applicable
Introduction	Research questions	• Are the research questions in alignment with the intended purpose? • Is the phenomenon under study identifiable in a broad research question?	☐ Strength ☐ Limitation ☐ Not evident ☐ Not applicable
Methods	Qualitative approach	• Is the rationale for using a qualitative approach explained? • Is the qualitative approach in alignment with the intended purpose (e.g., ethnography, biography, phenomenology, case study, grounded theory)?	☐ Strength ☐ Limitation ☐ Not evident ☐ Not applicable
Methods	Sample	• Was a sampling method or multiple methods used to identify participants who could inform the study (e.g., purposive sampling, snowball or network sampling, theoretical sampling)? • How did the researchers attempt to gain variation within the sample? • Were the inclusion and exclusion criteria clearly described, and were they appropriate for the purpose of the study?	☐ Strength ☐ Limitation ☐ Not evident ☐ Not applicable
Methods	Data collection protocol	• Were data collection methods appropriate for the intended purpose of the study (e.g., interviews, focus groups, observations, document review)? • Was the protocol for conducting the study described thoroughly and in enough detail? • Were data collection procedures consistently applied to the participants of the study • Did the data collector have sufficient qualifications and training? • Were data collected long enough to have saturation?	☐ Strength ☐ Limitation ☐ Not evident ☐ Not applicable

(continues)

Table 11–6 (continued)

Publication Section	Content	Questions	Appraisal (check one box)
		• Was the protocol ethical and approved by an Institutional Review Board (IRB)? • What steps were taken to ensure the confidentiality and anonymity of the participants? • What steps were taken to ensure credibility and objectivity during data collection?	
Results	Sample	• Were the participants' characteristics described in enough detail to understand how they contributed to the data? • Were the participants' experiences with the phenomenon varied?	☐ Strength ☐ Limitation ☐ Not evident ☐ Not applicable
Results	Data analysis	• What steps were taken to ensure that the interview or focus group data were transcribed verbatim? • How were the data coded? • How were categories and themes constructed? • How were interrelationships established and a theory constructed (i.e., grounded theory approach)? • What steps were taken to ensure credibility, dependability, and objectivity during data analysis?	☐ Strength ☐ Limitation ☐ Not evident ☐ Not applicable
Results	Findings	• Are the themes or theory presented in an understandable manner? • Are the findings supported by quotations from the participants to facilitate transferability? • Are findings presented relative to the intended purpose and each research question?	☐ Strength ☐ Limitation ☐ Not evident ☐ Not applicable
Discussion		• Did the researchers thoroughly explain their interpretation of the findings? • Were the explanations logical? • Did the researchers describe the contribution of their study to understanding the phenomenon? • Did the researchers discuss how their findings are related to previous studies and theories in their own discipline and, when appropriate, other disciplines? • Did the researchers thoroughly identify and discuss the limitations? • What are the implications for practice? • What future research recommendations are made?	☐ Strength ☐ Limitation ☐ Not evident ☐ Not applicable
Conclusions		• Are the conclusions in alignment with the intended purpose of the study? • Do the conclusions logically follow from the findings?	☐ Strength ☐ Limitation ☐ Not evident ☐ Not applicable

as their quantitative counterparts. Qualitative research articles tend to be exposed to greater levels of publication bias based on a preference for generalizable research results (which are native to quantitative research) among healthcare publications. In some health disciplines, qualitative research is not valued as much as in other disciplines; therefore, manuscripts reporting qualitative research might be rejected or their publication delayed. Other forms of publication bias result from word limits. A researcher who wants to provide richly detailed quotations from participants to support findings is severely limited by a low word count.

The critical appraisal questions to determine the trustworthiness of a qualitative research report were presented in Table 11–6. The first two items on the table, author information and funding source, are evaluated in the same manner as a quantitative study; therefore, refer back to the discussion on appraisal of quantitative studies. The introduction to the report generally states the intended purpose of the study and might include a broad research question. The phenomenon and population under study should be clearly identifiable in the purpose and research question. The following example states the purpose of a grounded theory inquiry and identifies the phenomenon ("how they consult with individuals with both diabetes and obesity and how they handle these concerns") and the population ("healthcare professionals").[21] The next example states the purpose of the study as well as a broad research question. Not all qualitative studies include a research question. The phenomenon under study is the "lived experience with diabetes" and the population is "Hispanic migrant farmworkers."[22]

> The aim of this study was to generate a theory grounded in empirical data derived from a deeper understanding of healthcare professionals' main concerns when they consult with individuals with both diabetes and obesity and how they handle these concerns.

> Through the use of the phenomenological approach, the researchers studied the lived experience of Hispanic migrant farmworkers with diabetes. In phenomenological inquiry, the researchers identify the meaning of human experiences concerning a phenomenon as described by the participants in the study (Moustakas, 1994). In this study, the research question was, "What is the lived experience of a Hispanic migrant farmworker diagnosed with diabetes?"

The next section in a qualitative research report to critically analyze is the methods section; this is where the researchers discuss the qualitative approach, the sampling strategies, and the data collection procedures. The rationale for selecting a qualitative approach should be explained, and this approach should be in alignment with the purpose of the study. The following excerpt from the grounded theory study provides the rationale for selecting this approach to study the phenomenon. Note that the methods are in alignment with the purpose stated in the previous example.[21]

> The method that was considered appropriate for this study was the classical version of grounded theory (GT; Glaser & Strauss, 1967). The method aims to inductively produce new knowledge to generate concepts, models, or theories that explain what is happening in the studied area. . . . The author's interest in diabetes care arose from her experience with the difficulties people with diabetes and obesity have with weight loss; she found that the situation was difficult for both individuals and health care professionals, e.g., nurses. This indicated a need for a better understanding of the main needs of the situation, and a qualitative approach seemed to offer the tools necessary to find new angles on the problem.

Sampling techniques for qualitative inquiries vary, and it behooves the researcher to describe the sampling methods used to identify and select the participants. **Purposive sampling** is a technique to recruit participants who have experience with the phenomenon being studied to thus provide valuable data. Another technique is **network sampling**, whereby others inform the researcher of potential participants. In addition, inclusion and exclusion criteria need to be clearly stated. Variation within the sample is the best way to provide a breadth of experiences on the phenomenon. The following description from a study on self-monitoring and diabetes contains these components.[23]

Patients with type 1 diabetes were recruited from the outpatient clinic of a general hospital in the Netherlands, and patients with type 2 diabetes from general practices in the same region (Isala Clinics Zwolle, the Netherlands). Eligibility criteria were: a diagnosis of type 1 or type 2 diabetes, treated with insulin, self-monitoring of blood glucose (SMBG) carried out for a minimum of 1 year, Dutch speaking, and over the age of 18. The initial selection focused on building a patient population with as much variation as possible in the factors relating to SMBG. Physicians and diabetes specialized nurses were asked to select patients who differed in age, gender, living status, education, type of diabetes, insulin therapy, duration of SMBG, and employment.

The data collection methods are another important component of the methods section to critically appraise. The reader needs to assess whether the methods used by the researchers were appropriate for the intended purpose of the inquiry and whether the protocol for conducting the study was described thoroughly and in enough detail to replicate the study. The data collection procedures should be consistently applied to the participants. Using a focus group or interview guide helps the researchers ask similar questions; however, probing questions are asked as a follow-up strategy to gain more depth to the participants' experiences. Taking notes during these sessions is a common practice; summarizing the session or having a debriefing meeting immediately following data collection is another strategy. The focus group facilitator and the interviewer need to have sufficient qualifications and training to gather the breadth and depth of experiences on which the analysis is

based. The following passage from a study of diabetes and depression exemplifies these criteria.[24]

Purpose: The co-occurrence of depression and diabetes is not only common but can influence symptom appraisal, explanatory models, help-seeking, self-care behaviors, and treatment adherence. In order to understand how Hispanics manage diabetes and depression and develop better services, it is important to examine how these individuals make sense and cope with these two conditions in their everyday lives.

Data Collection: Focus groups were held at participants' primary care clinics. Each focus group, ranging from 3 to 6 participants, lasted approximately an hour and a half. The first author, a bilingual researcher with a Ph.D. in social work and trained in qualitative methods, facilitated all focus groups. A trained bilingual doctoral student in social work served as note taker and observer for these focus groups. The focus group guide was informed by our review of the literature and consultations with experts in qualitative methods and mental health services research. . . .

Ten individual interviews were done either in person at the participants' primary care clinic (n = 7) or by telephone (n = 3) and lasted approximately an hour. Both the first and second authors conducted these interviews. The interview guide included themes explored in the focus group guide as well as new themes (i.e., stigma, attitudes and knowledge of depression and its treatments) that emerged from our preliminary analysis of focus group interviews. Focus group and interview guides are available upon request. Interviewers also completed interview summaries after each interview briefly describing their personal observations and interview process for both focus group and individual interviews.

Data collection needs to continue long enough for saturation to occur. The following excerpts are examples of continuing data collection until saturation is reached.[21,22,25]

After seven interviews, signs of similarities in the information appeared; however, another three interviews were conducted to reach saturation.

Theoretical sampling continued until no new ideas arose which were of value to the developing theory, and saturation was reached.

After the seventh focus group, no new themes were identified, suggesting a saturation of themes had been reached.

The protocol for the inquiry should be assessed to ensure that it was ethical and approved by an IRB, demonstrated in the first example below.[26] The researchers also should show that they took steps to ensure the participants' confidentiality and anonymity, as demonstrated by the second example.[22]

Before the discussion, the interview facilitators explained to the participants that information gathered in the elicitation interviews would be used for research purposes and that the discussion would be audio-recorded. Participants were assured that their names would not be associated with the tapes. The Institutional Review Board at the [Fred Hutchinson Cancer Research Center] FHCRC approved the interview questions and the methods. Written consent was obtained from all participants.

The Internal Review Board of the University of North Dakota approved the study, and participants received the usual assurances about anonymity, confidentiality, and the right to withdraw at any point without prejudice or an impact on the health care that they will be receiving at the migrant health center.

The data collection methods are appraised to determine the steps taken to ensure credibility, dependability, and objectivity. For example, the researcher addresses objectivity in the following statement: "To ensure that the first author's preconceptions would not affect the research process, reflexivity was used continuously throughout the process."[21]

The results of the qualitative inquiry include a description of the participants' characteristics (e.g., gender, age, ethnicity) in enough detail to understand how they contributed to the data. The participants' experiences with the phenomenon should be varied in order to inform the data collection.[22]

The sample consisted of 12 participants who migrated from southern Texas to the Upper Midwest for agricultural work. Participants ranged in age from 34 to 62 years of age with a mean age of 51 years. Of the participants, 6 were men, and 6 were women. Ten were married, 1 was single, and the marital status of 1 individual was unknown.

All of the participants were diagnosed with type 2 diabetes. The mean age of diagnosis for the participants was 40 years old. The mean years that they lived with this chronic disease was 10. Seven of the 12 participants were prescribed oral medications to control their diabetes, whereas 4 reported the use of insulin. The medication status of 1 individual was unknown.

The data analysis begins with the assurance that the data gathered during the interviews or focus groups was transcribed verbatim. The procedures used to code the data, to construct themes and categories, and to establish interrelationships and construct a theory (when using a grounded theory approach) are also provided, as demonstrated in the following excerpt.[21]

The analysis of the interviews took place as soon as each interview was transcribed, in accordance with the guidelines for [grounded theory] GT (Glaser & Strauss, 1967). Initially, each interview was read through to gain a sense of the wholeness of the content and its meaning. During the initial coding, which was done line-by-line close to the data, actions were identified and compared. By using the informants' words, we ensured that these codes were grounded in the data. Codes with similar meanings were then grouped together to form comprehensive categories, which were labelled on a more abstract level. Data were compared with data and categories with categories to develop their properties (subcategories). In the third step, the relationships between the categories were sought and organised into an emerging theory. Throughout the process, codes and preliminary categories were compared, modified, and eventually given new names.

The researchers need to establish credibility, dependability, and objectivity during data analysis. The decisions made during data analysis are documented to provide an audit trial to establish the dependability of the analysis. The following excerpt describes the use of memos, member check, and peer review to ensure credibility, dependability, and objectivity.[23]

> Memos were used in which the ideas were written down about the evolving theory. Validation was enhanced by member check and peer review. Four of the respondents were asked to verify the written summary of their interviews. All four confirmed that the summaries were a fair representation of their perspectives. Provisional conclusions and theoretical insights were discussed with a person from the Dutch Diabetes Association and a diabetes specialized nurse.

The results section of the research report discusses the themes established through the data analysis and provides direct quotations from the participants to support the themes. The quotations should be long enough for transferability by the reader. Some results are presented in tables with the themes and corresponding quotations. The results should be in alignment with the purpose and answer the research question.

The discussion section includes a thorough explanation of the researchers' interpretation of the findings, and this explanation needs to be logical. The researchers discuss the contribution of the findings to understanding the phenomenon and how their findings are related to previous studies and theories in their own discipline and, when appropriate, other disciplines. The discussion also identifies and explains the limitations of the inquiry, the implications for practice, and future research recommendations, in a similar fashion as a quantitative study.

The final section of the research report is the conclusions section. The conclusions need to relate to the intended purpose of the inquiry and logically follow from the findings and interpretation.

The following conclusions relate the results to the question examined.[22]

> The results of this study contribute to the body of literature of Hispanic migrant farmworkers and how they incorporate the meaning of this chronic disease into their day-to-day living. Based on the analysis of the interviews with the study participants, the individuals' explanations of this chronic disease are compiled within their own perceptions and cultural beliefs. For the Hispanic migrant farmworker, diabetes is an illness that affects their physical, psychological, emotional, and spiritual well-being.

Meta-Synthesis

When multiple qualitative studies have investigated a phenomenon (e.g., teenagers' experiences with motherhood[27], elderly patients' experiences with hope and chronic diseases[28], patients' experiences with undergoing hemodialysis[29]), a qualitative research synthesis can be conducted. This synthesis is "a process and product of scientific inquiry aimed at systematically reviewing and formally integrating the findings in reports of completed qualitative studies."[30] Therefore, the synthesis results in a higher abstract level of understanding the phenomenon and might include the formulation of a new model or the development of a theory. Data from each qualitative study are compared and synthesized into a novel interpretation. This new interpretation should be meaningful and should inform healthcare practice.[31] Thus, meta-syntheses can be viewed as more useful to a professional who is using EBP to inform their healthcare decisions.

Sandelowski and Barroso[30] outlined the process for conducting a meta-synthesis:

- Establish the purpose of the meta-synthesis
- Locate relevant qualitative studies
- Determine the quality of the research reports
- Compare the research reports and categorize the findings

- Synthesize the findings into a new interpretation of the phenomenon

Researchers who conduct a **meta-synthesis** are urged to maintain the integrity of the original study, to make their judgments transparent, and to use reflexivity to avoid a biased interpretation.[30] The validity of this process can be maintained by producing an audit trial and using a peer reviewer who is an expert in the discipline to confirm the interpretation. In addition, a minimum of two researchers should conduct independent searches for qualitative studies as well as determining the quality of the research reports. When assessing the quality of a meta-synthesis publication, make sure the researchers have taken steps to ensure the validity of this synthesized level of evidence.

In addition to ensuring validity, make sure the purpose of implementing this process is clearly identifiable. Sometimes broad objectives or questions are used to guide the meta-synthesis. The researchers should identify who conducted the literature searches and what databases, time frame, population (e.g., adults or children), and search terms were used in the search. The method to determine the quality of the research report should be clearly stated. Some researchers develop inclusion criteria and only select studies that meet these criteria. Likewise, exclusion criteria might be developed to eliminate research reports.

The studies are compared to one another, usually presented in a table to report each of the studies'

purposes, qualitative design, sampling method, data collection method, data analysis, and findings including categories and themes. Sometimes another table is provided to synthesize each study's findings into the new categories or themes of the new interpretation and show how the data from each study is interrelated with data from the other studies. The visual organization of these two steps makes the meta-synthesis process more transparent to the reader. When tables are not provided, these steps must be clearly delineated in the text.

Assess Relevance

Now that you have evaluated the trustworthiness of the evidence, it is time to assess its relevance to the first four components of the PPAARE question. **Table 11–7** has been provided for you to use to determine the relevance and usefulness of the evidence. In the first column of the table, identify the author of the publication or the source (e.g., PIER or DynaMed). Five fictitious pieces of evidence have been entered into the table as a point of discussion. RCT A and RCT B provide evidence on the *action* in the PPAARE question. RCT C and RCT D provide evidence on the *alternative* in the PPAARE question. SR is a systematic review, and EBR is an evidence-based review (e.g., practice guideline or point-of-care product, such as PIER or DynaMed).

The relevance of the evidence is rated in the next five columns using the following scale: 2 = highly

Table 11–7 Assess Relevance and Usefulness of Evidence

Identify Evidence, Authors, or Source	Relevance (2 = highly relevant, 1 = somewhat relevant, 0 = not relevant)					Total Score
	Problem	Patient or Population	Action	Alternative	Result	
RCT A	**2** 1 0	**2** 1 0	**2** 1 0	2 1 **0**	**2** 1 0	8
RCT B	**2** 1 0	**2** 1 0	**2** 1 0	2 1 **0**	**2** 1 0	5
RCT C	**2** 1 0	**2** **1** 0	2 1 **0**	**2** 1 0	**2** 1 0	5
RCT D	2 **1** 0	**2** 1 0	2 1 **0**	**2** 1 0	**2** 1 0	7
SR	**2** 1 0	2 **1** 0	**2** 1 0	2 **1** 0	2 **1** 0	7
EBR	**2** 1 0	2 **1** 0	2 **1** 0	2 **1** 0	**2** 1 0	7

relevant, 1 = somewhat relevant and 0 = not relevant. The healthcare professional needs to determine the relevance to the *problem* that the study was intended to address. The problem relates to the severity of the disease, condition, injury, or to understanding a patient's experiences. Likewise, the relevance of the demographics and risk factors of the patient or population needs to be assessed with the evidence. The demographics to consider are age, ethnicity, gender, educational level, and socioeconomic level, as well as any other factors appropriate to the situation.

Next, the relevance is determined by assessing whether the RCTs, the SR, and the EBR will be helpful in determining the *action*, *alternative* (if one was identified), and the *result* in the PPAARE question. Consider the usefulness of the action or alternative to your practice or public health setting. When deliberating on an intervention also determine whether the potential benefits outweigh the negative aspects (e.g., harm, cost) for the patient or community.

Practitioners new to EBP might find it useful to add the numbers from the table and get a total score for each piece of evidence in order to rank all of the evidence being used to make a decision. After this step has been completed, the practitioner can select an action before moving on to the final step of implementation and evaluation.

Select an Action

Selecting an action might be the most difficult step for students to perform based on their limited clinical or practical experiences. Healthcare professionals who have been practicing and have gained valuable experiences on which to base decisions are at an advantage. Experience in the field can be a valuable asset to help make decisions about what action to take because the practitioner can use both the evidence and his or her expertise.

Table 11–8 contains the five hypothetical pieces of evidence used in Table 11–7. When deliberating on an action, the first consideration is the level of evidence. Evidence is listed based on the hierarchical levels on the pyramid, as shown in the first column, with the systematic review being listed first, followed by the evidence-based review, and lastly the RCTs on the *action* and *alternative*. The following scoring method can be used to rank the level of evidence in the second column: 5 = meta-analysis or systematic review; 4 = evidence-based review; 3 = RCT; 2 = case-control series, case series, or case report; and 1 = textbook, review article, expert opinion, or laboratory research. The relevancy score can be carried over to this new table and the scores placed in the third column. The publication date is important to include in the decision-making process and can be placed in the fourth column. Finally, the consistency of the findings among the evidence is compared and noted in the last column.

Once you have completed the table, you should consider rearranging multiple pieces of evidence at the same level first by the publication date. Notice the two RCTs for the *action*; RCT B is listed first because its publication date is more current than RCT A. Now look at RCT D and C; both have

Table 11–8 The Five Fictitious Pieces

Author or Source	Level of Evidence	Relevancy Score	Publication Date	Consistency of Findings
SR	5	7	2010	RCT B
EBR	4	7	2012	RCT A, RCT C
RCT B	3	5	2013	SR
RCT A	3	8	2009	ER
RCT D	3	7	2011	
RCT C	3	5	2011	ER

Table 11–9 SWOT Analysis

Positive	Limitation
Personal Strengths	**Personal Weaknesses**
Knowledge to perform this action	Lack of knowledge to perform this action
Skills to perform this action	Lack of skills to perform this action
Values to perform this action	Lack of values to perform this action
Experience and expertise	Lack of experience and expertise
Any other items that will have a positive influence on performing the action	Any other items that will be limit the performance of this action
Outside Opportunities	**Outside Threats**
(related to the patient or community and health-care setting)	(related to the patient or community and health-care setting)
Knowledge to perform this action	Lack of knowledge to perform this action
Skills or resources to perform this action	Lack of skills or resources for this action
Values to perform this action	Lack of values to perform this action
Ability to pay for care (e.g., insurance)	Inability to pay for care (e.g., no insurance)
Presence of support system	Lack of support system
Any other items that will have a positive influence on performing the action	Any other items that will be limit the performance of this action

the same publication date and were ranked by the relevancy score.

Let's look at the table and discuss some decision-making strategies. The systematic review was published in 2010, and thus more current findings might be available. In fact, RCT B related to the *action* has consistent findings with the systematic review and was published in 2013; although, its relevancy score is relatively low. The evidence-based review was published in 2012 and is consistent with RCT A related to the *action* and RCT C related to the *alternative*. The relevancy score for the evidence-based review and RCT A are higher than the score for RCT C. RCT D is not consistent with any other evidence and can be eliminated from the decision-making process. There is no "cookbook" method for deciding on an action, and professional judgment needs to be applied as well.

Once all the evidence is weighed, practitioners can use their experience in the field to make a decision. If one is less experienced, a colleague can be consulted. Less experienced practitioners can use a SWOT analysis to help them make a decision on whether to choose the *action* or *alternative* in the PPAARE question. The SWOT analysis also

might be useful when there is no evidence or when there is conflicting evidence. SWOT refers to the practitioner's *personal* **S**trengths and **W**eaknesses and *outside* **O**pportunities and **T**hreats. Outside or external opportunities and threats relate to the patient, community, or the healthcare setting. **Table 11–9** contains information to think about when making an informed decision.

The practitioner chooses to implement the *action* or *alternative* as the preferred method of proceeding to the implementation and evaluation phase of EBP.

IMPLEMENTATION AND EVALUATION

The implementation of patient care or a community health program is a multifactorial, complex situation. **Figure 11–2** is a depiction of some of the factors in a patient care situation. At the center of the model is the patient, and implementation is based on many factors related to the patient. The patient's support system for the health intervention also is a consideration, especially for those individuals who have chronic debilitating diseases

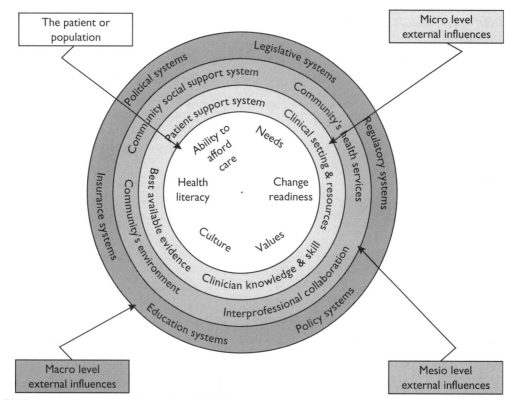

Figure 11–2 Patient-Centered Evidence-Based Model

and cognitive impairment. The practitioner's expertise and the use of evidence are only two factors in this complex situation. Other factors relate to the healthcare setting and the availability of resources and the community and the availability of health services for diagnostic and specialty care.

In a patient- or population-centered approach to health care, the action and alternatives are presented and the patient/population makes the decision as to which way to proceed. Whatever action is taken, the patient needs to understand the importance of follow-up care to determine the effectiveness of the intervention. The length of time needs to be carefully considered to make sure the intervention has had an adequate amount of time for results to be evident. Of course, the information needs to be thoroughly documented in the patient's record.

At the next appointment, the results of the intervention are evaluated. In the PPAARE question, the *results* of the intervention were specified. The

clinician needs to evaluate the progress toward the patient's achievement of the results. In addition, the patient's ability to manage the disease/condition and his or her satisfaction with the maintenance is important, especially when the management is on a long-term basis.

The last step in the evidence-based process is *reflection*: "Reflection is an invitation to think deeply about our actions so that we may act with more insight and effectiveness in the future."[32] Continual learning is necessary throughout healthcare professionals' careers to enable them to develop expertise in their discipline. The use of reflection-on-action is a strategy to enhance learning from experiences in the field.[33] Reflection-on-action requires retrospective critical thinking about actions to gain knowledge and refine frameworks on which decisions are based.[34] Reflection activities can be informal and as simple as thinking about the experience; however, reflections can be written

Table 11–10 Reflection Questions

- What have I learned as an individual from this experience? What have we learned as a collaborative interprofessional team?
- How will my future actions change based on this experience? How will our collaborative interprofessional team's actions change?
- What more do I need to learn related to . . . ? What more does our collaborative interprofessional team need to learn related to . . . ?
  - ○ Recognizing a need for information
  - ○ Establishing a purpose for the EBP
  - ○ Formulating a focused question
  - ○ Identifying target resources
  - ○ Performing a search
  - ○ Organizing findings
  - ○ Appraising trustworthiness of evidence
  - ○ Assessing the relevance of evidence
  - ○ Selecting an action
  - ○ Implementing and evaluating the action

or entries made into a journal. **Table 11–10** presents questions to help with the reflection process.

When healthcare professionals identify knowledge, skills, or values that need to be improved, a professional development plan can be created to assist the individual or the healthcare team in developing a concrete plan for learning. The learning plan includes setting goals, specifying actions to meet the goal, determining a date for completion, and recording completion of the action. **Table 11–11** provides an example of a professional development plan.

Lifelong learning is the continual development of a healthcare professional throughout one's career. Learning is based on experiences in the field that provide the mechanism to develop expertise. This level of professional practice is enhanced by the use of the best evidence available to assist the practitioner and the interprofessional collaborative team in their professional development and quest to provide quality care to patients in the community.

CHAPTER SUMMARY

The following exercises serve as a summary of this chapter, synthesizing the concepts and strategies in application to answering PPAARE questions.

Table 11–11 Components of a Professional Development Plan

Goal	Action	Date for Completion	Check Off when Completed
Locating more relevant evidence to PPAARE questions	• Meet with the librarian to review strategies for searching PubMed and Cochrane Library.	• Sept 30	☐
	• Practice searching on own.	• Oct 30	☐
Enhance critical appraisal of quantitative research	• Find a mentor to provide help with critical-appraisal skills.	• Nov 15	☐
	• Review four studies with mentor.	• Dec 1	☐

EXERCISE #1

For this exercise, you will develop a PPAARE question based on a patient scenario, retrieve a copy of an article related to the PPAARE question, read the article, and complete the Trustworthiness Appraisal Table for a Quantitative Study. We will provide our response to this exercise for comparison with yours.

Patient Scenario

Mr. Martinez, a 45-year-old male of Hispanic descent, visits his primary care provider as a follow-up to his previous employment-screening physical exam. He has been hired as a home construction site manager for a local company that required a medical release in order for him to start his job. At that time he was given a medical release to start the new job, but he agreed to return to your clinic to address his overall health needs. He returns today with an interest in avoiding a heart attack and living longer, adding that he is more interested in how to improve his health through nutrition than through medication. Specifically, based on something his coworker told him, he asks if eating walnuts and fatty fish can help improve his cholesterol levels as opposed to eating a regular healthy diet. He has started a healthy diet and is considering if he should make a point of eating walnuts and fatty fish. If so, he asks how much of these does he need and how often?

Mr. Martinez appears to be well, although overweight (height 70 inches, weight 202 pounds, waist 38 inches).* He has no health complaints. When asked about his family history, he reports that his father died recently at the age of 65 from a heart attack. He has a wife and two teenage sons. He does not want his family to lose him at a young age. Lab tests from his previous visit revealed that he has abnormal lipid levels: total cholesterol = 222 mg/dL; HDL = 30 mg/dL; LDL = 160 mg/dL; triglycerides = 160 mg/dL. He also admits to smoking one pack of cigarettes per day for the last 25 years. On physical exam he is found to have a heartbeat with regular rate and rhythm, without murmurs, rubs, or gallops. His pulse is 76 beats per minute. His blood pressure is 133/87 mm Hg. His lungs are clear to auscultation bilaterally.

*The CDC define overweight[6] in adults as those with a body mass index (BMI)[7] between 25 and 29.9.

There are many different focused PPAARE questions you could develop in response to this scenario. However, for this exercise we will focus on the question he has asked, if eating walnuts and fatty fish will improve his cholesterol levels compared to eating a healthy diet that does not include walnuts and fatty fish.

Instructions

1 Construct a PPAARE table for Mr. Martinez' question.
2 Locate and read (at least three times) the following article, which is available as of the writing of this text as a free full-text online article:
    Rajaram S, Hasso Haddad E, Mejia A, Sabaté J. Walnuts and fatty fish influence different serum lipid fractions in normal to mildly hyperlipidemic individuals: A randomized controlled study. *Am J Clin Nutr.* 2009;89(suppl):1S–7S.
    Note: be sure to download and save a copy of the article so that you can mark it up.
3 Complete the Trustworthiness Appraisal Table for a Quantitative Study
4 Determine if the article provides adequate information to address Mr. Martinez' question and formulate the response you will give him.

Resources to Use for Each Step in the Exercise

Step 1: Construct a PPAARE table for Mr. Martinez' question, filling in the information as indicated.

Use the PPARE question format based on the information you place in the table:

> What is the highest level of evidence available to determine whether a patient with P (= *disease or condition*) who is P (= *demographics or risk factors*) benefits from A (= *action*) as compared to A (= *alternative*) to produce, improve, or reduce the R (= *result*)?

PPAARE Table for Mr. Martinez' Nutrition Question

PPAARE Component	Case Example
Identify the problem related to the disease or condition (e.g., diabetes, rheumatoid arthritis, pregnancy).	
Identify the patient related to his or her demographics (e.g., age, ethnicity, gender) and risk factors (e.g., smoking, unhealthy eating practices).	
Identify the action related to the patient's diagnosis or diagnostic tests, etiology, prognosis, treatment or therapy, harm, prevention, patient education, or follow-up care.	
Identify the alternative to the action when there is one (not a required component).	
Identify the patient's result of the action to produce, improve, or reduce the outcomes for the patient.	
Identify the level of evidence available after searching (use the evidence hierarchy).	

Step 2: Locate the following article, which is available (as of the writing of this text) as a free full-text online article:

Rajaram S, Hasso Haddad E, Mejia A, Sabaté J. Walnuts and fatty fish influence different serum lipid fractions in normal to mildly hyperlipidemic individuals: A randomized controlled study. *Am J Clin Nutr.* 2009;89(suppl):1S–7S.

Step 3: Complete the Trustworthiness of the Quantitative Study table.

Step 4: Determine if the article provides adequate information to address Mr. Martinez' question and formulate the response you will give him.

No resource is needed for this step. Just write out your response.

Trustworthiness of the Quantitative Study

Publication Section	Content	Questions	Appraisal (check one box)
Located on the first and/or last page of the publication	Authors' names, credentials, affiliations, and conflict of interest	• Are the authors' credentials and educational background appropriate to conduct this type of study? • Are the authors affiliated with an educational program, health institution, or practice setting? • Do the authors report a conflict of interest?	☐ Strength ☐ Limitation ☐ Not evident ☐ Not applicable
Presented on the first or last page of the publication	Funding source	• Does the funding source have a vested interest in a beneficial outcome of the study?	☐ Strength ☐ Limitation ☐ Not evident ☐ Not applicable
Introduction	Purpose	• Is the intent of the study clearly stated? • Are the variables being investigated identifiable? • Are the outcomes of the study identifiable? • Is the population under study identifiable?	☐ Strength ☐ Limitation ☐ Not evident ☐ Not applicable

(continues)

Trustworthiness of the Quantitative Study

Publication Section	Content	Questions	Appraisal (check one box)
Introduction	Hypotheses and research questions	• Are the hypotheses in alignment with the intended purpose? • Are the variables under study identifiable in the hypotheses (e.g., independent and dependent variables)? • Is one hypothesis written for each dependent variable under study? • Are the research questions in alignment with the intended purpose? • Are the variables under study identifiable in the research questions? • Is one question written for each variable under study?	☐ Strength ☐ Limitation ☐ Not evident ☐ Not applicable
Methods	Research design	• Is the design selected in alignment with the purpose? • Is the design appropriate to reach the stated outcome? • Is a control or comparison group used when its use strengthens the validity of the outcome? • Are the researchers blind to the assignment of participants (when it makes sense)? • Are the participants blind to their assignment (when it makes sense)? • Does the design limit the number of extraneous variables?	☐ Strength ☐ Limitation ☐ Not evident ☐ Not applicable
Methods	Sample	• Did the authors describe the population that the sample is intended to represent? • Was the sampling frame used appropriate for the purpose of the study? • Was the inclusion and exclusion criteria clearly described, and was it appropriate for the intended outcome? • Was the assignment of participants to treatment and control/comparison groups random or nonrandom, and was the method appropriate? • Was the sample size sufficient to include all applicable variability? • Was a sampling calculation discussed?	☐ Strength ☐ Limitation ☐ Not evident ☐ Not applicable

Trustworthiness of the Quantitative Study

Publication Section	Content	Questions	Appraisal (check one box)
Methods	Research protocol	• Was the protocol for conducting the study described thoroughly and in enough detail? • Was the protocol followed appropriate for the purpose? • Did the study continue long enough to have valid outcomes? • Was the protocol consistently administered to the participants in each group? • Did the researchers take steps to control for extraneous variables? • Was the protocol ethical and approved by an Institutional Review Board (IRB)?	☐ Strength ☐ Limitation ☐ Not evident ☐ Not applicable
Methods	Data collection	• Were the data collection methods appropriate for the intended purpose of the study? • Were the data collection procedures consistently applied to the participants? • Was the validity and reliability of the data collection instrument established at a high enough level? • Was the reliability of the data collectors established at a high enough level?	☐ Strength ☐ Limitation ☐ Not evident ☐ Not applicable
Results	Sample	• Were important demographics of the intervention and control/comparison group similar and, if not, did it impact the results? • Were treatment and control groups similar at the baseline measurement of the outcome variables and, if not, did this difference impact the results? • How were eligible participants accounted for throughout the study? • Was the discontinuance rate comparable between the treatment and control or comparison group?	☐ Strength ☐ Limitation ☐ Not evident ☐ Not applicable
Results	Data analysis	• What did the power analysis indicate? • Were data analyzed using an on-protocol or intention-to-treat analysis, or both? • If intention-to-treat analysis was used, what method was used to input missing data?	☐ Strength ☐ Limitation ☐ Not evident ☐ Not applicable

(continues)

Trustworthiness of the Quantitative Study

Publication Section	Content	Questions	Appraisal (check one box)
		• Were the statistical analyses appropriate for the level of data (i.e., nominal, ordinal, interval, or ratio)? • Were the statistical analyses appropriate to test the hypotheses and answer the research questions?	
Results	Findings	• Are findings presented relative to each hypothesis and research question? • Are findings reported as statistically significant or not significant? • When confidence levels are reported, are the upper and lower limits acceptable to implement a change to your practice? • Do the findings have practical or clinical significance?	☐ Strength ☐ Limitation ☐ Not evident ☐ Not applicable
Discussion		• Did the researchers thoroughly explain their interpretation of the findings? • Were the explanations logical? • Did the researchers compare their findings to the findings of previous studies and provide a rationale on why they differ? • Did the researchers thoroughly identify and discuss the limitations? • What are the implications for practice? • What future research recommendations are made?	☐ Strength ☐ Limitation ☐ Not evident ☐ Not applicable
Conclusions		• Is a conclusion provided for the intended purpose of the study? • Do the conclusions logically follow from the findings and interpretation?	☐ Strength ☐ Limitation ☐ Not evident ☐ Not applicable

ANSWERS TO EXERCISE #1

Step 1: Develop a PPAARE question using the PPAARE table.
PPAARE Question:

What is the highest level of evidence available to determine whether a patient with *high cholesterol* who is *an overweight adult Hispanic male who smokes* benefits from *a healthy diet rich in walnuts and fatty fish* as compared to *standard healthy diet not rich*

in walnuts and fatty fish to reduce his *level of cholesterol* and *risk of heart attack, and to improve length of life*?

Step 2: Download and read the article three times.
We completed this step, choosing the most recent RCT available. Of the six articles we located, the one assigned with this exercise was the most recent and the highest level available for the PPAARE question.

Step 3: See table on next page.

PPAARE Table for Mr. Martinez' Nutrition Question

PPAARE Component	Case Example
Identify the problem related to the disease or condition (e.g., diabetes, rheumatoid arthritis, pregnancy).	High cholesterol
Identify the patient related to his or her demographics (e.g., age, ethnicity, gender) and risk factors (e.g., smoking, unhealthy eating practices).	Adult Hispanic male, 45 years old, who is overweight and a smoker
Identify the action related to the patient's diagnosis or diagnostic tests, etiology, prognosis, treatment or therapy, harm, prevention, patient education, or follow-up care.	Consuming a healthy diet rich in walnuts and fatty fish
Identify the alternative to the action when there is one (not a required component).	Consuming a healthy diet not rich in walnuts and fatty fish
Identify the patient's result of the action to produce, improve, or reduce the outcomes for the patient.	• Reducing cholesterol levels • Reducing risk of heart attack • Prolonging life
Identify the level of evidence available after searching (use the evidence hierarchy).	• Three opinion articles • One case-control study • Two RCTs

Trustworthiness of the Quantitative Study

Publication Section	Content	Questions	Appraisal (check one box)
Located on the first and/or last page of the publication	Authors' names, credentials, affiliations, and conflict of interest	• Are the authors' credentials and educational background appropriate to conduct this type of study? • Are the authors affiliated with an educational program, health institution, or practice setting? • Do the authors report a conflict of interest?	☒ Strength ☐ Limitation ☐ Not evident ☐ Not applicable

Reasoning:
+ All elements were provided, plus a statement regarding the specific contributions of each author to the manuscript.

| Presented on the first or last page of the publication | Funding source | • Does the funding source have a vested interest in a beneficial outcome of the study? | ☐ Strength
☒ Limitation
☐ Not evident
☐ Not applicable |

Reasoning:
− Yes. Also, the study was funded by the California Walnut Commission (CWC). One of the authors is a member of this organization and her travel to a national meeting was paid for by the organization. There is no mention in the conflict of interest statement of an agreement between the CWC and the authors. It is difficult to determine if publication bias is present.

(continues)

Publication Section	Content	Questions	Appraisal (check one box)
Introduction	Purpose	• Is the intent of the study clearly stated? • Are the variables being investigated identifiable? • Are the outcomes of the study identifiable? • Is the population under study identifiable?	☒ Strength ☐ Limitation ☐ Not evident ☐ Not applicable

Reasoning:

+ The objective was clearly stated.

+/− The outcome measures were stated in general terms in the introduction (serum cholesterol and total cholesterol) but the specific measures (Total Cholesterol, LDL, HDL, Triglycerides, Apolipoprotein A-1, and Apolipoprotein B) were not identified until later in the article.

+ The outcomes of the study are identifiable in the abstract for two of the measures. They are stated with confidence intervals.

+/− The population is partially identifiable in the Introduction as 25 adults with normal to mild hyperlipidemia. The Introduction did not specify the male/female ratio or the age range. The introduction did not define 'normal to mild hyperlipidemia.' The Subjects section of the article did provide the age range, but not the male/female ratio. The number of males and females was not stated until the Results section.

Publication Section	Content	Questions	Appraisal (check one box)
Introduction	Hypotheses and research questions	• Are the hypotheses in alignment with the intended purpose? • Are the variables under study identifiable in the hypotheses (e.g., independent and dependent variables)? • Is one hypothesis written for each dependent variable under study? • Are the research questions in alignment with the intended purpose? • Are the variables under study identifiable in the research questions? • Is one question written for each variable under study?	☐ Strength ☒ Limitation ☐ Not evident ☐ Not applicable

Reasoning:

− Neither the hypothesis nor the null hypothesis are directly stated. Based on the Introduction the null hypothesis would be that the three diets (with specific doses of n-3 fatty acids) are equivalent in terms of their impact on reducing cholesterol levels.

+ The study purpose aligns with the above hypothesis.

There is not a hypothesis written for each question. There should have been a question for each outcome measure.

+ The variables under study are identifiable.

Trustworthiness of the Quantitative Study

Publication Section	Content	Questions	Appraisal (check one box)
Methods	Research design	• Is the design selected in alignment with the purpose? • Is the design appropriate to reach the stated outcome? • Is a control or comparison group used when its use strengthens the validity of the outcome? • Are the researchers blind to the assignment of participants (when it makes sense)? • Are the participants blind to their assignment (when it makes sense)? • Does the design limit the number of extraneous variables?	☒ Strength ☐ Limitation ☐ Not evident ☐ Not applicable

Reasoning:

+ The design is well aligned with the study's purpose and achievement of the stated outcomes.

+ There is a control group. Also, a cross-over strategy was used to provide within-subject control.

− There is no mention of analyst blinding. Subject blinding is not mentioned, but was also not possible. The use of cross-over design helps overcome the lack of subject blinding.

+ Several strategies were used to limit extraneous variables. For example, the accuracy of the blood tests was validated by performing duplicate analyses. A sample size calculation was utilized (although the authors referred to it as a power calculation) to determine the needed sample size. The researchers verified subject compliance with the intervention through an objective clinical measure (fatty acid composition of the erythrocyte membrane). This does not, however, account for the possibility that subjects engaged in some other behavior that resulted in lower cholesterol. The feeding protocol was controlled by having the food prepared by a university's metabolic kitchen. Subjects ate meals at the facility Sundays through Fridays and were provided pre-packaged meals on Saturdays. Considering the control of the intervention and the use of a cross-over design, overall, this is a well-controlled design.

| Methods | Sample | • Did the authors describe the population that the sample is intended to represent?
• Was the sampling frame used appropriate for the purpose of the study?
• Was the inclusion and exclusion criteria clearly described, and was it appropriate for the intended outcome?
• Was the assignment of participants to treatment and control/comparison groups random or nonrandom, and was the method appropriate?
• Was the sample size sufficient to include all applicable variability?
• Was a sampling calculation discussed? | ☐ Strength
☒ Limitation
☐ Not evident
☐ Not applicable |

(continues)

Trustworthiness of the Quantitative Study		
Publication Section	**Content**	**Questions**	**Appraisal (check one box)**

Reasoning:

+/− The sample is described and the authors explain the need for dosing information related to n-3 fatty acids among adults with normal to mild hyperlipidemia. However, no other information is provided with regard to the intended population.

+/− The sampling frame was one university campus. The researchers used advertisements in and around the campus to recruit adult subjects.

− The researchers did not provide a demographics table, only the age range and number of subjects. It is possible that the sample was younger than the average population of adults with normal to mild hyperlipidemia.

− The researchers did not compare the sample to expected values based on an external data source. Internal comparisons were performed.

+ Exclusion criteria were explained and helped control for extraneous variables. The criteria were appropriate to the research question and intended outcome.

+/− Randomization was utilized for group assignments. They also used a stratification procedure to group according to age, gender, and baseline cholesterol. They did not describe the randomization procedure, however.

+ The sample size appears to be sufficient based on the reporting of a sample size calculation.

| Methods | Research protocol | • Was the protocol for conducting the study described thoroughly and in enough detail?
• Was the protocol followed appropriate for the purpose?
• Did the study continue long enough to have valid outcomes?
• Was the protocol consistently administered to the participants in each group?
• Did the researchers take steps to control for extraneous variables?
• Was the protocol ethical and approved by an Institutional Review Board (IRB)? | ☒ Strength
☐ Limitation
☐ Not evident
☐ Not applicable |

Reasoning:

+ The protocol was well described in terms of the administration of the intervention and the outcome measurement procedures.

+ The protocol was appropriate to the research question.

+ To answer this question the reader of the article needs to know how long it takes for a nutrition intervention to affect cholesterol levels. Each diet was 4 weeks in length with a week-long washout period between diets. Subjects were not followed after the study was complete, which would not have made sense for the research question.

+ The researchers took steps to control for extraneous variables.

+ The study was approved by an IRB.

Trustworthiness of the Quantitative Study

Publication Section	Content	Questions	Appraisal (check one box)
Methods	Data collection	• Were the data collection methods appropriate for the intended purpose of the study? • Were the data collection procedures consistently applied to the participants? • Was the validity and reliability of the data collection instrument established at a high enough level? • Was the reliability of the data collectors established at a high enough level?	☒ Strength ☐ Limitation ☐ Not evident ☐ Not applicable

Reasoning:

+ The data collection methods were appropriate to the research question and purpose of the study.

+ It appears that the data collection procedures were consistently applied, based on the use of an expert facility to provide the meals and another facility to perform the blood tests.

+/− The instruments used to measure blood levels, the primary outcome measures, were described, but no validity tests were reported. They used a duplicate testing procedure, but this might not overcome accuracy problems if there was a problem at the lab.

+/− The use of external experts for administration of the intervention and data analysis as well as duplicate testing procedures helps establish reliability. However, there is not enough detail to determine if different experts were consistent with one another.

| Results | Sample | • Were important demographics of the intervention and control/comparison group similar and, if not, did it impact the results?
• Were treatment and control groups similar at the baseline measurement of the outcome variables and, if not, did this difference impact the results?
• How were eligible participants accounted for throughout the study?
• Was the discontinuance rate comparable between the treatment and control or comparison group? | ☒ Strength
☐ Limitation
☐ Not evident
☐ Not applicable |

Reasoning:

+/− Comparisons were made between the groups regarding outcome measures, and a randomization procedure as well as a stratification procedure were used to assign subjects to groups. However, the groups were not compared statistically in terms of demographics.

− The authors made no mention of the number of potential subjects. They did not provide a sampling fraction.

+ Only two subjects dropped out. The reason reported for dropping out was time conflicts. The sample size did not drop below the minimum number needed for statistical power. The authors did not explain the use of per-protocol analysis, but it is evident from the data table and reported statistics that they used this method.

(continues)

Trustworthiness of the Quantitative Study			
Publication Section	**Content**	**Questions**	**Appraisal (check one box)**
Results	Data analysis	• What did the power analysis indicate? • Were data analyzed using an on-protocol or intention-to-treat analysis, or both? • If intention-to-treat analysis was used, what method was used to input missing data? • Were the statistical analyses appropriate for the level of data (i.e., nominal, ordinal, interval or ratio)? • Were the statistical analyses appropriate to test the hypotheses and answer the research questions?	☒ Strength ☐ Limitation ☐ Not evident ☐ Not applicable

Reasoning:

+/− The authors reported an excess of 90% power to detect changes in the outcomes of interest. However, they did not report power in terms of each outcome measure.

+/− The per-protocol (also known as on-protocol) analysis procedure was used. However, the authors did not state this. This fact had to be deduced from the article.

+/− A mixed linear model was used to test differences in treatment means. This model assumes that random effects have a normal distribution. They did not report results of tests for normality of the data. The authors did not provide a justification for the use of this procedure. They did use a correction for multiple comparisons (Tukey-Kramer).

+ The statistical analysis is appropriate to the data types for the outcome measures, which were continuous scale.

Results	Findings	• Are findings presented relative to each hypothesis and research question? • Are findings reported as statistically significant or not significant? • When confidence levels are reported, are the upper and lower limits acceptable to implement a change to your practice? • Do the findings have practical or clinical significance?	☒ Strength ☐ Limitation ☐ Not evident ☐ Not applicable

Reasoning:

+ There are results for each outcome measure.

+ The CI's were sufficiently narrow for the statistically significant findings.

− However, the actual effect sizes for the significant outcomes were small. For example, the walnut diet reduced total cholesterol by 0.47 mmol/L. The desired level of total cholesterol is less than 5.2 mmol/L. It is not clear if a change of 0.47 mmol/L is a minimal clinically meaningful effect. Similarly, the fatty fish diet reduced total cholesterol by 0.28 mmol/L, which is even less clear an outcome.

Trustworthiness of the Quantitative Study

Publication Section	Content	Questions	Appraisal (check one box)
Discussion (this section included the Conclusions section as well)		• Did the researchers thoroughly explain their interpretation of the findings? • Were the explanations logical? • Did the researchers compare their findings to the findings of previous studies and provide a rationale on why they differ? • Did the researchers thoroughly identify and discuss the limitations? • What are the implications for practice? • What future research recommendations are made?	☐ Strength ☒ Limitation ☐ Not evident ☐ Not applicable

Reasoning:
+ The discussion is complete, addressing the study's findings in light of the literature.
− The authors did not discuss the limitations of the study. This is a significant deficiency.
− The authors go so far as to state, "Every 1% decrease in LDL cholesterol results in a 2% decrease in risk of CHD [coronary heart disease]," but the reference they provide for this statement is not an actual study. The authors did not test the subjects' risk of CHD and provided an opinion as the defense of this claim. This is a fairly significant weakness, considering the absence of a statement regarding minimal clinically meaningful effect. Reducing risk of CHD is an important outcome that matters and statements related to it need to be carefully considered.

Conclusions (incorporated into the Discussion section)		• Is a conclusion provided for the intended purpose of the study? • Do the conclusions logically follow from the findings and interpretation?	☒ Strength ☐ Limitation ☐ Not evident ☐ Not applicable

Reasoning:
+ The conclusions do follow from the research question and the purpose of the study.
+ The conclusions also follow from the findings and the authors' interpretations.

Step 4: Recommendation to Mr. Martinez

This article was well-written. It was fairly easy to locate information related to the various trustworthiness questions. It would be possible to replicate the study on a larger scale and address some of the limitations. However, there were two important flaws in the article. First, the authors did not discuss the limitations of the study. Second, the authors included an important statement about reduction of CHD in association with reduction of cholesterol. They provided no information on minimal clinically meaningful effect with regard to cholesterol levels, nor did they measure an outcome that mattered.

When considering Mr. Martinez and his question about following a diet rich in walnuts and fatty fish, the decision is not crystal clear. The intervention is unlikely to be harmful, and there is some evidence that the diet presented in this study could be beneficial in terms of cholesterol lowering. It is possible to suggest to Mr. Martinez that there is one study showing that this particular diet might be effective. We need to consider his cholesterol levels and other factors that might influence the outcome for him as an individual.

Here are three of Mr. Martinez' cholesterol levels, followed by the reference ranges for each.

TC = 30 mg/dL		LDL = 160 mg/dL		Tg = 160 mg/dL	

Total Cholesterol (mg/dL)		LDL (mg/dL)		Triglycerides (mg/dL)	
< 200	Desirable	< 100	Optimal	< 150	Normal
200–239	Borderline high	100–129	Near optimal/above optimal	150–199	Borderline high
240	High	130–159	Borderline high	200–499	High
		160–189	High	500	Very high
		190	Very high		

Mr. Martinez' cholesterol levels place him in the Borderline High category for Total Cholesterol, the High category for LDL, and the Borderline High category for triglycerides (Tg). In this presented study, the subjects had normal lipids or were mildly hyperlipidemic. The authors did not define 'mildly hyperlipidemic.' As such, it is unclear if Mr. Martinez matches the subjects in terms of lipids. We might, nonetheless, describe him as mildly hyperlipidemic. The researchers did not describe the ethnicities of the subjects. As such, we cannot determine if the intervention is different among people with different ethnicities. Mr. Martinez is within the target age range of the study, however. It would be important to provide all of this information to him to help him make his decision.

Lastly, the diet administered in the study is described in highly scientific terms. If Mr. Martinez were to choose to follow the diet, it might be necessary to provide a menu showing combinations of foods that would satisfy the requirements of the diet. It would be important to schedule regular follow-up with Mr. Martinez to monitor his progress. Based on the design of the study, a four-week follow-up seems appropriate.

EXERCISE #2

Critically appraise the trustworthiness for a qualitative study using the questions provided in Table 11–6. Use the reading strategy discussed in the beginning of the chapter to make sure you have a complete understanding of the research report before you proceed to the critical appraisal. The

following research report can be found in PubMed Central; therefore, you have free access to it. Once you are on the PubMed home page, place the PubMed Central index number (PMCID) in the search box and it will take you directly to the article.

PMCID: PMC1468411

Title: "I really should've gone to the doctor": older adults and family caregivers describe their experiences with community-acquired pneumonia

Authors: Caralyn Kelly, Paul Krueger, Lynne Lohfeld, Mark Loeb, and H. Gayle Edward

ANSWERS TO EXERCISE #2

In order to determine the overall trustworthiness of the qualitative study, you would compare the number of criteria judged as strengths with the number of limitations. In this example, 10 of the 12 criteria were rated as strengths and none were identified as limitations. Another consideration to judge the trustworthiness is the number of criteria marked "Not evident." It is important to look at the items marked as "Not Evident" to determine if these missing items are, in fact, limitations. For example, the research question was not evident in the article for this exercise. The article would have been more understandable for the reader if the authors had stated the research question, thus this is a limitation. The second item that was not evident was the specific qualitative approach utilized. The study appeared to be a phenomenology. The reader is able to understand the research purpose and findings even though the specific method was not identified. This is a flaw, but not truly a limitation.

Trustworthiness of the Qualitative Study

Publication Section	Content	Questions	Appraisal (check one box)
Located on the first page of the publication	Authors' names, credentials, affiliations, and conflict of interest	• Are the authors' credentials and educational background appropriate to conduct this type of study? • Are the authors affiliated with an educational program, health institution, or practice setting? • Do the authors report a conflict of interest?	☒ Strength ☐ Limitation ☐ Not evident ☐ Not applicable

Reasoning: The authors Kelly, Krueger, Lohfeld, and Loeb are affiliated with the Department of Biostatistics at McMaster University in Canada. Authors Krueger, and Loeb are also affiliated with the Department of Pathology and Molecular Medicine at McMaster University. The author Edward is affiliated with the Department of Family Relations and Applied Nutrition at University of Guelph in Canada. The authors represent an interprofessional research team representing well respected universities. None of the authors reported a conflict of interest. No credentials are provided for the authors. At the end of the research report the authors' contributions to this scholarly work are provided.

Presented on the first or last page of the publication	Funding source	• Does the funding source have a vested interest in a beneficial outcome of the study?	☒ Strength ☐ Limitation ☐ Not evident ☐ Not applicable

Reasoning: At the end of the research report under the "Acknowledgements," the funding source is identified as the Canadian Institutes of Health Research Interdisciplinary Health Research Team. This entity is a governmental agency and has no vested interest in the outcome for financial gain.

Introduction	Purpose	• Is the intent of the study clearly stated? • Is the phenomenon being investigated identifiable? • Is the population identifiable?	☒ Strength ☐ Limitation ☐ Not evident ☐ Not applicable

Reasoning: In the "Background" section of the research report, the authors review the literature surrounding seniors' experience with illnesses and how they make healthcare decisions. An understanding of how seniors make healthcare decisions related to community-acquired pneumonia is based solely on anecdotal evidence; therefore this study is warranted. The purpose of the study is stated in the last sentence, "The qualitative component was designed to collect rich and detailed descriptions of pneumonia experiences from a small, purposively selected sample of older adults and their family caregivers using both in-depth interviews and focus groups." From this statement, we can determine that the phenomenon being investigated is "pneumonia experiences" and the populations include seniors and their caregivers.

Introduction	Research questions	• Are the research questions in alignment with the intended purpose? • Is the phenomenon under study identifiable in a broad research questions?	☐ Strength ☐ Limitation ☒ Not evident ☐ Not applicable

(continues)

Trustworthiness of the Qualitative Study

Publication Section	Content	Questions	Appraisal (check one box)
Methods	Qualitative approach	• Is the rationale for using a qualitative approach explained? • Is the qualitative approach selected in alignment with the intended purpose (e.g., ethnography, biography, phenomenology, case study, grounded theory)?	☐ Strength ☐ Limitation ☒ Not evident ☐ Not applicable
Methods	Sample	• Was a sampling method or multiple methods used to identify participants who could inform the study (e.g., purposive sampling, snowball or network sampling, theoretical sampling)? • How did the researchers attempt to gain variation within the sample? • Was the inclusion and exclusion criteria clearly described, and was it appropriate for the purpose of the study?	☒ Strength ☐ Limitation ☐ Not evident ☐ Not applicable

Reasoning: The participants were recruited for the qualitative study after they had participated in a quantitative telephone survey. The inclusion criteria were established to recruit older adults (60 years and older) and their family caregivers who spoke English and were able to provide "rich details about their experiences." In addition, the seniors had to have a chest x-ray confirmation of pneumonia. A purposive sampling strategy was employed by the researchers to ensure the participants represented "a variety of pneumonia experiences on the basis of symptom severity and site of treatment and convalescence." The sampling strategy was appropriate based on the populations being studied as described in the purpose.

Publication Section	Content	Questions	Appraisal (check one box)
Methods	Data collection protocol	• Were data collection methods appropriate for the intended purpose of the study (e.g., interviews, focus groups, observations, document review)? • Was the protocol for conducting the study described thoroughly and in enough detail? • Were data collection procedures consistently applied to the participants of the study • Did the data collector have sufficient qualifications and training? • Were data collected long enough to have saturation? • Was the protocol ethical and approved by an Institutional Review Board (IRB)?	☒ Strength ☐ Limitation ☐ Not evident ☐ Not applicable

Trustworthiness of the Qualitative Study

Publication Section	Content	Questions	Appraisal (check one box)
		• What steps were taken to ensure the confidentiality and anonymity of the participants? • What steps were taken to ensure credibility and objectivity during data collection?	

Reasoning: The researchers used a combination of interviews and focus groups to gather data. Semi-structured interviews were conducted individually with seniors and individually with family caregivers using an interview guide to gain data about their experiences with the pneumonia episode. Seven pairs of interviews with seniors/family members were conducted. Saturation was achieved on the theme of delayed treatment-seeking behaviors during the individual interviews. Two focus groups of seniors and two focus groups of family caregivers were used to confirm this theme as a form of member checks (to establish confirmability). Two members of the research team were "trained interviewers." The questions on the interview guide were modified as new results were revealed through the procedures of concurrent data collection and data analysis. When considering all aspects of the previous discussion, the data collection procedures were in alignment with the purpose of the study, were described in enough detail to replicate, and were completed until saturation occurred.

Two entities approved the study: McMaster University and the Brant Community Healthcare System. Written informed consent was gained before data collection. The researchers do not mention how objectivity was maintained during data collection.

Publication Section	Content	Questions	Appraisal (check one box)
Results	Sample	• Were the participants' characteristics described in enough detail to understand how they contributed to the data? • Were the participants' experiences with the phenomenon varied?	☒ Strength ☐ Limitation ☐ Not evident ☐ Not applicable

Reasoning: Table 1 contains information about the older adults' characteristics related to the severity of the pneumonia experience, whether they were admitted to the hospital, age, sex, marital status, education level, and income. The characteristics of the participants were varied and it is understandable how they contributed to the data. Minimal details about the family caregivers were provided, including their relationship to the older adult and their gender. This limited information seems appropriate because the role of the family member was to provide additional information about the pneumonia experience.

Publication Section	Content	Questions	Appraisal (check one box)
Results	Data analysis	• What steps were taken to ensure that the interview or focus group data were transcribed verbatim? • How were the data coded? • How were categories and themes constructed?	☒ Strength ☐ Limitation ☐ Not evident ☐ Not applicable

(continues)

Trustworthiness of the Qualitative Study

Publication Section	Content	Questions	Appraisal (check one box)
		• How were interrelationships established and a theory constructed (i.e., grounded theory approach)? • What steps were taken to ensure credibility, dependability, and objectivity during data analysis?	

Reasoning: During the interview, each of the two interviewers wrote field notes to record their insights about the data obtained during the interview and record nonverbal communication. The interviewers reviewed the transcripts to verify the content was verbatim. At the same time, the interviewers inserted their field notes into the transcript. Each interviewer "independently coded the transcripts line by line" and discrepancies were resolved by the two interviewers. Weekly team meetings were held to discuss the data analysis and interpretation. Common themes were continuously compared among the transcripts (constant comparison method). Data analysis was confirmed by the four focus groups. Researcher triangulation was evident by the entire team confirming the data analysis and interpretation. Dependability was established by an audit trial of decisions made throughout the process. Objectivity was maintained by having the two interviewers independently code the transcripts and resolve their differences before presenting the analysis at the weekly team meetings.

Publication Section	Content	Questions	Appraisal (check one box)
Results	Findings	• Are the themes or theory presented in an understandable manner? • Are the findings supported by quotations from the participants to facilitate transferability? • Are findings presented relative to the intended purpose and each research question?	☒ Strength ☐ Limitation ☐ Not evident ☐ Not applicable

Reasoning: The researchers developed a three-stage model of delay in seeking medical care by older adults with pneumonia. Each stage is explained and is understandable. Quotations for the first stage of the model are reported in Table 2; quotations for the second stage are shown in Table 3; and quotations for the third stage are reported in Table 4. These quotations provide support for each stage and articulate the participants' experiences with pneumonia. The three-stage model is the outcome of this qualitative inquiry, and is aligned with the intended purpose of describing pneumonia experiences of seniors and their family caregivers.

Publication Section	Content	Questions	Appraisal (check one box)
Discussion		• Did the researchers thoroughly explain their interpretation of the findings? • Were the explanations logical? • Did the researchers describe the contribution of their study to understanding the phenomenon? • Did the researchers discuss how their findings are related to previous studies and theories in their own discipline and, when appropriate, other disciplines?	☒ Strength ☐ Limitation ☐ Not evident ☐ Not applicable

Trustworthiness of the Qualitative Study

Publication Section	Content	Questions	Appraisal (check one box)
		• Did the researchers thoroughly identify and discuss the limitations? • What are the implications for practice? • What future research recommendations are made?	

Reasoning: The researchers interpreted the findings of delayed care and the key factors of decision making to seek medical intervention. The model of delay is compared to a similar model developed by another researcher. Limitations are presented in light of the participants including those who received an x-ray, the small sample size and problem related to the recruitment of the initial participants. The researchers explained the steps taken to strengthen the older adults' recall of the experience. Suggestions for future research are provided. The context of this study was explained as being within the Canadian healthcare system. The implication for healthcare professionals is discussed in the Conclusions section (e.g., education of older adults on the consequences of delayed action in seeking medical treatment).

Conclusions		• Is a conclusion provided for the intended purpose of the study? • Do the conclusions logically follow from the findings?	☒ Strength ☐ Limitation ☐ Not evident ☐ Not applicable

Reasoning: Yes, the researchers start this section by reviewing the purpose of the study and presenting the conclusions based on the pneumonia experiences of older adults. The conclusions are related to the delay in decision making for seeking medical treatment for pneumonia.

REFERENCES

1. Lincoln YS, Guba EG. *Naturalistic inquiry*. Newbury Park, CA: Sage; 1985.
2. Polit DF, Beck CT. The content validity index: Are you sure you know what's being reported? Critique and recommendations. *Res Nurs Health*. 2006;29:489–497.
3. Polit DF, Beck CT, Owen SV. Is the CVI an acceptable indicator of content validity? Appraisal and recommendations. *Res Nurs Health*. 2007;30:459–467.
4. Pelander T, Leino-Kilpi H, Katajisto J. The quality of paediatric nursing care: Developing the child care quality at hospital instrument for children. *J Adv Nurs*. 2008;65(2):443–453.
5. Portney LG, Watkins MP. *Foundations of clinical research*. Upper Saddle River, NJ: Pearson Education; 2009.
6. Keogh KM, Smith SM, White P, McGilloway, Kelly, Gibney J, O'Dowd T. Psychological family intervention for poorly controlled type 2 diabetes. *Am J Manag Care*. 2011;17(2):105–113.
7. McCarrier KP, Ralston JD, Hirsch IB, Lewis G, Martin DP, Zimmerman FJ, Goldberg HI. Web-based collaborative care for type 1 diabetes: A pilot randomized trial. *Diabetes Technol Ther*. 2009;11(4):211–217.
8. Bogner HR, Morales KH, de Fries HF, Cappola AR. Integrated management of type 2 diabetes mellitus and depression treatment to improve medication adherence: A randomized controlled trial. *Ann Fam Med*. 2012;10(1):15–22.
9. Keogh KM, White P, Smith S, McGillowway, O'Dowd T, Gibney J. Changing illness perception in patients with poorly controlled type 2 diabetes, a randomised controlled trial of family-based intervention: protocol and pilot study. *BMC Fam Pract*. 2007;8:36–45.
10. Khunti K, Gray LJ, Skinner T, Carey ME, Realf K, Dallosso H, et al. Effectiveness of a diabetes and self-management programme (DESMOND) for people with newly diagnosed type 2 diabetes mellitus: Three year follow-up of a cluster randomized controlled trial in primary care. *BMJ*. 2012;344:e2333

11. Patten ML. *Understanding research methods*. Glendale, CA: Pyrczak Publishing; 2012.

12. Shea BJ, Grimshaw JM, Wells GA, Boers M, Anderson N, Hamel C, et al. Development of AMSTAR: A measurement tool to assess the methodological quality of systematic reviews. *BMC Med Res Methodol*. 2007;7:10.

13. Shea BJ, Mael C, Wells GA, Boulter LM, Kristjansson E, Grimshaw J, et al. AMSTAR is a reliable and valid measurement tool to assess the methodological quality of systematic reviews. *J Clin Epidemiol*. 2009;63(10):1013–1020.

14. Moher D, Liberati A, Tetzlaff J, Altman DG. The PRISMA Group. Preferred reporting items for systematic reviews and meta-analyses: the PRISMA statement. *PLoS Med*. 6(6):e1000097.

15. Creswell JW. *Research design: qualitative, quantitative, and mixed methods approaches*. Thousand Oaks, CA: Sage Publications Inc.

16. Strauss A, Corbin J. *Basics of qualitative research. Techniques and procedures for developing grounded theory*. 2nd ed. Thousand Oaks, CA: Sage; 1998.

17. Creswell JW, Miller DL. Determining validity in qualitative inquiry. *Theory Pract*. 2000;39(3):124–130.

18. Denzin NK. *The research act: A theoretical introduction to sociological methods*. New York: McGraw-Hill; 1978.

19. Glaser BG, Strauss AL. *The discovery of grounded theory: Strategies for qualitative research*. Hawthorne, NY: Aldine Publishing; 1967.

20. Patton MQ. *Qualitative research and evaluation methods*. 3rd ed. Thousand Oaks, CA: Sage; 2002.

21. Svenningsson I, Hallberg LLR-M, Gedda B. Health care professionals meeting with individuals with type 2 diabetes and obesity: Balancing coaching and caution. *Int J Qualitative Stud Health Well-being*. 2011;6:7129.

22. Heuer L, Lausch C. Living with diabetes: Perceptions of Hispanic migrant farmworkers. *J Community Health Nurs*. 2006;23(1):49–64.

23. Hortensius J, Kars M, Wierenga WS, Kleefstra N, Bilo HJG, van der Bijl JJ. Perspectives of patients with type 1 or insulin-treated type 2 diabetes on self-monitoring of blood glucose: A qualitative study. *BMC Public Health*. 2012;12:167–177.

24. Cabassa LJ, Hansen MC, Palinkas LA, Ell K. Azucar y Nervios: Explanatory models and treatment experiences of Hispanics with diabetes and depression. *Soc Sci Med*. 2008;66(12):2413–2424.

25. Cherrington A, Ayala GX, Sleath B, Corbie-Smith G. Examining knowledge, attitudes, and beliefs about depression among Latino adults with type 2 diabetes. *Diabetes Educ*. 2006;32:603–613.

26. Livaudais J, Thompson B, Islas I, Ibarra G, Godina R, Coronado G. Type 2 diabetes among rural Hispanics in Washington State: Perspectives from community stakeholders. *Health Promot Pract*. 2010;11(4):589–599.

27. Clemmens D. Adolescent motherhood: a meta-synthesis of qualitative studies. *MCN Am J Matern Child Nurs*. 2003;28(2):93–99.

28. Duggleby W, Hicks D, Nekolaichuk C, Holtslander L, Williams A, Chambers T, Eby E. Hope, older adults, and chronic illness: a metasynthesis of qualitative research. *J Adv Nurs* 2012; 68(6):1211–1223.

29. Bayhakki, Hatthakit U. Lived experiences of patients on hemodialysis: a meta-synthesis. *Nephrol Nurs J* 2012; 39(4):295–304.

30. Sandelowski M, Barroso J. *Handbook for synthesizing qualitative research*. 2009. New York, NY: Springer Publishing Co.

31. Zimmer L. Qualitative meta-synthesis: a question of dialoguing with texts. *J Adv Nurs*. 2006; 53(3):311–318.

32. Northwest Service Academy. Reflection toolkit. 2003. Available at: www.nationalserviceresources.org/filemanager/download/615/nwtoolkit.pdf. Accessed July 27, 2012.

33. Schon DA. *The reflective practitioner: How professionals think in action*. London: Temple Smith; 1983.

34. Craik J, Rappolt S. Theory in research utilization enhancement: a model for occupational therapy. *Can J Occup Ther*. 2003;70(5):266–275.

Glossary

absolute risk (AR)—Another way of stating the event rate or incidence rate of a group. The event rate in the control group (CER) is the absolute risk of the condition for that group. Similarly, the event rate in the exposed group (EER) is the absolute risk of the condition for that group.

absolute risk increase (ARI)—When the *absolute risk* (AR) among the exposed group is greater than the AR among the control group. Also referred to as *attributable risk*.

absolute risk reduction (ARR)—When the *absolute risk* (AR) among the exposed group is less than the AR among the control group. Also referred to as *attributable risk*.

abstract—A brief overview of a publication that outlines the major topics. Abstracts are limited in terms of the number of words that can be included. The word limit varies from one publisher to the next, although 250 to 350 words are typical. Abstracts are usually structured according to required elements, such as background, problem, purpose, methods, results, and discussion (or conclusions). Publishers vary in the expected topics and headings for their abstracts. Often abstracts are available for free, even with subscription-only articles.

action phase of change—In the transtheoretical model of change, at this stage the patient is actively engaged in changing behavior less than 6 months.

adherence—The degree to which patients are able to sustain a treatment regimen according to how it was prescribed.

administration of treatment—Administration of treatment includes the issues of mode (also known as route), method, and dose.

adverse event (AE)—Any undesirable experience associated with the use of a medical product in a patient.

Adverse Event Reporting System (AERS)—An online database administered by the FDA in which researchers report adverse events. AERS is available to the public.

AE—*See* adverse event (AE).

AERS—*See* Adverse Event Reporting System (AERS).

affective objectives—Patient outcomes that focus on changing a patient's attitudes or values.

AHRQ (Agency for Healthcare Research and Quality)—An agency within the Department of Health and Human Services charged with improving the quality, safety, and effectiveness of health care for all Americans.

alpha—The probability of a Type I error. It is selected during the design of the research and represents the researchers' risk of incorrectly rejecting the null hypothesis (of saying there is a difference when in fact there is not). Alpha is sometimes referred to as *probability (p)*. The most common levels of alpha used in research are 0.05, 0.01, and 0.001; that is to say a 5% chance of making a Type I error, a 1% chance of making a Type I error, or a 0.1% chance of making a Type I error.

alpha-halves—The risk of a Type I error when a test of equality is performed. If equality is tested, the researchers assume that either group could turn out to be superior, in which case alpha should be divided in half. When a test of equality is performed it is referred to as a *two-tailed test*, meaning that there are two sides.

ANOVA—An abbreviation for *Analysis of Variance*. It is a test for differences between two or more variables. It is similar to the *t*-test and can substitute for a *t*-test when only two groups are compared. It will show if there is a difference in the mean between multiple groups. However, it will not show which group differs from which. In many cases, an additional test must be performed to determine which group(s) differ.

AR—*See* absolute risk (AR), attack rate (AR), or attributable risk (AR).

area under the curve (AUC)—The ratio of the false positive rate to the true positive rate produces a proportion called the area under the curve. An AUC of 0.50 (50%) means the diagnostic test is no better than chance. An AUC of 1.0 (100%) means the diagnostic test is perfectly accurate.

ARI—*See* absolute risk increase (ARI).

assessment—Collecting the data upon which a diagnosis can be based. The process of identifying the signs and symptoms of disease and recording the associated data for the purpose of informing a diagnosis. An assessment is not a diagnosis; it is a process of data collection and the collected data itself. For example, the presence of calculus on teeth can be observed and noted on a clinical assessment, but the diagnosis of periodontal disease would require additional information.

assumptions—Characteristics that must be satisfied in order for a statistical test to be accurate and robust.

attack rate (AR)—Similar to incidence, an attack rate represents an increased occurrence of disease among people over a short period of time.

attributable risk (AR)—A difference in the absolute risk (AR) between the experimental and the control group. Either group can have the higher attributable risk. *See also* absolute risk reduction (ARR) and absolute risk increase (ARI).

attributable risk percent (AR%)—Attributable risk (AR) calculated as a proportion. AR% is the percent of the incidence of a disease in the exposed population that is due to the exposure. In other words, it is the percent of the incidence of a disease in the exposed that would be eliminated if the risk factor was removed. The AR% is calculated by dividing the AR by the exposed event rate (EER) and then multiplying the product by 100 to obtain a percentage.

AUC—*See* area under the curve (AUC).

audit trail—A record of decisions made throughout a naturalistic (qualitative) study that can be referenced by a peer reviewer or an external auditor in assessing the trustworthiness of the study.

bar graph—A chart that reports the frequencies of observations in groupings (called *bins*) of qualitative data. The gaps between the columns in the chart indicate that the data are qualitative (nominal, categorical, or ordinal).

bias—Something other than the predictor variable influencing the response variable in a quantitative study.

bin—In a frequency table or chart, the bins are the ranges of values used to group data (e.g., the number of patients between the ages of 18 and 25, the number of patients between 26 and 32, etc.). In most cases, the range for each bin should be equal between all bins. The bins must be mutually exclusive, meaning no observation can be counted in more than one bin.

binary data—A type of nominal or categorical data that includes only two discrete categories, such as true/false, yes/no, or male/female.

biography—The study of an individual and her or his experiences as told to the researcher or found in documents and archival material.

biologics—Products used for the treatment, prevention, or cure of disease in humans. In contrast to chemically synthesized small molecular-weight drugs that have a well-defined structure and can be thoroughly characterized, biologics are generally derived from living material and are complex in structure, and thus are usually not fully characterized.

biostatistics—Statistics applied to biological research.

blinding—A procedure through which individuals (subjects, clinicians, and/or data analysts) are kept uninformed of the designation of subjects to study groups. In single-blind studies, the subjects are blinded to which group they are assigned. In a double-blind study, subjects as well as those who provide the interventions are blinded. In a triple-blind study, the subjects, the providers, and the data analysts are blinded.

BMI (Body Mass Index)—A measure of body fat based on height and weight that applies to adult men and women.

Boolean operator—A word that functions in a search engine as a command. The three most common Boolean operators are AND, NOT, and OR. These operators are used to focus search results. Not all search engines utilize Boolean operators, nor do all engines utilize them in the same way.

box-and-whisker plot—A chart used to show a five-number summary. Often displays outliers.

calculators—In health care there are numerous calculators that are available online or as downloadable computer or smartphone applications. Some calculators are free of charge and others require a fee for use. There are many different types of calculators, such as conversions between metric and standard measurement, decision trees, medication dosing, diagnostic algorithms, etc.

case-control study—A retrospective study in which subjects are divided into cases (those with the outcome of interest) and controls (those without the outcome of interest), and associations are sought between exposures and the outcome(s) of interest.

case definition—A set of standard criteria for classifying whether a person has a particular disease, syndrome, or health condition. It is a working definition that researchers have agreed upon as the basic unit of study. A case definition provides parameters for comparing cases across time and place.

case report—Another term used for case study research. The term *case report* is more common in healthcare research and publications.

case study—An exploration of a bounded system (a case or multiple cases) over time through detailed, in-depth data collection involving multiple sources of information rich in context. The bounded system is bound by time and place such that the case or cases of interest might be an event, an activity, or the individuals themselves.

categorical data—In positivistic research, categorical data are designated as qualitative because they are not measurable. Categorical data are observations that can each be assigned to one unique category, similar to nominal data. There can be many categories, such as city of birth, or only two categories, such as male/female. Categorical data are converted into numerical data by counting the number of observations in each category.

Centers for Disease Control and Prevention (CDC)—Part of the Department of Health and Human Services. Its mission is to enhance health promotion; prevent disease, injury, and disability; and prepare for new health threats.

central tendency—A single number that represents the typical value for the data set, expressed as a mean, median, and/or mode.

CER—*See* control event rate (CER).

chi square—A nonparametric statistical test most often used to test for differences in frequencies between two or more groups. It is symbolized by χ^2.

CI—*See* confidence interval (CI).

CINAHL—The Cumulative Index to Nursing and Allied Health Literature (CINAHL) is an online index of literature about nursing, allied health, biomedicine, and other healthcare topics. It is provided by EBSCO Publishing and requires a license to access it, although some CINAHL resources are available for free to the public. Many colleges and universities purchase site licenses so that all students can access the full version of CINAHL.

citation—Details of the bibliographic information of a source, such as a book, website, or journal article. It includes the title of the document, the name(s) of the authors(s), the title of the source it came from (such as a journal), and other helpful details, such as the volume and issue number, as well as page numbers of the article.

Clinical Queries—In PubMed, Clinical Queries are filtered sets of resources that have been grouped together into three major clinical research areas: clinical studies, systematic reviews, and medical genetics. Searches performed in the Clinical Queries section of PubMed produce only publications that fall into one of these three areas. The Clinical Queries tool shows the number of results that fall into each area and allows users to further reduce results by subcategories if any are applicable.

clinical trial—Clinical trials take various forms and can combine styles, including case series, surveys, control trials, cohort studies, and randomized control trials. Clinical trials either directly involve a particular person or group of people or use materials from humans. Researchers observe subjects and/or collect data to answer a health-related question about the safety or efficacy of an intervention.

Clipboard—In search engines such as PubMed, the Clipboard is a place where selected search results can be retained. In PubMed, users have to create a MyNCBI account in order for the system to be able to retain Clipboard information after the window has been closed.

Cochrane Collaboration—The leading research organization for systematic reviews and meta-analyses, setting the standards for design and quality of these types of studies. This international network provides information to help healthcare providers, policy makers, patients, their advocates, and care providers make well-informed decisions about health care by preparing, updating, and promoting the accessibility of Cochrane Reviews. Cochrane reviews are the *gold standard* for the highest level of evidence.

Cochrane Library—An online collection of databases that brings together in one place rigorous and up-to-date research on the effectiveness of healthcare treatments and interventions, as well as methodology and diagnostic tests.

Cochrane Systematic Review—A systematic review of primary research in human health care and health policy. Cochrane Reviews are internationally recognized as the highest standard in evidence-based health care. They investigate the effects of interventions for prevention, treatment, and rehabilitation. They also assess the accuracy of a diagnostic test for a given condition in a specific patient group and setting.

coefficient of determination—The square of r (Pearson's product-moment correlation coefficient). The coefficient of determination tells us the proportion of the variability in the response variable that is explained by the variability in the predictor variable. The higher the percentage, the stronger the association.

cognitive objectives Outcomes that focuses on changing a patient's knowledge.

Cohen's *d*—A statistic that shows effect size. A d score of 0.80 is considered a large effect. 0.20 is a small effect, 0.50 is a medium effect, 1.10 is a very large effect, and 1.40 or higher is an extremely large effect.

Cohen's kappa—A statistic that shows inter-rater reliability for categorical data. A score of 0.80 or higher is generally considered an indication of a high level of consistency, meaning the data are reliable. *See also* inter-rater reliability.

cohort study—Cohort studies are observational, prospective studies (usually large in size and longitudinal in duration) in which the groups in the study are determined by a given exposure, characteristic, or risk factor. Patients are followed forward in time to monitor for the development of a given outcome. Group assignment is not random in cohort studies. These studies can include comparisons of various levels of exposures, and numerous factors that might influence the frequency of outcomes and their severity.

common-source outbreak—When an agent or toxin from a single source simultaneously affects exposed individuals.

community—Community can be defined several ways, such as being in the same geographic location (country, state, public health district, county, city, or neighborhood); having shared interests; having a common culture, religion, or background; or having a shared experience (e.g., a community of individuals who experience diabetes as patients or as caregivers). *See also* subcommunity.

community health initiative—A program or project aimed at improving health at a community or subcommunity level. *See also* community; subcommunity.

complete history—A process for collecting information about a patient designed to elucidate a patient's entire health status. A complete history covers all body systems.

compliance—Degree of constancy and accuracy with which a patient follows a prescribed regimen, as distinguished from adherence or maintenance.

complications—Unintended adverse events, such as injury or death, resulting from treatment, diagnostic, prevention, or screening interventions.

concurrent EBP—Looking up information in response to clinical questions and using that information to make decisions regarding an individual patient. This practice can occur while the patient is in clinic.

confidence interval (CI)—The range in which the true parameter can be found, within a given percentage likelihood. The most frequently used value is 95%. A 95% confidence interval tells us that 95% of the time the test statistic will fall within the given range; some might say we are 95% confident that the true value of the population falls within the given range. The range of the confidence interval is useful because it helps determine if the outcome is sufficiently narrow.

constant comparative method—Interview data are analyzed after each participant's interview and the data from one interview are compared to the data from the other interviews; therefore, data collection and analysis occur simultaneously.

contemplation phase of change—In the transtheoretical model of change, at this stage the patient is considering action to change behavior in the next 6 months.

contingency table—A relationship table used for organizing data to support calculations. The most common form of a contingency table is a 2 × 2 table, which is a table that has four cells for data. The contingency table can be used to calculate sensitivity, specificity, PPV, NPV, CER, EER, RR, RRR, AR, and OR.

continuous data—Interval and ratio data are continuous; there is an infinite number of possible values when measuring on a continuous scale. Also, continuous data are ordered, have no natural categories, might contain a true zero (making them ratio) or no true zero (making them interval), and have a measurable/equivalent distance between each increment in the scale.

contraindications—The circumstances in which a given treatment should *not* be used.

control event rate (CER)—The rate of the event of interest among the control group. In a 2 × 2 table the formula for CER is $a/(a + b)$.

control group—A set of subjects in a trial that acts as the basis of comparison for the treatment group. The control group can receive no intervention, a placebo, or the usual care intervention.

control trial—A prospective study in which a control group receiving no intervention, placebo, or usual care is compared to a treatment group that receives an intervention of interest. Subjects are not randomly assigned to treatment or control groups in a control trial.

convenience sampling—Selecting the subjects of a study based on ease of access (convenience).

correlation study—A study that identifies statistically significant relationships between variables.

credibility—The degree to which data collection and interpretation are plausible. This concept is generally applied to naturalistic (qualitative) research.

critical appraisal—A process of evaluating the trustworthiness and relevance of a resource within the context of a given clinical situation. Appraisal involves questions such as potential sources of bias, representativeness of a study's sample, consistency of a study's methods, accuracy of the data collected, duration of the research in light of the question explored, and even just the common sense of a study.

cross-over trial—A prospective study, similar to pre/post studies, in which patients are moved from one group to another. They are in the control group for a period of time and then moved to one or more treatment groups. This differs from pre/post studies in that the subjects can be in multiple treatment groups. There might not even be a control group in a cross-over trial, although that would weaken the study.

cross-sectional research—Studies that collect data at a single fixed point in time. Studies of prevalence are perhaps the most common type of cross-sectional research. Cross-sectional research is noninterventional and observational in nature.

CT (computed tomography)—A type of imaging procedure.

culturally competent care—According to the Office of Minority Health, culturally competent care is a set of congruent behaviors, attitudes, and policies that come together in a system, agency, or among professionals. Culturally competent care enables effective work in cross-cultural situations.

data transformation—*See* transformation of data.

defensive medical practice—Excessive use of diagnostic procedures to avoid lawsuits by

showing that every available measure was employed.

dependability—The degree to which the interpretations in a naturalistic (qualitative) study are consistent with the data collected.

dependent variable—A measured variable that responds to the predictor (i.e., independent variable). A dependent variable is also referred to as a *response variable*. Dependent variables are associated with the outcomes of interest in a study. For example, mortality from heart disease can be dependent of predictors (independent variables) such as age, sex, smoking, body mass, etc.

descriptive statistics—Numerically describing a phenomenon.

df (degrees of freedom)—The number of observations minus 1.

differences—In statistics, differences are mathematical variations between variables. When the difference is sufficient, the variables can be declared statistically significant in difference, which usually means the null hypothesis can be rejected.

differential diagnosis—Systematically comparing and contrasting results of diagnostic measures in order to determine which one of two or more diseases or conditions a patient is suffering from.

disease surveillance—An epidemiological activity that involves tracking the number of people afflicted with a particular illness.

distribution—A ranking of observations in a data set from lowest to highest showing the number of observations in each grouping, usually plotted on a graph to show the shape of the distribution.

dose—The amount and frequency of administration and quantity of a treatment or other type of intervention.

dot plot—A graph that shows frequencies of observations. Dot plots are similar to histograms in that they are used to show frequencies, but they have the advantage of making it somewhat easier to see how many items are in each column.

double-blind randomized control trial—A randomized control trial in which the allocation of subjects to treatment and control groups is concealed from both the subjects themselves and from the clinicians who treat them.

Dx—A clinical abbreviation that stands for *diagnosis*.

EBP—*See* evidence-based practice (EBP).

EER—*See* experiment or exposed event rate (EER).

effect size—In a statistical power calculation, effect size is the expected amount of effect that is considered a minimal clinically meaningful effect. Effect size is often reported as a Cohen's *d* statistic.

efficacy—The degree to which an intervention produces the desired beneficial outcome.

e-health—The use of technology to communicate information to improve health and health services.

endemic—A disease that is persistently stable in a specific locale.

epidemic—When there is an incidence of disease that exceeds what is normally expected.

epidemiological triad—A theory that explains disease outbreak in terms of the relationships and interactions among the host, the agent, and the environment.

epidemiology—The study of the occurrence and distribution of health-related states or events in specified populations. Epidemiology includes the study of the determinants influencing disease states, and the application of knowledge to control health problems.

ethnography—A description and interpretation of a cultural or social group or system. The researcher examines the group's observable and learned patterns of behavior, customs, and ways of life. Involves prolonged observation of the group, typically through participant observation in which the researcher is immersed in the day-to-day lives of the people or through one-on-one interviews with members of the group.

etiology—Literally, the science and study of causes. In health care, the term relates to the causes of illness, also referred to as *pathogenesis*.

evaluation phase of care—A stage in the patient care process, following the implementation phase, in which the goal is to determine the patient's progress with the intervention. This phase uses subjective information gained from the patient as well as objective measurements of the outcome based on tests.

evidence-based practice (EBP)—The process of combining the best available research evidence with your knowledge and skill to make collaborative, patient- or population-centered decisions within the context of a given healthcare situation.

evidence pyramid—A visual representation and system for categorizing healthcare information according to level of evidence. In most systems, the top of the pyramid represents the highest level of evidence, those resources that are considered to be the most trustworthy.

exclusion criteria—Characteristics (such as age, diagnosis, comorbidities, gender, etc.) that result in an individual being excluded from participating in a study. In many cases, exclusion criteria relate to risks of harm from the study intervention.

experiment event rate (EER)—The rate of the event of interest among the exposed (or treatment) group. In a 2 × 2 table the formula for EER is $c/(c + d)$. Also referred to as *exposed event rate*.

experimental research—In biomedical research, experimental research includes studies that involve randomly selecting subjects from the entire population or randomly assigning participants into intervention and control groups and measuring differences between them or associations between predictor and response variables. Researchers are able to control variables in this type of study.

exposed event rate (EER)—*See* experiment event rate.

external validity—The degree to which the findings of the study are generalizable to the population and to a similar healthcare context.

extraneous variables—Undesirable variables that interfere with the intended purpose of the investigation by introducing error to the study and affecting the dependent variable or outcome. Also known as *intervening variables*.

factor analysis—A procedure for combining items in a survey instrument to represent a single concept (called a *construct* or *domain*). A survey is broken down into domains (also called *sub-scales*) that include multiple questions. A certain number of items should be included in each domain in order for the domain to be considered valid. Each of the items in a domain must be conceptually as well as statistically related.

FDA (Food and Drug Administration)—A federal agency that regulates most medications, many medical devices, as well as other products (such as vaccines, blood and biologics, and radiation-emitting products).

filters—Another term for *limiters* or *limits*. In PubMed, the filter options appear along the left column of the home search page. Filters include text availability (e.g., full-text, free full-text, etc.), publication date, species, article type, language, and more. There is a link called "Show additional filters" that offers a pop-up menu with more filter options.

5E model—A model of learning that promotes active rather than passive patient education. The model includes the following five stages: Engage, Explore, Explain, Elaborate, and Evaluate.

five-number summary—A shorthand way of reporting five commonly used descriptive statistics (minimum, lower quartile, median, upper quartile, and maximum). The values in a five-number summary can be calculated on ordinal, interval, or ratio data.

focused clinical question—A question formulated around a clinical information need, including three major elements: (1) a specific condition or outcome (e.g., treatment of LDL cholesterol); (2) patient demographics (e.g., age, ethnicity, gender); and, (3) patient risk factors (e.g., smoking, overweight).

focused history—A process for collecting information about a patient designed to elucidate a specific problem and differentiate between critical and noncritical causes. A focused history covers only the relevant body systems.

forest plot—A forest plot is a special usage of box-and-whisker plots. It includes a series of these graphs with a trend line across the different plots.

FPG—Fasting plasma glucose.

frequency—A descriptive statistic showing the number of observations or the proportion of observations (if expressed as a percentage).

full-text—The complete version of a publication. Full-text publications can be free or can be available only for a fee.

funding bias—A type of publication bias in which a study is not published at the behest of the funding agency for reasons other than the quality of the research or the relevance of its findings.

generalizability—The positivistic assumption that an inference can be drawn from a sample of patients that will hold true with the population represented by the sample.

gold standard test—The test that is known to be the most accurate, regardless of cost, invasiveness, or other considerations.

goodness-of-fit test—A type of chi-square test that can test if the sample distribution fits with a theoretical distribution. Such tests are often employed in making comparisons between groups with regard to demographic factors, such as the age distribution of the sample, compared to the population and compared to the control group.

grounded theory—The study of abstract problems and their processes. It is a general methodology of analysis linked with data collection that uses a systematically applied set of methods to generate an inductive theory about a substantive area. The research product constitutes a theoretical formulation or integrated set of conceptual hypotheses about the substantive area under study.

hazard ratio (HR)—A measure of how often a particular adverse event occurs in one group compared to another group over time. The element of time is the primary distinguishing characteristic of a hazard ratio. It is essentially a relative risk calculation weighted according to time across a survival curve during the course of a study. The hazard is the slope of the survival curve, and the hazard ratio compares the slope between two groups.

health belief model—An approach to behavior change designed to influence individuals to take action to engage in healthy behaviors.

health communication—The study and use of communication strategies to inform and influence individual and community decisions that affect health. It links the fields of communication and health and is increasingly recognized as a necessary element of efforts to improve personal and public health.

health literacy—The degree to which individuals have the capacity to obtain, process, and understand basic health information and services needed to make appropriate health decisions. Health literacy is critical to achieving the objectives set forth in *Healthy People 2020*.

Healthfinder.gov—An online database sponsored by the National Health Information Center that contains health topics and other databases to locate physicians and other providers and healthcare centers, including long-term care or nursing home facilities, hospitals, community health centers, home health services, and hospice care.

histogram—A frequency chart used with continuous data (interval and ratio).

history—In Internet browsers and other search tools (such as PubMed) the history is a record of searches that have been performed. In some cases, depending on settings, the history is deleted as soon as the window is closed. In other cases, the history is stored on the computer. Some systems have features that allow you to save the history under a specific title so you can retrieve or return to a prior search.

HR—*See* hazard ratio (HR).

hypothesis—A positivistic statement about what is believed to be true.

icon display—A visual representation that utilizes icons to represent concepts. Examples include Cates plots and visual analog scales.

implementation phase of patient care—The implementation phase of care encompasses the actions the clinician and patient take to maintain or improve health.

incidence—The number of new cases of a disease or condition during a specified time frame.

inclusion criteria—Characteristics (such as age, diagnosis, comorbidities, gender, etc.) that must be satisfied in order for an individual to be included in a study.

independent variable—A measured variable that influences the outcome of a dependent variable. An independent variable is also referred to as a *predictor variable*. An independent variable can affect a response (i.e., dependent) variable, such as age, sex, smoking, or body mass being a predictor of heart disease.

indications—The circumstances in which a given treatment should be used.

inferences—A deductive prediction made about a population based on observations of a sample. With inferential statistics researchers attempt to generalize a phenomenon measured in a sample to the population represented by the sample.

inferential statistics—Deriving inferences about a population based on a representative sample.

Institutional Review Board (IRB)—An organization that reviews research proposals and regulates research activities. IRBs can be internal or external and must be approved by the Office for Human Research Protections (OHRP). The OHRP is an agency within the U.S. Department of Health and Human Services that provides oversight of IRBs.

intention-to-treat analysis—Also referred to as *intent-to-treat*. A procedure in which the data analyzed from a study include participants who completed at least one follow-up. There are several ways to perform intent-to-treat analysis. It is generally considered a more rigorous analytic procedure than per-protocol analysis because it accounts for the effect of dropouts on study outcomes. The most rigorous approach is to utilize both per-protocol (on-protocol) and intent-to-treat and compare the results to see if they differ. *See also* per-protocol analysis; on-protocol analysis.

interaction—In the context of healthcare provision, a mutual or reciprocal action or influence. Interactions can increase the effect of a treatment (positive interaction) or reduce the effect of a treatment (negative interaction).

internal validity—A characteristic of research design that relates to the degree to which the outcomes of the study can be attributed to the interventions.

interprofessional collaborative practice (ICP)—The development of a cohesive practice between professionals from different disciplines. It is the process by which professionals reflect on and develop ways of practicing that provides an integrated and cohesive answer to the needs of the client/family/population.

interquartile range (IQR)—The difference between the upper quartile and the lower quartile.

inter-rater reliability—The degree to which the data collected are consistent between different researchers. Inter-rater reliability is often measured through a Cohen's Kappa test. It is often used in systematic reviews and meta-analyses to assess the level of consistency across reviewers in their procedures for selecting and for critically appraising studies.

interval data—Interval data are measurable observations that have natural order and equivalence, but whose scale has no true zero point. While there is a value of 0 degrees F (for example), even at that temperature there is still some warmth. Zero represents the absence of something, but 0 degrees F does not mean there is an absence of temperature. Interval data are similar to ratio data in that each observation is an equivalent distance from the next (e.g., the distance from 2 to 3 is equal to the distance from 136 to 137). Values in an interval scale can be added and subtracted, but not multiplied or divided.

intervening variables—*See* extraneous variables.

intervention—In biomedical research, an intervention is an activity that is intended to alter an outcome, such as a risk reduction strategy, a pain management procedure, a drug therapy, or a diagnostic tool.

intra-rater reliability The degree to which the data collected on one participant are consistent with the data collected on the other participants.

IRB—*See* Institutional Review Board (IRB).

left skew—A visual description for a non-normal data set in which values trail off to the left side of the bar chart, creating a "tail" on that side.

likelihood ratio (LR)—A statistical test that evaluates the accuracy of a diagnostic procedure. Likelihood ratios can be positive or negative.

Likert scale—A survey response list that is ordinal in nature, e.g., 5 = Strongly Agree; 4 = Agree; 3 = Neutral; 2 = Disagree; 1 = Strongly Disagree. Between 5 and 10 response options are most common.

limitations—In positivistic research, aspects of a study that reduce its generalizability. Limitations are also referred to as *bias*.

limiters or limits—With regard to using online search tools, limiters are settings or options to reduce/focus the results of a search. Common limiters include date range, file type, file size, language, etc. Nearly every search tool has its own limiters that users can select.

LR—*See* likelihood ratio (LR).

maintenance phase of change—In the transtheoretical model of change, at this stage the patient has sustained the behavior change for more than 6 months.

maximum—The highest value in an ordered data set.

MCID—*See* minimal clinically important difference (MCID).

MCSD (minimal clinically significant difference)—*See* minimal clinically important difference (MCID).

mean—The average of a data set. Usually the arithmetic mean is calculated. Other types of means include the harmonic mean and the geometric mean. Usually, unless otherwise stated, a mean is an arithmetic mean, rather than one of the other types.

measurement bias—Limitation(s) to the procedures used for quantifying information in a quantitative study. Measurement bias can include inaccurate measurement tools, calculation errors, mistakes in recording measurements, participant bias, recall bias, and more.

median—The middle observation in an ordered data set. It is the point at which the data set can be cut in half. When there is an odd number of observations, the median is the one that has an equal number of observations above and below.

When there is an even number of observations, then the two middle observations are averaged in order to determine the median.

medical geography—Studies of the land, atmosphere, and the inhabitants in a specific area, addressing the physical environment and the people, with the goal of understanding disease processes in order to improve health.

medical statistics—Another term for *biostatistics*.

MedlinePlus—A consumer health information website developed and maintained by the National Library of Medicine and the National Institutes of Health. The information provided is free.

member check—A procedure utilized in naturalistic (qualitative) research in which the researchers present interpretations to participants to verify that the researcher's interpretations are consonant with the participants' experiences. It is a strategy used to establish the credibility of the findings.

MeSH—An abbreviation that stands for Medical Subject Heading. MeSHs are used in PubMed as well as other publication indexing systems. MeSHs are a type of controlled vocabulary that are used for categorizing and grouping publications. Searching PubMed by MeSHs can significantly improve the accuracy of search results compared to performing key word searches.

MeSH Database—In PubMed, the MeSH Database is where users can search for MeSH terms as well as bring up the MeSH tree for the selected term.

MeSH tree—In PubMed, a MeSH tree is a relational list of Medical Subject Headings (MeSH) that categorize MeSHs within one another, creating a branching structure (e.g., morbid obesity falls in the category of obesity, which is within the category of overweight, which is in the category of body weight, etc.). These branches show the hierarchies within MeSHs. Each level of the hierarchy represents a change in the generality of the topics contained. A MeSH tree can help users expand or narrow searches to improve the relevance of results.

meta-analysis—An added step to a systematic review in which a statistical analysis is performed to quantify the findings of multiple studies in the review. Statistical analysis of results from separate studies is performed, leading to a quantitative summary of the results.

meta-search engine—A search engine capable of searching for information in multiple databases at the same time, resulting in one list of results. TRIP is an example of a meta-search engine.

meta-synthesis—A research procedure in which all prior qualitative studies on a given topic are brought together and analyzed collectively.

method of administration—The technique for performing the treatment (e.g., holding an instrument at a specific angle, using a specific amount of pressure, at a particular location) as well as who will administer the treatment (the patient or a clinician).

minimal clinically important difference (MCID)—The smallest difference in score in an outcome of interest to patients that is perceived as beneficial and would mandate a change in treatment. Also referred to as *minimal clinically significant difference* (MCSD).

minimum—The lowest value in an ordered data set.

mixed-method research—Research that combines naturalistic (qualitative) and positivistic (quantitative) research strategies.

mode—The most frequently occurring value in an ordered data set. Data sets can have more than one mode (multimodal).

mode of administration—How the treatment reaches its target location (e.g., absorption through the skin).

modifiable risk factor—An exposure, attribute, or behavior people can change that is associated with but not the cause of a given outcome of interest.

morbidity—A diseased state/illness.

mortality—Death or rate of death associated with a given health problem or intervention.

motivational interviewing (MI)—A treatment modality that identifies and utilizes the intrinsic motivation of individuals. MI is a strategy for clinicians to collaborate with patients to identify their health-related goals and make self-directed changes toward achieving these goals.

MRI (magnetic resonance imaging)—A type of imaging procedure.

multimodal—A data set with more than one mode (more than one value that occurs most frequently). Multimodal distributions are non-normal by definition.

multistage sampling—A procedure in which sampling occurs in one or more steps (stages). Often this procedure is used when dealing with very large sampling frames and researchers want to ensure that every subgroup is included.

n—A lowercase letter n stands for *number* and represents the number of subjects in a sample.

National Health Education Standards (NHES)—National standards for health education that articulate the framework for promoting health at the personal, family, and community levels for students in pre-kindergarten, elementary school, middle school, and high school. The standards are developed through a collaboration between the Centers for Disease Control and Prevention (CDC) and the American Cancer Society. The NHES are available on the CDC website.

naturalistic research—Also referred to as *qualitative research*. It is a paradigm through which knowledge is viewed as stemming from the internal reality of an individual or a group. Naturalistic studies focus on open-ended questions; utilize small, purposeful samples; follow emergent designs; occur in uncontrolled settings; rely on observational data; employ inductive reasoning and thematic, narrative, and content analytic procedures; and, include the researcher as an active participant as well as source of data.

negative case—In naturalistic (qualitative) studies, a negative case is an example of a subject whose experience differs from other subjects or from the expected experience. Some qualitative researchers seek negative cases in order to ensure the research question has been thoroughly investigated.

negative likelihood ratio (NLR)—The relative likelihood of having the disease if the patient has a negative test result. Symbolized as −LR.

negative predictive value (NPV)—The likelihood someone with a negative test result will actually not have the disease. It is expressed as a proportion. NPV is the percentage of those with a negative test result who actually do not have the disease. In a 2 × 2 table the formula for NPV is $d/(c + d)$.

network sampling—*See* snowball sampling.

NLM (National Library of Medicine)—An entity within the National Institutes of Health. It is the world's largest biomedical library. The NLM administers PubMed, Clinicaltrials.gov, MedlinePlus, and other health information resources.

NLR (or −LR)—*See* negative likelihood ratio (NLR).

NNH—*See* number needed to harm (NNH).

NNS—*See* number needed to screen (NNS).

NNT—*See* number needed to treat (NNT).

nominal data—In positivistic research nominal data are designated as qualitative because they are not measurable. Nominal data are observations that are assigned names, such as male or female. The word *nominal* comes from the Latin word *nominalis,* which means "of a name."

nonmodifiable risk factor—An exposure, attribute, or behavior people cannot change that is associated with but not the cause of a given outcome of interest.

nonparametric statistics—Statistical procedures designed to be used with data that do not meet the assumptions of normality and/or data that are qualitative. Nonparametric statistics require fewer assumptions than parametric statistics.

nonprobability sampling—A procedure in which subjects are purposely selected in order to ensure that they represent/experience the phenomenon of interest. This is often used with rare conditions or with small populations.

normal distribution—A set of data with a single center point that represents the mean, median, and mode whose values are equally distributed over both sides of the mean. The values must be interval or ratio scale. When drawn, a normal distribution looks like a bell curve.

NPV—*See* negative predictive value (NPV).

number needed to harm (NNH)—The average number of persons who need to be treated in order to produce one more adverse event; NNH = 1/ARI.

number needed to screen (NNS)—The number of persons, on average, who must undergo a screening test and related diagnostic and therapeutic procedures in order to prevent one case of the disease of interest; NNS = 1/ARR.

number needed to treat (NNT)—The average number of persons needed to be treated in order to prevent one more adverse event; NNT = 1/ARR.

numeracy—Application of numbers and measurement into daily tasks such as medication dosing.

nursing assessment—According to the U.S. Library of Medicine, nursing assessment is the evaluation of the nature and extent of nursing problems presented by a patient for the purpose of patient care planning.

nursing diagnosis—Clinical judgment about actual or potential individual, family, or community experiences/responses to health problems/life processes that provides the basis for selection of nursing interventions. The goal is to achieve outcomes for which the nurse has accountability.

objective data—Information you observe or measure.

objectivity The conscientious practice among researchers of remaining unbiased, honest, and precise in order to avoid making unconscious choices when planning, conducting, and reporting the results of the study.

observation—A single data point representing a phenomenon of interest.

observational research—A type of quantitative (positivistic) research in which a phenomenon is quantified but no intervention is employed by researchers to alter an outcome.

odds—The ratio in a group of those with an event to those without the event. In a 2 × 2 table, the odds for the exposed group are *a/b*; the odds for the control group are *c/d*.

odds ratio (OR)—The ratio of the odds of an event occurring in one group to the odds of an event occurring in another group. In a 2 × 2 table the formula is *ad/bc*. An OR significantly less than 1.0 indicates a protective factor. An OR equal to 1.0 indicates a nonfactor; an OR significantly greater than 1.0 indicates a risk factor.

one-sample *t*-test—A quantitative test that compares the mean score of a sample to the known mean (normative or expected) value from a trustworthy source. This test is used when a normative value derived from a previously known, and trustworthy, source is the basis of comparison for a variable measured among the experimental group. The normative value takes the place of a control or placebo group. Typically, the normative value is based on a measure that is regularly performed by an authoritative organization such as the CDC or the WHO (World Health Organization). The central question in a one-sample *t*-test is if there is a difference between the experimental group(s) and the known normative value.

on-protocol analysis *See* per-protocol analysis

open-label design—Researchers, subjects, providers, and analysts all know to which group each subject has been assigned. Also referred to as *nonblinded research*. Open-label approaches are sometimes necessary due to the nature of the research (e.g., comparing a surgical intervention to a medication would be very difficult to create blinding).

OR—*See* odds ratio (OR).

oral diagnosis—Assessment of the oral cavity and the structures contained therein in order to diagnose and differentiate intraoral disease or identify manifestations in the oral cavity of systemic conditions.

ordinal data—In positivistic research ordinal data are designated as qualitative because they are not measurable. Ordinal data are observations that can be placed into a specified order, such as responses to a Likert scale, where the lowest number represents the lowest level of agreement and the highest number represents the highest level of agreement. Even though the observations have a value relative to one another, there is no natural measurement between them (e.g., you cannot subtract "Strongly Agree" from "Agree").

outcomes of care—The measurable or observable results of illness or treatment.

outcomes that matter—Clinically relevant outcomes that provide direct measures of disease.

It encompasses more than clinical data, including other outcomes that patients and providers care about, such as the patient's ability to function or the cost of care. Outcomes that matter include such factors as quality of life as well as mortality.

outlier—An outlier is an extreme value. An outlier can, by itself, alter the determination of significance. An outlier might also indicate an error has been made. In a box-and-whisker plot, an outlier is a value that falls above or below the whiskers.

overweight—In adults, overweight is defined by the Centers for Disease Control and Prevention (CDC) as those with a BMI between 25 and 29.9.

p-**value**—The probability that the test statistic represents normal variation. A *p*-value is reported with each test statistic. The test statistic *p*-value is compared to the level of alpha selected for the study. If the test statistic is less than alpha (or alpha-halves), then the result is deemed statistically significant.

paired-samples *t*-test—Also known as the dependent-samples *t*-test, this parametric statistical test is used to determine if a significant difference exists between the means of two dependent (or related) measures that have a similar sample size and degree of variation.

pandemic—When an epidemic is widespread over several countries or continents.

PAR—*See* population attributable risk (PAR).

parameter—A descriptive measure of a population, such as the number of people in the population, the mean, or the standard deviation. In most cases, a parameter cannot be known or measured and a sample must be drawn. The symbols used to represent parameters differ from those used to represent sample statistics. For example, the symbol μ (mu) is used to represent the mean of a population where x̄ represents the mean of a sample.

parametric statistics—Statistical procedures designed to be used with data that meet the assumption of normality and are quantitative.

patient-centered health care—A model for health care in which the needs, preferences, goals, capabilities, and resources of the patient or population are at the center of healthcare decisions. Patient-centered care contrasts with the traditional (biomedical) healthcare model, which focuses on the healthcare provider as the expert and authority in healthcare decisions. The clinician's role is transformed from one of being an expert and making decisions for the patient or population to that of being a facilitator and helping people make informed decisions.

Pearson's correlation coefficient—*See* Pearson's product-moment correlation coefficient.

Pearson's product-moment correlation coefficient—Symbolized by a lowercase *r*. A test for relationship between two variables that are interval or ratio data types. A rule of thumb employed with correlation tests is that an *r* of at least 0.755 is considered a strong positive association (whereas −0.755 would be a strong negative association). Also referred to as *Pearson's correlation coefficient*.

peer-reviewed publications—Publications that are reviewed by experts in the discipline who judge whether articles are worthy of publication.

peer reviewer—In a naturalistic (qualitative) study, a peer reviewer serves as an external analyst to critique the interpretations of the researchers. This procedure helps establish the credibility of the study.

period prevalent—A health issue that is specific to an intermediate period of time (months or up to a few years).

per-protocol analysis—A procedure in which the data analyzed from a study include only those subjects who completed the study, dropping data from subjects who did not complete. It is generally considered less rigorous than intent-to-treat analysis because per-protocol analysis does not account for the effect of dropouts on study outcomes. The most rigorous approach is to utilize both per-protocol (also known as on-protocol) and intent-to-treat and compare the results to see if they differ. *See also* intent-to-treat analysis.

persistent observation—Researchers being in the field for an extended period of time to establish rapport and gain the trust of participants so that they feel comfortable disclosing their experiences during data collection.

pertinent negatives—Diagnostic or assessment findings that are pertinent to other diagnoses and are negative for a particular diagnosis. Pertinent negatives help rule out items in the differential.

Phase I clinical trial—According to the FCA: a clinical trial in which researchers test an experimental drug or treatment in a small group of people (20–80) for the first time to evaluate its safety, determine a safe dosage range, and identify side effects.

Phase II clinical trial—According to the FCA: a clinical trial in which the experimental study drug or treatment is given to a larger group of people (100–300) to see if it is effective and to further evaluate its safety.

Phase III clinical trial—According to the FCA: a clinical trial in which the experimental study drug or treatment is given to large groups of people (1,000–3,000) to confirm its effectiveness, monitor side effects, compare it to commonly used treatments, and collect information that will allow the experimental drug or treatment to be used safely.

Phase IV clinical trial—According to the FCA: a postmarketing clinical trial that delineates additional information, including the drug's risks, benefits, and optimal use.

phenomenology—A study of the lived experiences of several individuals centered on a single phenomenon. A phenomenology is similar to a biography in its procedures, differing primarily in terms of the examination of a group as opposed to an individual.

phenomenon—A lived experience that is observable or unobservable. Phenomena experienced by patients and/or observed by clinicians become the focus of healthcare research. For example, this can include the experience of living with HIV or weight gain as a consequence of illness.

phocomelia—A birth defect in which the long bones of the arms and legs do not form properly such that the hand or foot attaches to the body by a short stump resembling a flipper.

PICO—An acronym that stands for Patient or Problem, Intervention, Comparison, Outcome. The acronym was created to guide physicians and medical students in the development of focused clinical questions.

pie chart—A circular graph which includes 100% of the observations in a sample. The chart divides up a sample into proportions.

planning phase of patient care—During this phase of patient care, the patient shares in the decision-making process when the clinician presents his or her findings during the case presentation and gains informed consent to proceed with care. A care plan is collaboratively developed with the patient.

PLR (or LR +)—*See* positive likelihood ratio (PLR).

POEM—An abbreviation that stands for Patient Oriented Evidence that Matters. POEMs are high-level information sources, usually published in print journals, online journals, or online point-of-care resources. POEMs are focused on a single clinical question and provide a careful review of the best available evidence to address the question.

point estimate—A single number such as a sample mean or incidence rate.

point-of-care products (or resources)—Health information search tools that contain synthesized evidence useful to the practitioner while treating the patient. A few examples include UpToDate, MD Consult, Essential Evidence Plus, ACP-PIER, DynaMed, Nursing Reference Center, Rehabilitation Reference Center, Patient Education Reference Center, GIDEON, British Medical Journal Point-of-Care, PEDro, Medscape Reference, and Mosby's Nursing Consult.

point prevalent—A health issue that is specific to a short period of time, such as a day or a week.

point-source outbreak—When one source of infection results in a very rapid increase in the number of cases, such as in the cholera epidemic during John Snow's time in London.

population attributable risk (PAR)—The proportion of disease cases among the population, both exposed and not exposed. It represents the reduction in incidence of a disease in the population if the exposure were eliminated. The PAR is calculated by subtracting the incidence in the unexposed (CER) from the incidence in the population (exposed + unexposed groups).

population attributable risk percent (PAR%)—The percent of the incidence of a disease in the population (exposed + unexposed) that is due to exposure. It is the percent reduction in incidence of disease in the population if the exposure were eliminated. Divide the PAR by the incidence in the total population and then multiply the results by 100 to obtain the PAR%.

positive likelihood ratio (PLR)—The relative likelihood of having the disease if the patient has a positive test result. Symbolized by +LR.

positive predictive value (PPV)—The likelihood someone with a positive test result will actually have the disease. It is expressed as a proportion. PPV is the percentage of those with a positive test result who actually have the disease. In a 2×2 table the formula for PPV is $a/(a + b)$.

positivistic research—Also referred to as *quantitative research*. It is a paradigm through which knowledge is viewed as stemming from the external reality of individuals or groups. Positivistic studies focus on objective questions, looking for causal relationships to make predictions; utilize large, preferably random samples; follow predetermined and fixed designs; rely on numerical, measurable, objective data; employ deductive reasoning and descriptive or inferential statistics; and exclude the researcher as a source of data.

power calculation—A statistical procedure to determine the probability that the effect of interest will be observed when it occurs. A power level of 0.8 is generally accepted as a sufficient level of power. Power is utilized in a sample size calculation in order to determine the necessary number of subjects needed in order to attain the desired level of power.

PPAARE—An acronym that stands for Problem, Patient or Population, Action, Alternative Action, Result, Evidence. The acronym is used to guide the development of focused questions.

PPV—*See* positive predictive value (PPV).

practice guideline—A document related to a specific disease or disorder put together by an expert working group with recommendations for diagnosis and treatment. Some practice guidelines employ the procedures of a systematic review and represent the best available evidence. Other practice guidelines are expert opinion only.

preclinical trials—As defined by the National Institutes of Health, studies that involve testing of experimental drugs in test tubes or in animals. It includes testing that occurs before human trials are permitted.

precontemplation phase of change—In the transtheoretical model of change, at this stage the patient is not willing or ready to change behavior within the next 6 months.

predictor variable—Also referred to as an *independent variable*, which is a variable that can affect a response variable, such as sex or age being a predictor of heart disease.

preparation phase of change—In the transtheoretical model of change, at this stage the patient is preparing for the change within the next month and is partially engaged in changing.

pre/post study—A trial in which the same group serves as both the control and intervention group. Subjects receive the control intervention (no treatment, placebo, or usual care) for a period of time and then receive the experimental treatment. This is also referred to as an *A-B design*. The studies sometimes include a third stage, with a return to the A status, in which the subjects again receive no intervention, placebo, or usual care. This is referred to as an *A-B-A design*. This type of study is also often referred to as a *self-controlled design*.

prevalence—The proportion of a population with a given disease at a single point in time.

primary literature—Original sources of information that have not been filtered through interpretation, such as an historical document, description of a laboratory experiment, an eye-witness account (e.g., case study), or the proposal of an original idea or other original work (publications written by the researcher who conducted a study).

primary outcome measures—End points that are intended to be directly impacted by the intervention.

primary prevention—Strategies that aim to reduce the incidence of disease by personal and communal efforts, such as decreasing environmental risks, enhancing nutritional status, immunizing against communicable diseases, or improving water supplies. It is a core task of public health.

probability sampling—*See* random sampling.

prognosis—The predicted outcome of a disease or disorder, usually expressed in terms of length of time until a specific outcome, such as full recovery, limited recovery, or mortality.

prolonged engagement—Researchers being immersed in data collection long enough to provide depth to the data collected on the phenomenon.

proof-of-concept experiment—A single-group study in which the plausibility of an underlying principle is tested.

propagated epidemic—When an infectious agent infects one person, who then transmits the disease to another person.

proportion—A descriptive statistic showing the percentage of a value in terms of the whole. Proportions are also often referred to as *relative frequency*.

prospective EBP—Seeking information in advance, rather than only in response to patient encounters. Developing your fund of knowledge and being able to draw on that knowledge in clinical situations. Making a habit of searching for the latest developments in your areas of interest and practice (also known as *scanning*).

prospective research—Studies that involve the formulation of a hypothesis, followed by the collection of data and subsequent analysis of findings. Data are collected over a defined period of sufficient duration to draw reliable inferences about a population based on the sample represented by the population. It is possible for prospective research to be observational, quasi-experimental, or experimental in design. The defining characteristic is its forward orientation in time. An outcome is predicted based on a predetermined set of characteristics, a specified experience, or a chosen intervention.

protective factor—An exposure or attribute that is associated with a decreased risk of disease; the risk ratio (RR) is less than 1.0.

PSA test—Prostate specific antigen test. It is used as a diagnostic tool for prostate cancer. The test is controversial due to its poor sensitivity.

PSR—A pharmaceutical sales representative.

psychomotor objectives—Outcomes that focus on changing a patient's motor skills.

publication bias—When the determination about whether to publish a study is based on factors other than the quality of the research and the relevance of its findings.

PubMed—PubMed is an online database administered by the National Library of Medicine. It can be used to search millions of publications in biomedical literature, life science journals, and online books. PubMed is an excellent tool for locating primary biomedical literature, although not all publications are available full-text online for free. Even though not all resources are available for free, PubMed makes it easy to locate the citations for a vast array of publications.

PubMed Health—A website maintained by the National Center for Biotechnology Information for consumers to access summaries on clinical effectiveness research published in systematic reviews.

purpose statement—A statement in a publication that explains the reason the study was undertaken.

purposive sampling—Typically used in qualitative research studies, such as grounded theory, phenomenology, ethnography, or biography. A purposive sampling procedure is often necessary when there are few cases of a specific problem, such as with a rare diagnosis or when researchers are interested in the experiences of specific subjects.

qualitative data—In positivistic research, quantitative data are values that are categorical, nominal, or ordinal scales. For statistical analysis, qualitative data points are counted and, thereby, converted to numerical values. Nonparametric statistics apply to qualitative data collected through positivistic research. In naturalistic research, nearly all data are qualitative (non-numerical) taking the form of text, images, observations, etc. Qualitative data are not statistically analyzed in purely naturalistic studies.

qualitative research—Also known as *naturalistic research*. It is a paradigm of research focused on describing phenomena as experienced by those who live them. There are many different methods and products of qualitative research.

quantitative data—In positivistic research, quantitative data are values that are interval or ratio scales. In order to utilize parametric statistical strategies, data must (at a minimum) be quantitative in type and satisfy other assumptions associated with the statistical procedure of interest.

quantitative research—Quantitative research is also known as *positivistic research*. Quantitative research utilizes numerical data to measure and explain observable phenomena. There are many quantitative research methods.

quartile—The division of the distribution into four equal parts.

quasi-experimental research—Studies in which researchers cannot randomly select subjects or randomly assign subjects to treatment and control groups; however, researchers are able to control some independent variables.

quaternary prevention—Strategies that aim to identify patients at risk of overdiagnosis or overmedication and that protect them from excessive medical intervention.

Quick Response (QR) codes—Bar codes that can be scanned with a smartphone that lead to websites, online videos, telephone numbers, maps, and other health information. QR Codes can be read by smartphones using a free application that can be downloaded to a smartphone.

r—The correlation coefficient.

r^2—The correlation coefficient of determination.

random sampling—A process through which every member of a population has equal probability of being selected for a study. Also known as *probability sampling*.

randomization—A procedure for assigning subjects to intervention groups (placebo group, control group, experimental group, etc.) that ensures that every subject has an equal chance of being assigned to any group.

randomized control trial (RCT)—A study in which the allocation of patients to treatment or control groups is random and concealed. At least one control group must be utilized. Preferably patients as well as providers are not informed (blinded) regarding which intervention that patients receive.

range—The difference between the highest and lowest values in an ordered data set.

ratio data—Measurable observations that have a natural order and equivalence. Each observation is an equivalent distance from the next (e.g., the distance from 2 to 3 is equal to the distance from 136 to 137). There is also a true zero point. For example, height is typically measured on a ratio scale, be it inches or centimeters. You can divide one ratio value by another and achieve a meaningful result. This is the reason the term ratio is used.

RCT—*See* randomized control trial (RCT).

readiness ruler—A visual analog scale used with patients to assess their willingness for changing their behaviors.

recall bias—A flaw in research data caused by poor recall among research subjects. When patients with an outcome are asked to remember exposures or behaviors in their past, they are much more likely to respond positively than patients who do not have the outcome.

receiver operating characteristic (ROC)—A plot that compares the true positive rate to the false positive rate. The ROC curve is a visual representation of the area under the curve (AUC) statistic. The greater the true positive rate compared to the false positive rate the stronger the diagnostic test.

refereed publications—Publications that are not only peer-reviewed but also come from journals that include primary research, systematic reviews, or meta-analyses.

reference standard test—The current standard or the gold standard. It is the test that is normally used or the test that has been shown to be the most accurate.

reflexivity—A practice of critical self-reflection through which researchers, especially naturalistic (qualitative) researchers, become conscious of how their views and perspectives might influence their inquiry.

regression analysis—Test that focuses on relationships among several variables that best explain a specific response. A regression analysis determines the line that best fits within a set of coordinates. It is the line that comes the closest to all of the dots on a scatter diagram. Regression analysis can include multiple variables and often includes the identification of a model that accounts for multiple variables at one time. The goal of regression analysis is to identify the combination of predictor variables that best explain the variability in the response variable.

rehabilitation—A health professional field that encompasses numerous types of health professionals who provide care designed to facilitate recovery or improvement from injury, illness, disease, or other disorder to as functional a condition as possible.

rehabilitative care—Care designed to facilitate recovery or improvement from injury, illness, disease, or disorder to as functional a condition as possible. Several health professions focus on rehabilitative care, such as physical therapy, occupational therapy, speech therapy, cancer rehabilitation, audiology, rehabilitative nursing, and many more. Rehabilitative care is also a part of all health professions.

relationships—In statistics, relationships are mathematical associations between variables, usually predictor and response variables.

relative risk (RR)—Also referred to as the *risk ratio*. It is the event rate among those exposed to a factor divided by the event rate among those not exposed to the same factor. The formula for RR is EER/CER. *See also* exposed event rate (EER); control event rate (CER).

relative risk increase (RRI)—Similar to relative risk reduction (RRR), but representing a higher event rate among the exposed group than the control group; RRI = (CER − EER)/CER.

relative risk reduction (RRR)—An extrapolation from relative risk. RRR is the difference in event rates between the exposed and unexposed groups expressed as a proportion of the event rate in the unexposed group; RRR = (CER − EER)/CER.

reliability—The consistency, or reproducibility, of the manner in which the data were collected.

repeated measures tests—Pre/post, within-subject, self-controlled, and correlated group designs are all types of repeated measures tests. When a test for differences is used to compare variables that are from different groups that do not influence one another, the measures are said to be independent, whereas repeated measures tests are used when the variables being compared are not independent. Usually this means the same subjects are in both groups, making the groups dependent rather than independent.

representativeness—In a quantitative study, the degree to which subjects in the sample match the population they represent. The sample should match the population in terms of characteristics such as the distribution of people by sex, age, race/ethnicity, severity of disease, and so on.

response variable—Also referred to as a *dependent variable*, a response variable is affected by a predictor (i.e., independent) variable. For example, mortality from heart disease is a response variable that is affected by age, sex, smoking, or body mass.

retrospective EBP—Looking up information subsequent to a clinical encounter.

retrospective research—Retrospective research examines an outcome or exposure that has already occurred and utilizes numerical data to test for relationships between variables, or differences between groups, which can be associated with the phenomenon.

right skew—A visual description for a non-normal data set in which values trail off to the right side of the chart, creating a 'tail' on that side.

risk—The probability or chance that an individual will develop a disease or condition over a specified period of time.

risk factor—An exposure or attribute that is associated with but *not* the cause of a given outcome of interest.

risk ratio (RR)—*See* relative risk (RR).

ROC—*See* receiver operating characteristic (ROC).

RR—*See* relative risk (RR).

RRI—*See* relative risk increase (RRI).

RRR—*See* relative risk reduction (RRR).

s—The symbol for the standard deviation in a sample.

sample size—The number of subjects who enter into a study.

sample size calculation—A statistical procedure that should be calculated *prior* to the start of a study that tells researchers how many subjects are needed in order to accurately answer the research question based on the type of data to be collected, the level of Type I error risk (alpha), and the amount of effect of the intervention.

sampling bias—Limitation(s) to the process of selecting and recruiting subjects in a study that results in the study sample not being representative of the population from which it is drawn and is intended to represent.

sampling fraction—The proportion that a sample is of the population it represents. For example, if a population was known to have 100,000 people and the sample drawn for the research is 425 people, the sampling fraction would be 0.425%. The researchers would report that the sample represented approximately 0.425% of the population.

sampling frame—The source from which the subjects are drawn, usually a list of some kind that has been deemed to include a sufficient number of potential subjects that can represent the population and allow for a representative, random sample to be drawn.

sampling strategy—A procedure or set of procedures for identifying and recruiting subjects.

saturation—The point at which participants are not providing new data to contribute to the analysis and the analysis is well defined and demonstrates variation. This concept is generally applied to naturalistic (qualitative) research.

scatter plot—A graph that shows relationships (also known as associations or correlations) between variables (similar to a line graph). The closer the dots are in a scatter plot to forming a line, the stronger their association.

scientific method—The process of formulating a hypothesis, performing objective experiments, and engaging in sound reasoning supported by the collected data.

screening—Procedures used to identify early signs and symptoms of a disease or health problem associated with a population at risk for a specific disease or event.

secondary literature—A summary, interpretation, or evaluation of primary literature, such as a traditional literature review. Practice guidelines and position papers might also fall in this category depending on the sources used.

secondary outcome measures—Additional end points (beyond primary outcome measures) that are evaluated but are not the specific focus of the intervention.

secondary prevention—Strategies that aim to reduce the prevalence of disease by shortening the duration of disease.

selection bias—A type of sampling bias in which there is a systematic procedural error in the selection of subjects or when a nonrandom (nonprobability) sample is utilized.

self-efficacy ruler—A visual analog scale used to determine a patient's self-efficacy with making a behavior change.

self-management—The process of monitoring an existing disease, such as taking medications and other interventions, to maintain or improve a disease or condition and dealing with the emotions that accompany the illness.

self-reporting bias—A type of measurement error in which subjects inaccurately report data about themselves.

sensitivity—The ability of the test to be positive given the person tested has the disease/problem. Sensitivity is expressed as a proportion. It is the percentage of those who are known to have the disease/problem who test positive. Also known as the proportion of true positives. In a 2 × 2 table the formula for sensitivity is $a/(a + c)$.

side effects—Unintended symptoms from treatment, prevention, diagnostic, or screening procedures.

σ (sigma)—The standard deviation of a population.

simple random sample—A form of probability sampling (which means each individual has a known probability of being selected) that allows every member of the population to have an equal chance of being selected for the study.

Snow, John—A physician who lived in the 1800s who is credited with one of the first epidemiological studies. He identified the well in London of a specific water company—(the Broad Street pump) as the source of a cholera outbreak.

snowball sampling—A type of nonprobability sampling used in quantitative research when the researchers are interested in studying a population that is difficult to identify, such as gang members, IV drug users, or illegal aliens, to name a few. Also known as network sampling. Those identified initially are asked to identify others who might be able to provide data. The researchers then contact them and determine if they fit the research question. If they are a good fit they are added to the sample, and then those added are asked to identify other acquaintances, and so on, until a sufficient sample size is accomplished to achieve statistical power.

social cognitive theory—A theory of behavior that proposes behavioral factors, cognitive factors (knowledge, expectations, and attitudes), and environmental factors (including social norms and interaction with other individuals) influence human behavior.

specificity—The ability of the test to be negative given the person does not have the disease/problem. Specificity is expressed as a proportion. It is the percentage of those who are known not to have the disease/condition who test negative. Also known as the *proportion of true negatives*. In a 2 × 2 table the formula for specificity is $d/(b + d)$.

standard deviation—A measure of variability. It is the square root of the variance (average distance of all observations in a data set from the mean) of the data set.

standard of care—The usual practice utilized by other clinicians and experts in the region.

statistics—The theory, study, and practice of quantitatively summarizing data. There are two general categories of statistics: descriptive and inferential.

stratified random sample—A procedure in which the sampling frame is divided into strata (groupings) and a random sample is drawn from each stratum.

studies of harm—Observational, retrospective studies with the purpose of identifying harmful exposures (e.g., case-control studies) as well as observational, prospective studies with the purpose of identifying harmful exposures (e.g., cohort studies, systematic reviews, meta-analyses).

studies of prevention—Interventional, prospective studies with the purpose of preventing patients from developing a condition (e.g., case studies, case series, control trials, randomized control trials, cohort studies) as well as observational, prospective studies with the purpose of determining whether patients develop a given condition (e.g., case studies, case series, cohort studies, systematic reviews, meta-analyses).

studies of treatment—Interventional, prospective studies with the purpose of treating a diagnosed condition (e.g., case studies, case series, control trials, randomized control trials, cohort studies) as well as observational, prospective studies with the purpose of determining outcomes of patients with a diagnosed condition who are already receiving a specific treatment (e.g., cohort studies, systematic reviews, meta-analyses).

subcommunity—A smaller group within a community that shares a separate community within itself. *See also* community.

subjective data—The patient's perceptions.

surrogate outcomes—An indirect outcome (such as a physiological measure) that reflects another type of outcome, usually an outcome that matters. Surrogates are selected based on the association of a physiological or biological measure with another known clinical end point (e.g., morbidity, mortality).

surveillance—The ongoing, systematic collection, analysis, and interpretation of health data.

survival curve—A survival curve is a graph used to show the length of time until a bad event, such as death. It can have one line or multiple lines. The x-axis shows the length of time until the bad event, and the y-axis shows the percentage of the group or groups.

syndemic—When two or more afflictions, interacting synergistically, contribute to excess burden of disease in a population.

systematic review—A research procedure in which all prior positivistic studies on a given topic are brought together and analyzed collectively.

t-test—Also known as the Student's t-test or independent-samples t-test, this parametric statistical test is used to determine if a significant difference exists between the means of two independent groups that have a similar sample size and degree of variation.

teach-back method—A strategy used during the implementation phase of care in which patients are asked to teach the procedure back to the practitioner by demonstrating the use of equipment or explaining medication dosing.

temporal style—The time-orientation of research: retrospective, cross-sectional, or prospective.

tertiary literature Distilled collections of primary and secondary sources, such as a textbooks, dictionaries, or encyclopedias.

tertiary prevention—Strategies that aim to soften the impact of long-term disease and disability by eliminating or reducing impairment, disability, and handicap; reducing suffering; and maximizing potential years or useful life. It is mainly a task of rehabilitation.

test-retest method—A procedure for testing the reliability of an instrument in which the instrument is administered to a small group of participants at one time and then the same instrument is administered a short time later (such as one week). The level of agreement between the test and retest are compared using a correlation coefficient. The higher the correlation coefficient, the higher the reliability of the instrument.

tests for differences—Comparison of a statistic, such as a mean or a proportion, between two or more groups.

tests for relationships—Used to determine if variables change in relationship to other variables (e.g., arthritis incidence increases with age or heart disease increases with incidence of diabetes). A positive relationship exists when an increase in one variable is associated with an increase in another. A negative relationship exists when an increase in one variable is associated with a decrease in another. The stronger the association between variables, the more likely the relationship is significant, meaning that it cannot be explained by random chance.

test statistic—The value produced by a statistical test.

thalidomide—A sedative hypnotic drug originally used as a treatment for morning sickness and to help pregnant women sleep. However, it causes phocomelia (seal limb) in infants. As such, it was never approved in the United States for pregnant women. It is now approved in the treatment of leprosy and certain forms of cancer.

theoretical sampling—A procedure for selecting participants in a naturalistic (qualitative) study that ensures participants can provide data to inform the research question.

therapeutics—According to the U.S. Library of Medicine: procedures concerned with the remedial treatment or prevention of diseases.

time-to-event curve—Another name for a survival curve. It indicates that a survival curve can be used to measure time until any type of event, not just a bad event.

transferability—A characteristic of a naturalistic (qualitative) study that represents the degree to which the findings of the study are viewed as applicable to other situations. Transferability is usually established by the reader of a study and cannot be ascertained by the researcher. The researcher must provide a sufficiently rich/thick description of the study so that readers can make the determination of transferability.

transformation of data—A procedure that converts data points into another form that has a normal distribution (e.g., logarithmic transformation).

translational critical thinking—An application of critical thinking in which the theoretical skills and concepts of critical thinking are enacted to solve real-world, ill-structured problems. Translational critical thinking requires self-awareness, intellectual humility, self-direction, and active learning.

triangulation—Procedures utilized to compare findings via different data sources. This concept is generally applied to naturalistic (qualitative) studies.

triple-blind randomized control trial—A randomized control trial in which the allocation of subjects to treatment and control groups not only is concealed from the subjects and the clinicians but also from the researchers who analyze the data.

truncated trial—A trial (study) that ends early. Usually this happens for one of two reasons: (1) the results indicate an unexpected adverse outcome and the study is stopped for safety purposes or (2)—the results indicate a strongly positive outcome, making it unnecessary to continue. When a positive outcome is the cause of a truncated trial, usually the control group is given the experimental treatment so that they may benefit from it.

Tuskegee syphilis study—A study performed between 1932 and 1972 in which the Public Health Service of Alabama denied treatment for syphilis to over 400 African Americans, mostly adult males. It is one of the reasons for human subjects' protections in U.S. law and regulation.

Tx—A clinical abbreviation that stands for *treatment*.

unimodal—A data set with one mode (a single value that occurs most frequently). Unimodality is one of the required characteristics for a distribution to be considered normal.

USPSTF (U.S. Preventive Services Task Force)—An agency within AHRQ. According to the USPSTF, it is an independent group of national experts in prevention and evidence-based medicine that work to improve the health of all Americans by making evidence-based recommendations about clinical preventive services such as screenings, counseling services, or preventive medications.

validity—The accuracy of measurements. It is the degree to which an instrument measures what is it supposed to measure.

variability—The dispersion of data points within a set.

variance—The average distance of all observations from the mean in a normally shaped distribution (data set).

visual analog scale (VAS)—A graphic used to assess pain severity and duration in patients or experimental animals.

web of causation—A theory that posits that there is no singular reason for the occurrence of a disease. Rather a compendium of factors predisposes an individual to meet criteria for a particular case definition.

WHO (World Health Organization)—The coordinating authority for health within the United Nations system.

WOMAC Scale—Western Ontario and McMaster Universities Osteoarthritis scale used to assess pain, stiffness, and physical function in hip or knee osteoarthritis.

$\bar{x}$—Referred to as x-bar. The symbol used to designate the mean of a sample.

Index